The Medical Detectives

BY THE AUTHOR

THE
MEDICAL
DETECTIVES

Volume II

*Berton
Roueché*

•

A Truman Talley Book
E. P. DUTTON, INC.
New York

•

Published in the United States by Truman Talley Books • E. P. Dutton, Inc. 2 Park Avenue, New York, N.Y. 10016

Library of Congress Catalog Card Number: 84-70904
ISBN: 0-525-24270-8

Published simultaneously in Canada
by Fitzhenry & Whiteside Limited, Toronto

COBE

10 9 8 7 6 5 4 3 2
First Edition

*For
Brad,
Lillian
&
Kira Victoria*

All diseases of Christians are to be ascribed to demons.

—St. Augustine
354–430 A.D.

Contents

The Medical Detectives

CHAPTER 1

The Alerting
of Mr. Pomerantz

————————————————

A VIOLENT, BODY-RACKING, infectious fever called rickettsialpox is the newest of known diseases. Its onset is abrupt, it is as prostrating as a kick in the stomach, and its course is a trying one, but it is not fatal. Although medical authorities are of the uneasy opinion that thousands of new diseases would afflict mankind if all the microörganisms potentially capable of causing illness were to become sufficiently virulent to break down the body's resistance to them, the outbreak of just one such disease is happily an unusual occurrence. The first known case of rickettsialpox in medical history turned up some eighteen months ago, in Queens. Cases of it have since been reported elsewhere in the city. No other disease has ever made its initial appearance here. It is, in fact, practically unheard of for one to originate in any metropolis. Nobody knows why.

Almost everything about rickettsialpox is peculiar. It is among the few identified ailments that bear scientifically illuminating names. A disease usually is named for its discoverer (Bright's disease), for the geographical area in which it was first observed (Asiatic cholera), or for its predominant symptom (whooping cough). Sometimes a disease is named for its cause or, as often as not, for what was once erroneously *thought* to be its cause (malaria, which is not caused by bad air, and the common cold, which is not caused by low temperatures). Rickettsialpox, as a name, not only gives a good idea of one of the disease's most notable manifestations, a spotty rash, but indicates its cause, a microörganism of the genus *Rickettsia.* Such etiological exactitude in the naming of a disease is uncommon because the discovery of the existence of a disease generally precedes by many years the discovery of its cause. In certain instances—that of syphilis, for one—a cure has been found before the cause of the disease has been determined. The causes of numerous familiar ailments, including several of the most malignant, are still unknown. Smallpox, for example, dates back to at least the third century B.C., yet science is still unable to say exactly what causes it or exactly how it is transmitted. The dispatch with which the *Rickettsia* microörganism was identified made it possible to give the disease a definitive name. As a jig-time medical project, the investigation was probably unique. The cause of rickettsialpox and its means of transmission were established just seven months and seven days after its first known victim, an eleven-year-old boy, came down with it on the afternoon of February 23, 1946.

The boy was Edmund Lohr, Jr., the son of Mr. and Mrs. Edmund Lohr, of 141-12 Seventy-eighth Road, in the Kew Gardens section of Queens. Mr. Lohr is the head night auditor of the Shelton Hotel, at Lexington Avenue and Forty-ninth Street. The family occupies a third-floor apartment in an attractive, moderate-priced housing development called Regency Park, which was completed in 1939. Regency Park consists of sixty-three three-story buildings, in which there is a total of five hundred and forty-five more or less identical flats, and covers three large blocks. It is bounded by Union Turnpike, Seventy-eighth Avenue, Main Street, and 141st Street, and it is trisected by Seventy-ninth Avenue and Seventy-eighth Road. The apartment in which the Lohrs live is in the middle block. Mrs. Lohr clearly recollects the start of her son's illness. "Edmund came in from playing, looking sick and grippy," she told me not long ago when I called on her in the course of talking to a number of people who were involved in tracking down rickettsialpox. "He said he hurt all over. Well, I put him to bed and took his temperature. It was over a hundred and one, so I telephoned our doctor and he came around as soon as he could. Before he left, he began to look very serious, and I remember he said, 'I've got a case on my hands.' "

The physician who was thus candidly disturbed is Dr. Benjamin Shankman, a young general practitioner with a warm bedside manner, whose office is a block north of Regency Park. He recalls that when he reached the Lohr apartment, Edmund's temperature was a hundred and three. Upon examining the child, Dr. Shankman found a pimple-like lesion on his back and a somewhat swollen gland near the right armpit. He tentatively diagnosed the illness as chicken pox. It was a plausible diagnosis, and it might have stuck if Mrs. Lohr had not pointed out, with reasonable surprise, that Edmund had already *had* chicken pox, some years before. This disclosure naturally unsettled Dr. Shankman, but he sought to reassure himself with the thought that the earlier diagnosis, which had been made by another man, might not have been accurate. There was no getting around the fact, however, that the boy seemed to be a lot sicker than the average chicken-pox sufferer. Dr. Shankman decided that he'd better wait awhile to ascertain if more lesions would develop, and then see.

Two or three days later, there was a generous rash of lesions for Dr. Shankman to study. Careful examination convinced him that they were not precisely like the pox of chicken pox. He therefore discarded the chicken-pox theory and took a blood count. It revealed the presence of a high percentage of white cells, a characteristic of cases of severe infection. Meanwhile, Edmund's temperature was fluctuating eccentrically. At one time, it climbed as high as a hundred and six—a blisteringly high fever, even for a child. Dr. Shankman concluded that his patient had better be put in a hospital, if only for observation. "I was beginning to get scared," the physician told me frankly. Mr. and Mrs. Lohr were even less composed. On February 28th, they and Dr. Shankman took Edmund in a taxi to the Kew Gardens General Hospital, the nearest to their home, where the boy was at first refused admittance, because the examining physician, falling into Dr. Shankman's earlier error, thought that he had chicken pox, and the institution was not equipped to care for patients suffering from a contagious disease. After appealing to several of the authorities there, however, Dr. Shankman succeeded in getting Edmund admitted, and the boy was put to bed in a remote and isolated room. Then Dr. Shankman prescribed a regimen of penicillin therapy. Edmund was given tests for various illnesses during the next few days. The results were all negative. Presently, he began to get well. He was released on March 4th, as good as new. Dr. Shankman closed his record of the case with the cautiously generalized, though not inaccurate, diagnostic notation, "Sepsis, with a rash."

Most physicians recover promptly from the distress of uncertainty. They are accustomed to it. Within a week or so, Dr. Shankman had almost managed to forget his unnerving experience. Then, one morning in the middle of March, having been summoned for what sounded over the telephone like a routine case, he found himself confronted by another unruly fever, with glandular swelling and a small, pimplish lesion. Later, he came to recognize lesions of this nature as an unmistakable symptom of the strange disease. The patient on this occasion was a woman of thirty-four who lived a few doors from the Lohrs. Dr. Shankman's heart sank as he examined her, but also his interest quickened, for he strongly suspected that he was up against the same freakish thing again. He still had no idea of what it was, but he did have a pretty good idea of what it *wasn't*. The tests made on the Lohr boy had shown that it wasn't any of the diseases it most resembled —chicken pox, typhus, endemic typhus, dengue fever, Japanese river fever, Rocky Mountain spotted fever, smallpox, or infectious mononucleosis. Dr. Shankman checked back over his records of the Lohr case and realized that he had no reason to be certain that the penicillin had been responsible for the boy's recovery. This time, therefore, he tried one of the sulfonamides. It seemed to be no more and no less effective than the penicillin. Since the powers of these two drugs are not identical, the Doctor was inclined to suspect that the disease he was confronted with was not affected by either.

This hunch of Dr. Shankman's was strengthened when, before

the month was out, another of his Regency Park patients, a middle-aged woman, came down with the same illness. Treated only with aspirin, codeine, and reassuring conversation, she recovered in about the same length of time as the others had. Four or five more cases came to the Doctor's attention during April. They, too, responded favorably to non-medicinal therapy. Dr. Shankman reached the conclusion that the disease was at least self-limiting. Moreover, it appeared to be accompanied by no complications or troublesome aftereffects. "Those were very comforting things to know," he told me, "especially as it was beginning to turn up all over the place. Also, people in the neighborhood were naturally getting a little upset about it. It was nice to be able to assure them that it wasn't anything fatal, or even very serious. As a matter of fact, it's been nice to know that ever since, for we have yet to find a cure." At around this time, some residents of Kew Gardens got into the habit of calling the ailment Shankman's disease. Dr. Shankman laughed modestly as he recalled that brief promise of lasting fame. "Well," he said, "I guess I did see all the very first cases." Meanwhile, other Kew Gardens physicians had begun to encounter the same affliction. They were not tempted to call it Shankman's disease. They did, however, tend to agree with him that it was probably something disconcertingly new. Talking with these colleagues and reviewing his records, Dr. Shankman found that the disease was occurring only among residents of Regency Park. That struck him as odd, since there was nothing singular about the place that he could see. There were a dozen new cases in May, still all in Regency Park. Toward the end of that month, Dr. Shankman, feeling that the time had come for official action, reported the existence of the new disease and his perplexities concerning it to the Department of Health, which for a while seemed to show a depressing lack of interest.

As summer came on, more and more cases of rickettsialpox appeared in Regency Park. In spite of the assurances of Dr. Shankman and other physicians that the disease was not dangerous, an understandable apprehension spread through the three blighted blocks. People began to feel trapped. Several gave up their flats and moved away, preferring the agonies of homehunting to illness. Their apartments did not remain vacant long; there were plenty of other people who evidently preferred the risk of illness to homelessness. Many residents of Regency Park began to experience a kind of social ostracism. Their acquaintances elsewhere in the city, after hearing rumors of the pestilence, hesitated to visit them. "It got so our oldest and best friends would hem and haw and act perfectly hateful when I asked them over to dinner," a woman who was an early victim of the disease remembers. "Why, even my own mother wouldn't come and see me."

Presently, after some intramural fumbling, the Health Department started its own inquiry by sending two of its most expert investigators to Kew Gardens. They interviewed a few of the sick, the convalescent, and the recovered, made some blood tests, conferred inconclusively with the neighborhood doctors, and hospitalized several patients for close, if rather fruitless, examination. Nearly a hundred cases, all among residents of Regency Park, had been reported by then, and the incidence of the disease was nearing epidemic proportions. A few days later, the newspapers got wind of the trouble. On Friday morning, July 19th, the *Times* carried a not entirely unruffled story in which Dr. Shankman was quoted as saying that the illness somewhat resembled Rocky Mountain spotted fever. The following Thursday evening, Dr. Shankman received a telephone call at his office from a man named Charles Pomerantz, who said that he had a theory about what the shriller newspapers had taken to referring to as the "Kew Gardens Mystery Fever," and asked if he could pay the physician a visit. Dr. Shankman had never heard of Mr. Pomerantz, but he told him to come right over, for at that point he was ready to listen to anyone with a fresh approach to the subject. What Mr. Pomerantz, who spoke guardedly, wanted, it turned out, was to inspect the Regency Park basements, and he hoped that Dr. Shankman could arrange it for him. The Doctor encouraged his visitor to be a bit more specific. Then, though more startled than convinced by what Mr. Pomerantz had to say, Dr. Shankman agreed to help. He is thankful that he did.

Mr. Pomerantz, a small, pink-and-white, highly combustible man of fifty who came to this country from Poland at an early age, is the president of the Bell Exterminating Company, on Hudson

Street. He is also a gifted, self-taught entomologist, and something of an authority on ticks. He became an exterminator in 1936, after spending nearly twenty remunerative, but spiritually unreward-ing, years in the jungles of Seventh Avenue as a manufacturer of ladies' coats. A brother-in-law, David Cantor, at that time a jaded pharmacist, wheedled Mr. Pomerantz into joining him in the exterminating business. "I was unhappy and restless and ripe for almost anything," Mr. Pomerantz told me, "but when David suggested we become exterminators, I recoiled. Cockroaches! Bed-bugs! Rats! That went against my aesthetic sense. I am a man who keeps a volume of Keats on my bedside table, and I have pro-gressed in fiddle playing to Mendelssohn. But then I thought, 'But pest control is science, and science enjoys a kinship with the arts. Why should I find it more repulsive than ladies' ready-to-wear?' So I assured David I was with him, and we hired a couple of experienced operators." Mr. Pomerantz let his fiddle-playing slide, abandoned Keats, and embarked on a course of technical reading. "It was a challenge to me," he said. "My blood raced with enthusiasm. First, I learned the façade, and finally I began to learn the marrow of the subject. I began to specialize in everything, especially ticks."

When Mr. Pomerantz opened his *Times* on the morning of July 19th and learned what was happening at Regency Park, his blood raced again. "I was intensely fascinated," he said. "Here was a disease resembling Rocky Mountain spotted fever. Rocky Moun-tain spotted fever is transmitted by the bite of a *tick!* And the tick is my specialty. I said to myself, 'If even the *Herr Doktors* are baffled, then Charles Pomerantz has a moral right to look into it.' " Mr. Pomerantz exercised his moral right on the afternoon of the following day by going out to Regency Park and thoughtfully casing the buildings from the street. He disclosed his identity to no one, not wishing his mission to be suspected of being tainted with commercialism. "I walked and walked," he said, "studying the outside economy, getting the feel of the problem. I asked people I met if many ticks had been found in the neighborhood, but nobody had ever heard of any. Even the owners of two dog kennels just across the street from the south block of apartments told me they had seen no ticks. And yet the disease had appeared in almost every building. With my knowledge of the mechanism and habits of ticks, I found it fantastic to believe that enough ticks —it would take hundreds, thousands—to cause so many people to become ill could suddenly invade an area without anybody finding a single one, not even kennelmen. Ticks are not so small that they are invisible, and when they are gorged with the blood of the necessary host, they are as big as a kidney bean. Besides, New York is not known for anything but the brown dog tick, which is not thought to carry infection to man. A puzzle!" Mr. Pomerantz went home that night as baffled as the doctors.

He was not, however, disheartened. He returned to Regency Park the next day, Sunday, and resumed his sharp-eyed, reflective strolling. Nothing came of it. On Tuesday morning, he trotted back for another look. By that time, he was convinced that the outside economy of the place was immaculate. He prepared to consider the inside economy. "I reasoned that if the cause of the trouble was inside," he recalled, "then there must be some loco-motive mechanism that could go here, there, and everywhere through the buildings, thus spreading the infection. I asked my-self, 'What is the most obvious such mechanism?' The answer came at once—a rat or mouse. But rats or mice are not known to *transmit* any rash-producing disease. So the rat or the mouse, whichever it is, must be merely the host—or, more entomologi-cally, the reservoir—to a disease-bearing parasite that can bite and infect man. I worked the relationship out in my mind. The rat or mouse—and probably the mouse, because I had learned that there were many mice in the buildings but few rats—would be what we call the usual host, with man just the accidental host. But what kind of parasite? Then I had the answer. It flashed into my mind, and I said to myself, 'Ticks out! Mites in!' "

The lack of intense conviction entertained by Dr. Shankman when Mr. Pomerantz presented this hypothesis to him is not surprising. From a medical viewpoint, it was a fairly eccentric notion. Most of the doctors who had treated cases of the peculiar disease were almost certain by then that the characteristic initial lesion was the bite of some minute creature, but they had little reason to suspect mites of being the guilty parties. At the time, it was generally believed that mites could transmit only two serious febrile diseases —Japanese river fever and endemic typhus. Both of these are rarely found in the United States, and anyway both had been eliminated from consideration in this instance by laboratory tests. Moreover, the mouse, unlike the rat, had never been proved to be a reservoir for disease-bearing parasites. Mr. Pomerantz admits that hitting upon the mouse as the probable host was largely intuitive. He is persuaded, however, that in singling out mites as the carriers—or vectors, as such agents are known—of the disease he was guided entirely by deduction.

Mites are insectlike organisms, closely related to ticks. Both are members of the Arachnida, a class that also includes spiders and scorpions. Compared to a tick, a mite is a minute animal. A mite, when fully engorged, is about the size of the strawberry seed. In that state, it is approximately ten times its usual, or unfed, size. So far, science has classified at least thirty families of mites, most of which are vegetarian and indifferent to man and all other animals. The majority of the parasitic, bloodsucking mites have to feed once in every four or five days in order to live. Most mites of this type attach themselves to a host only long enough to engorge, and drop off, replete, after fifteen or twenty minutes. No one ever feels the bite of a mite—or of a tick, either, for that matter —until the animal has dropped off. (Entomologists believe that both creatures, at the instant they bite, excrete a fluid that anesthetizes a small surrounding area of the body of the host.) Mites are only infrequently found in this country and until recently were practically unknown in New York City. Consequently, very few Americans, even physicians and exterminators, have ever seen a mite. Mr. Pomerantz is one of those who have. He came across some in line of duty on three occasions in 1945. His first encounter was with cheese mites, a nonparasitic variety, in a private house at Hastings-on-Hudson. Some months later, in two widely separated Manhattan apartment buildings, he found infestations of the Oriental rat mite, a suspected vector of endemic typhus. These successive discoveries made a deep impression on Mr. Pomerantz. "Three distinct infestations all of a sudden," he reminded me. "Three warnings that New York and vicinity were no longer immune. I became alerted on mites."

Sponsored by Dr. Shankman, Mr. Pomerantz received permission from the building superintendent at Regency Park to explore the basements of the development on Sunday, July 28th. At one o'clock that afternoon, equipped with a flashlight, a magnifying glass, a couple of two-ounce specimen bottles, and a fine-pointed camel's-hair brush, he ducked resolutely into a cellar on Seventy-ninth Avenue. "I had that Stonewall Jackson feeling," he told me. "I *knew* there were mites somewhere in those buildings and I was determined not to go home until I'd found them. Of course, I wasn't a damn fool and didn't just look anywhere. If a detective is looking for a shady character, he looks where it is probable the criminal would hide. I searched the usual haunts of mites. Mites like to be cozy and sandwiched in. Thigmotropism, this instinct is called. So I examined the little cracks in the walls, and especially the tops of the incinerator doors." Mr. Pomerantz had trudged in and out of a dozen basements, and aroused scores of mice, before he spotted his first mite. It was overfed and sluggish, and, using the tip of his brush, he had no trouble flicking it into one of his bottles. By six o'clock when he knocked off, he had bagged forty-five specimens, some unfed, some bloated. Success had left him shaken. "I, a humble pest-control operator, had found something to relieve the uncertainty of men of scientific learning," he said. "I can't describe my sensation of glory."

Mr. Pomerantz is happily married, but he had not discussed his theory with his wife. He did not do so even now. "There was still a chance that my mites might turn out to be physiologically or morphologically incapable of transmitting such a disease," he said to me. "I didn't want to raise her false hopes." When Mr. Pomerantz got home, he merely remarked, "Vera, I have something in these bottles that may make medical history." "I don't doubt it," replied Mrs. Pomerantz, a woman in whom, I gathered, the inquisitive instinct is blunted. "Supper is almost ready."

Mr. Pomerantz ate a light supper, read a few chapters of "Medical Entomology," by William B. Herms, and went to bed early. Before he got to sleep, he had decided to take his mites down to Washington the next day and get an authoritative opinion on them from a professional acquaintance, C. F. W. Muesebeck, who is the head of the Division of Insect Identification of the United States Department of Agriculture.

It was midafternoon when Mr. Pomerantz reached Mr. Muese-beck's office. Mr. Muesebeck, after hearing the mite theory, examined the specimens with interest and then dispatched them to one of his colleagues, Dr. E. W. Baker, a mite specialist, for identification. An hour or so later, Dr. Baker reported that the mites were members of a rather rare species, *Allodermanyssus sanguineus,* discovered and classified in Egypt in 1913, and that, although they had no medical history, they had always been looked upon by parasitologists as possible transmitters of disease. Mr. Pomerantz assured me that he received this stimulating news with a scientist's urbanity. "But I was all electricity inside," he added. "I was vibrating. I felt wonderful. Mr. Muesebeck even asked me to collect some more specimens for them." Mr. Pomerantz left his mites in the hands of the government and hopped the next train back to New York. That night, he told his wife everything. "You are to be congratulated," he remembers her saying calmly, to which he replied, throbbing with hope and prophecy, "Something has been accomplished, but greater events are coming."

By this time, the more general investigation of the new disease conducted by the city health authorities was well under way. It embraced the clinical, etiological, and epidemiological aspects of the malady. Among those called in to help was a senior assistant surgeon in the United States Public Health Service named Robert J. Huebner. It is customary for municipal authorities to ask the Public Health Service for assistance with troublesome cases. The Service welcomes such invitations, especially because it likes to show what can be accomplished by its National Institute of Health at Bethesda, Maryland, where it maintains a high-powered staff and superb laboratory facilities. Dr. Huebner, who is young, tough-minded, and carefully unenthusiastic, is a staff worker at the Institute. His assignment in this instance was to try to determine the cause of the disease. He suspected, as did several other investigators, that some member of the genus *Rickettsia* was responsible for the infection. That would account for the resemblance of the disease to Rocky Mountain spotted fever and to typhus, both of which are rickettsial ailments. The rickettsiae, which are named for the late Dr. Howard T. Ricketts, the American pathologist who discovered them, in 1909, are a class of minute bacteria-like organisms, much smaller than real bacteria and generally very elusive. Dr. Huebner buckled down to his job without much expectation of success.

The usual method of isolating a disease organism, and the one that Dr. Huebner followed, involves inoculating a group of highly susceptible laboratory animals whose reactions to disease are known to be similar to man's with a specimen of blood obtained from a person suffering from the disorder. Only if an animal becomes sick and exhibits the symptoms of the disease, as happens with exasperating infrequency in the case of so mild an affliction as rickettsialpox, is the transmission considered a success. The next step is simply to check to make certain that the results of the first were not a fluke. It consists of inoculating another group of animals with a fluid made from diseased brain tissue of the infected animals. If any animals in the second group come down with the disease, the organism is presumed to have been isolated, and fluid made from the brain tissue of these animals is then injected into the yolk sac of a fertile chicken egg. There the organisms multiply with exceptional alacrity, and thus a denser concentration of them is obtained. Smears of the yolk sac are next placed on slides—a very delicate operation—and at last, if everything has gone right, the organisms become visible under the microscope and, with luck, identifiable. For weeks, checking and rechecking in the Institute's laboratories, Dr. Huebner tried in this way to isolate the organism responsible for the Regency Park epidemic. He travelled tirelessly back and forth between Kew Gardens and Bethesda, conferring with Dr. Shankman on the clinical aspects of the illness, procuring new specimens of blood, and supervising the inoculation of hundreds of animals—white rats, cotton rats, rice rats, guinea pigs, rabbits, monkeys, and Syrian hamsters, which are a cross between a rat and a guinea pig. In all, he took specimens of blood from about twenty patients.

Only one specimen turned out to be of strength sufficient to produce infection in any of the animals. Dr. Huebner had hardly counted on even that. It was obtained, on July 26th—by which time about a hundred and twenty cases of the disease had been reported—from one of Dr. Shankman's many patients, a twenty-two-year-old woman named Marjory Kaplan. Miss Kaplan has since achieved a kind of immortality in medical literature as the donor of what is called, as a rather stark tribute to her, the M.K. Organism. For a while, it looked to Dr. Huebner as if her morbid gift, like those from the other patients, had been made in vain. "Then a fortuitous incident occurred in the laboratory on August 4th, nine days after we had inoculated five mice and two guinea pigs with Miss Kaplan's blood," he told me. "The guinea pigs and three of the mice hadn't reacted at all to the serum. One of the other mice had reacted, all right, but it had got sick and died at night, when nobody was around. By the time we found it, it was of no use to us. Well, I happened to be standing beside the cage where we were keeping those mice and I noticed that one of them was lying down. Then, all of a sudden, it rolled right over and died. Very obliging. We had the organism transferred from it to another group of animals within fifteen minutes. The test went along very nicely from there on. It was a fine, strong strain, apparently. We were able to keep passing it from one animal to another for weeks and weeks." This was the organism that eventually was isolated and recognized as a rickettsia. Later, several other tests revealed that the organism was a previously unknown species of the genus.

Mr. Pomerantz, in the meantime, had dispatched another batch of Regency Park mites to the Division of Insect Identification. They, too, were *Allodermanyssus sanguineus,* Mr. Muesebeck reported. He didn't ask for any more, and, feeling a little let down, Mr. Pomerantz returned halfheartedly to exterminating. He couldn't think of anything else to do. Then, on August 16th, he was exhilarated all over again by a telephone call from Dr. Huebner, whose activities he had been wistfully following in the newspapers. Dr. Huebner, it developed, had been informed of Mr. Pomerantz's discovery by Mr. Muesebeck. "It was an interesting piece of information," Dr. Huebner said to me. "We were beginning to get somewhere in our isolation tests and we knew that

Regency Park was crawling with mice, but we didn't know what was actually carrying the organism. Pomerantz's mites sounded like the missing link. If we could produce the disease in a laboratory with mites and then trace its cause back to the same organism, we'd have a very illuminating cycle. Also, if we could definitely establish it as a mouse-borne and mite-transmitted disease, we'd have not only the cause but the preventative as well. It would simply be a matter of keeping down the mouse population." Dr. Huebner's telephone call to Mr. Pomerantz was to ask if he would care to catch some mites for *him.* Mr. Pomerantz didn't have to be urged. That very day, he abandoned his business, for what turned out to be the rest of the summer, and raced out to Regency Park. The next morning, he met Dr. Huebner there and happily handed him a generous sample of mites. His impression of Dr. Huebner was favorable. "I saw he was a true scientist," Mr. Pomerantz assured me. "He knew how to say, 'I don't know.' We got along fine. I had been afraid that he might think I was a smart alex who was just seeking commercial publicity, but he understood right away that I was as much above reproach as Caesar's wife."

Mr. Pomerantz spent seven weeks in the basements of Regency Park, blissfully gathering mites. Dr. Huebner was insatiable. The days flew by. Occasionally, at Dr. Huebner's suggestion, Mr. Pomerantz varied his work by trapping mice, and to his delight he found most of them to be ridden with disease-carrying mites. Once, he had the satisfaction of capturing a mouse on which ten mites were feeding. Toward the end of August, when Dr. Huebner began to give most of his attention to the mite phase of his study, a field laboratory, staffed by Public Health Service operatives, was set up in the basement of one of the apartment houses, in order to expedite the processing and shipping of Mr. Pomerantz's catches. On September 10th, one of the Service's foremost parasitologists, Dr. William L. Jellison, who is engaged in research at an experimental station at Hamilton, Montana, was called to Regency Park to lend an experienced hand in the conduct of the laboratory. He, too, impressed Mr. Pomerantz as a true scientist. "Dr. Jellison never remembered to eat," Mr. Pomerantz informed me. "I always had to keep reminding him that we'd missed lunch and that it was now past dinnertime. He subsisted on love of work. I found his attitude very contagious. And yet somehow I gained five pounds."

On the morning of Tuesday, October 1st, Dr. Huebner, who had spent the weekend at Bethesda, sauntered into the basement field laboratory. Mr. Pomerantz was alone in the room. Dr. Huebner grinned at him. "Well, Charlie," he said casually, "we've made it." "Bravo!" Mr. Pomerantz shouted. It was his last utterance for several minutes. "I was suddenly stricken dumb," he told me. "I turned pale and weak. I realized that he had said more than that the investigation was a success. That 'we' included *me!* Dr. Huebner of the United States Public Health Service was calling Charles Pomerantz of the Bell Exterminating Company his scientific colleague. Who can describe my wonderful feelings? It was like meeting Mischa Elman and I had my fiddle and he had his fiddle and we sat down and played together Mendelssohn's Concerto in E minor."

[1947]

CHAPTER 2

A Man from Mexico

SMALLPOX IS AN ANCIENT and immoderately ferocious disease of Oriental origin that shares with plague, cholera, and epidemic typhus the distinction of having once or twice in the past five hundred years come fairly close to eradicating the human race. It is less unmanageable now. A full-fledged smallpox epidemic has been nearly unheard of since the late nineteenth century. Except in a few parts of the world—most of them easy-going—the appearance of even a handful of cases is an unusual occurrence. The only countries in which serious outbreaks have been at all frequent in recent years are India, Japan, Siam, Korea, British East Africa, Venezuela, and the United States.

About the best that can be said for smallpox is that it is somewhat less barbaric than plague. Plague is almost invariably fatal. Smallpox strikes with varying degrees of intensity and in some epidemics there have been so many mild cases that a large majority of the victims have recovered, but the disease is by no means always so benign. At its worst—when it is known as black, or hemorrhagic, smallpox—it is almost always lethal. Victims of even the blandest attacks of smallpox occasionally succumb to one or another of several complications to which the disease is hospitable, among them septic poisoning and bronchopneumonia, and those fortunate enough to survive an attack are often crippled for life. Blindness is a possible, though uncommon, consequence. Few have ever emerged scot-free from an attack of smallpox. Because of the pustular eruptions which characterize the disease, and from which its name is derived, it is almost certain to be permanently disfiguring. It can also be one of the most unnerving and repulsive of ailments. "The patient often becomes a dripping, unrecognizable mass of pus by the seventh or eighth day of eruption," Dr. Archibald L. Hoyne, medical superintendent of the Chicago Municipal Contagious Disease Hospital, has noted in a clinical study. "The putrid odor is stifling, the temperature often high [107° has been authoritatively reported], and the patient frequently in a wild state of delirium." Moreover, unlike plague, cholera, typhus, and many other deadly infections, the transmission of which is usually limited to either a carrier insect or contaminated drinking water, smallpox is abundantly contagious. Some epidemiologists consider it the most contagious of all diseases, including measles and the common cold.

The cause of smallpox is a durable virus. It enters the body through the respiratory system and is present in the exhalations of its victims for hours, and very likely days, before the apparent onset of illness. It is prolifically communicable during the entire course of the disease and may even be contracted from a victim some hours after his death. It can be conveyed by clothing, books, or letters, and there is good reason to believe that it is as readily airborne as dust. Nobody is naturally immune to smallpox, survival of one attack is no absolute assurance of future immunity, and, since both nonagenarians and unborn babies have been stricken, susceptibility is seemingly unrelated to age. A specific cure has yet to be discovered, and medical treatment, while desirable, is merely palliative. However, smallpox is not unavoidable. It is, in fact, among the few diseases against which certain immunization is possible. "There is no more certain truth in all the world," Dr. Hoyne has written, "than that an individual properly vaccinated with potent lymph [living virus] cannot contract smallpox in any manner whatsoever."

Many physicians are inclined these days to regard smallpox as an anachronism. This assumption, though infirm, is by no means unreasonable. The development of a reliable method of preventing the disease is not only one of scientific medicine's loftiest triumphs but one of its earliest; by illuminating the mechanics of disease in general, vaccination, which dates from the eighteenth century, inspired the immunological discoveries of Pasteur, von Behring, Ehrlich, and others. Long before the discovery of vaccination, it was possible to exert some preventive control over smallpox. In the third century before Christ, pioneering healers in India became aware that the injection of a minute quantity of virulent smallpox matter into a healthy person often produced a painless seizure and subsequent immunity. Inoculation, as this procedure came to be known, was introduced into Europe, by way of Turkey, in 1717, or thereabouts, and was widely practiced on the Continent and elsewhere until vaccination turned up, a couple of generations later. The first deliberate vaccination was performed by an English dairy farmer named Benjamin Jesty in 1774. Jesty had observed that milkmaids who had suffered an attack of vaccinia, or cowpox—a harmless occupational malaise of bovine derivation —seemed to be impervious to smallpox. He conceived the useful notion of relating that barnyard phenomenon to the technique of inoculation, and, using lymph from an ailing cow, immunized himself and his wife and children, at least to his own satisfaction. As a vaccinator, Jesty apparently confined his efforts to the family circle. It is possible that Dr. Edward Jenner, a British physician who is more commonly celebrated as the discoverer of vaccination, never heard of him. Dr. Jenner vaccinated his first patient in 1796, with the same sort of lymph Jesty had employed. Two years later, he published his revolutionary treatise "An Inquiry into the Causes and Effects of the Variolæ Vaccinæ, a Disease Discovered in Some of the Western Counties of England, Particularly Gloucestershire, and Known by the Name of the Cowpox." Inoculation has two drawbacks as a smallpox preventive. In addition to being uncomfortably speculative, the seizure it brings on is as contagious as the real thing. Since the virus of cowpox, though the disease is probably a form of smallpox, is consistently effective but innocuous, vaccination has neither of these imperfections. Its only flaw, an easily remedied one, is that the immunity conferred by it diminishes with the passage of time.

The model efficiency of vaccination was almost at once recognized throughout the world. The first American vaccinator, Dr. Benjamin Waterhouse, professor of physics at the Harvard University Medical School, immunized his first patient in 1800. Not long after, in England, the Bishop of Worcester set a clerical precedent by commending the practice to his communicants. In 1805, Napoleon made vaccination compulsory in the French Army, a precaution that has since been taken by the military authorities of nearly all nations, and persuasively urged it upon civilians, not only in France but in Italy as well. Compulsory vaccination of everybody was presently instituted in many countries—Bavaria (1807), Norway, Denmark, and Iceland (1810), Sweden (1814), the German states (1818), Great Britain (1853), Rumania (1874), Hungary (1876), and Austria (1886). Other countries have since become equally thorough, but the United States is not among them. Compulsory vaccination has always been considered unnecessary here, except for the armed forces. In some states and in some cities (New York City is one), it is required only as a prerequisite to attending elementary school. Even this gentle bit of coercion has occasionally been opposed by patriots as tyrannical.

In spite of this country's somewhat indulgent attitude toward smallpox prevention, the disease is no longer, at least statistically, a very active menace here. A visitation in 1901-02 that centered upon New York City and caused seven hundred and twenty deaths in this area is usually cited as the last high-velocity epidemic. However, smallpox still turns up; generally, more than a hundred cases of it occur in the United States every year, and in one recent year, 1930, nearly forty-nine thousand were reported —an incidence, considering the ease with which the disease can be prevented, of almost astronomical proportions. Ordinarily, the cases are widely scattered, but there have been numerous concentrated outbreaks ever since the First World War. A hundred and sixty people died in one, in 1921, in Kansas City. Another, later that year, in Denver, caused thirty-seven deaths. In 1924, in Detroit, out of sixteen hundred and ten cases a hundred and sixty-three were fatal. There were twenty deaths during an outbreak in the Puget Sound area around Seattle in 1945. In the spring of 1947, to the unnatural astonishment of the press, the public, and most physicians, smallpox reappeared, after an absence of not quite eight years, in New York City. It struck, altogether, twelve men, women, and children. Two of them died. Largely because of a combination of dazzling good luck and the dispatch with which the Department of Health tracked down and sequestered several hundred people presumed to have been exposed to the disease, the outbreak proved to be one of the mildest on record. It could have been hair-raising. Dr. Morris Greenberg, director of the Department's Bureau of Preventable Diseases, has estimated that at the time the first victim died, only about two million of the city's nearly eight million inhabitants had any degree of immunity whatever to smallpox.

The New York City Health Department, to which the appearance of a serious communicable disease anywhere in the city must be promptly reported, learned of the 1947 outbreak toward noon on Friday, March 28th. Its informant was Dr. Dorothea M. Tolle, medical superintendent of Willard Parker Hospital, a municipal institution for the treatment of contagious diseases, at the foot of East Fifteenth Street. Her report, which she made by telephone, as is customary when a potentially fast-moving contagion is involved, was inconclusive but disheartening. Two patients, whose trouble was at first believed to be chicken pox, had overnight developed eruptions that looked alarmingly like those of smallpox. Dr. Edward M. Bernecker, Commissioner of Hospitals, and Dr. Ralph S. Muckenfuss, director of the Bureau of Laboratories, had both been apprised of the occurrence, she added, and the latter was arranging for a definitive laboratory analysis of material taken from the patients. Dr. Tolle's lack of certainty, which was shared by her deputy, Dr. Irving Klein, and the other members of the Willard Parker staff, was not surprising. Smallpox has always been an elusive disease to diagnose in its early stages, the symptoms that mark its onset—chills, fever, headache, and nausea—being indistinguishable from those of influenza, malaria, and typhoid fever. Bedside recognition of it at any stage is difficult now, for contemporary physicians generally find even the rash peculiar to the disease—a rash that emerges on the third or fourth day of illness and becomes pustular by the eighth—more confusing than enlightening. One reason for this diagnostic stumbling is that many doctors currently in practice have never seen a case of smallpox. Another is that several other rashy disorders—among them chicken pox, measles, scarlet fever, scabies, acne, impetigo, syphilis, and ulcerative endocarditis—are more insistently prevalent and, consequently, come more readily to mind. The thought of smallpox forced itself upon Dr. Tolle and Dr. Klein that Friday morning in 1947 mainly because the rash displayed by the two invalids was, providentially, of an almost classic clarity.

By one o'clock, copies of Dr. Tolle's report had been distributed to all administrative officers of the Department and an investigation of the cases was briskly under way. Its pattern, despite the unusual nature of the alarm, was routine and confidential. As a preliminary defensive measure, Dr. Bernecker and Dr. Israel Weinstein, then Commissioner of Health, ordered a speedy vaccination of everybody at Willard Parker—doctors, nurses, lay employees, and patients—and instructed the authorities there not to admit any visitor who declined to be vaccinated on the spot. A summary clinical inquiry was at the same time, and as a matter of course, undertaken by Dr. David A. Singer, chief diagnostician of the Manhattan division of the Bureau of Preventable Diseases. He lit out for the hospital the moment the notification reached him. He found both suspected victims flushed, feverish, freshly vaccinated, and tucked away in individual, glassed-in cubicles in a remote corner of an isolation building. One of them was a twenty-six-year-old Puerto Rican, who, because of the turn events took in his instance, can be specifically identified as Ismael Acosta. The other was a Negro infant, Patricia G—, aged twenty-two months, whose name, like the names of most patients under such circumstances, can be given only in part. Dr. Singer's diagnosis, which he presently telephoned to Dr. Greenberg, his superior, tentatively confirmed the suspicions of Dr. Tolle and Dr. Klein. Dr. Muckenfuss, meanwhile, within an hour after being alerted by Dr. Tolle, had obtained some fluid from the lesions of the two patients and dispatched the samples by plane to Dr. Joseph Smadel, director of the United States Army Medical School Laboratory, in Washington, for full-scale examination. His choice of the Army Laboratory was instinctive; at the time, it was the closest to New York of the few laboratories in the country that were equipped to perform the intricate and time-consuming tests by which the presence of smallpox virus can be detected. Then, before turning his attention to other things, Dr. Muckenfuss got in touch with Dr. Weinstein. He told him that a dependable yes-or-no answer from Dr. Smadel should be along in about a week.

The cheerless uniformity of the clinical opinions of Dr. Tolle, Dr. Klein, and Dr. Singer gave Dr. Weinstein little reason to hope for a relaxing word from Dr. Smadel, but he felt restrained by the lack of absolute certainty from authorizing at the moment a far-reaching investigation. He preferred, so long as there was any doubt, to shield the city from the shrieks and speculations of the press. His discretion did not, however, encourage departmental idleness. The next morning, Saturday, March 29th, as part of the undercover investigation, a couple of the most inquisitive operatives in the Bureau of Preventable Diseases were quietly assigned to assist Dr. Singer. Their job was to discover where and how, if Acosta and Patricia did have smallpox, the disease had been contracted. To this end, with the lively coöperation of Dr. Tolle and Dr. Klein, they fixed their attention on the hospital records. Taken together, the dossiers of the two patients made provocative reading. Acosta was married, lived in the East Bronx, was employed as a porter at Bellevue Hospital, and had reached Willard Parker on Thursday, March 27th, having first spent two days in the dermatologic ward at Bellevue. The baby had been admitted to Willard Parker six days before Acosta. She had fallen sick on March 19th. Two days later, her parents had taken her to a clinic near their home, in Harlem, and from there she had been sent at once to Willard Parker. What quickened the interest of the investigators was that neither of the patients was a newcomer to the hospital. Both had been there previously, and at the same time. Less than a month before, Acosta had spent a couple of weeks— from February 27th to March 11th—at Willard Parker, with the mumps. Patricia's earlier visit, the outcome of an attack of croup, had lasted from February 28th to March 13th. Dr. Singer and his colleagues, mindful that the incubation period of smallpox is generally around twelve to fourteen days and never more than twenty-one, made themselves comfortable and began to absorb this instructive set of coincidences. By Saturday evening, they had been led to the somewhat reassuring suspicion that Acosta and Patricia had acquired the disease from the same source. Over the weekend, a third and equally probable case of smallpox was uncovered in Willard Parker. The new victim was a boy of two and a half, named John F—, who had been in the hospital, suffering from whooping cough, since March 6th. The fact that his had been an uninterrupted confinement strengthened the investigators' hunch to a near certainty. They concluded that Acosta, Patricia, and John had contracted smallpox at the hospital, from somebody who had been there between March 6th and March 13th.

The unflattering implications of this conclusion embarrassed Dr. Tolle and Dr. Klein, but only momentarily. They calmed themselves with the reflection that diagnostic infallibility is more often the aspiration than the achievement of any hospital staff. To Dr. Klein, the experience was even salutary, and he emerged from it both unruffled and inspired. Memory revived in him with the abruptness of revelation. Early in March, he now recalled, there had been a patient at Willard Parker in whom one physician had fleetingly thought he detected indications of smallpox. Dr. Klein guided the investigators back to the files and, after some digging, produced the record of the patient he had in mind. It was that of a man named Eugene La Bar, and the case it described was morbid, chaotic, and dismaying. La Bar, an American, had lived since 1940 in Mexico City, where he had desultorily engaged in exporting leather goods. He was forty-seven years old, married, and childless. Toward the end of February, he and his wife had left Mexico City and headed for New York, travelling by bus. It was their intention to go right on to Readfield, Maine, to view a farm that Mrs. La Bar had just inherited near there, but La Bar became ill during the journey. His discomfort, which he attempted to relieve by frequent doses of aspirin, codeine, Nembutal, and phenobarbital, consisted of a headache and a severe pain in the back of the neck. By the time the couple reached New York, La Bar felt too unwell to go any farther. As far as could be ascertained from the record, he had gone at once to the clinic at Bellevue, where an examining physician, observing that he had a fever of 105° and an odd rash on his face and hands, admitted him to the hospital's dermatologic ward. The date of his admittance was March 5th, a Wednesday. Three days later, on March 8th, La Bar was transferred to Willard Parker, his condition having baffled and finally frightened the Bellevue dermatologists. He arrived there more dead than alive. The rash by then covered his entire body, and it was pustular and hemorrhagic. It was this rash that prompted one of the Willard Parker doctors to offer a half-hearted diagnosis of smallpox. It also impelled him to vaccinate Mrs. La Bar when she called at the hospital that afternoon to inquire about her husband. Then the physician dropped the theory. His reasons were plausible. A freehand analysis of material taken from the lesions did not appear to support his guess; the rash, upon closer scrutiny, was not strikingly typical of smallpox; La Bar had an old but well-developed vaccination scar; and Mrs. La Bar insisted that her husband could not possibly have been in recent contact with anybody suffering from the disease. Three other diagnoses that had also been more or less seriously considered were enumerated in the record. One, suggested by the vigor and variety of the painkillers with which La Bar had stuffed himself, was drug poisoning. Another was Kaposi's varicelliform eruption, a kind of edema complicated by pustules. The third was erythema multiforme, an acute skin infection, and this had seemed the likeliest. La Bar lay in an agony of delirium for two days. On Monday morning, March 10th, his fever suddenly vanished and he felt almost well. Late that afternoon, he died. An autopsy disclosed, among other internal dishevelments, an enlarged spleen, a friable liver, and multiple hemorrhages in the viscera and the lungs. The final entry on the record was the cause of death: "Erythema multiforme, with laryngo-tracheo-bronchitis and bronchopneumonia." It was not a deduction in which Dr. Klein and the Health Department physicians, whose wits had been sharpened by hindsight, were tempted to concur. Their persuasion was that they had just read a forceful account of an unusually virulent attack of black smallpox.

On the morning of Friday, April 4th, the report from Dr. Smadel came through. It was affirmative; both Acosta and Patricia had smallpox. (Subsequently, Dr. Smadel was able to say the same of John and several others, including the deceased La Bar; some material taken from the latter's lesions for the test made at the hospital had, it developed, fortunately been preserved.) Dr. Weinstein received the report without marked consternation. His reaction was almost one of relief. It delivered him from the misery of retaining an increasingly unreasonable doubt. It also propelled him into rapid motion. He notified the United States Public Health Service of the outbreak. Then he had a word of counsel with Dr. Bernecker. After that, he assembled the administrative officers of the Departments of Health and of Hospitals for a briefing on tactics. Next, waving Dr. Greenberg's agents out into the open, he set a full-dress investigation in motion. At two o'clock Dr. Weinstein broke the news to the press at a conference in his office. His statement included an exhortation. "It is not surprising that smallpox has reappeared in this city," he said. "The Health Department has stated many times that we are exposed to communicable diseases occurring in this and neighboring countries. The danger of a widespread epidemic is slight, because our population is for the most part protected by vaccination. Smallpox is one of the most communicable of all diseases, and the only known preventive measure is vaccination. Anyone in the city who has never been vaccinated, or who has not been vaccinated since early childhood, should get this protection at once. Smallpox is a serious disease that may cause permanent disfigurement, damage to vital organs, and even death. With vaccination, a simple and harmless procedure, available to all, there is absolutely no excuse for anyone to remain unprotected." Dr. Weinstein was aware, as he spoke, that his advice was somewhat sounder than his optimism.

The public investigation, like the plainclothes reconnaissance that had preceded it, was accompanied by a quarantine measure; the dermatologic ward at Bellevue was closed to visitors who could not give convincing assurance that they had recently been vaccinated. In addition, vaccination of the entire population of the hospital commenced—a considerable task in itself, which was entrusted to the Department of Hospitals and the Bellevue staff.

The rest of the undertaking was handled, without complaint, by the Bureau of Preventable Diseases. It involved the tracking down, the vaccination, and the continued surveillance during the smallpox period of incubation of every person who was known to have been exposed to the disease. Dr. Greenberg's medical staff consists of, in addition to himself and Dr. Singer, three full-time inspectors and thirty-five part-time men. He put them all to work on the task. By nightfall on Friday, less than twelve hours after the arrival of Dr. Smadel's report, Dr. Greenberg's men had called upon, examined, and vaccinated some two hundred potential victims and were on the trail of several hundred others. These two groups comprised all the residents of the apartment buildings in which the Acostas and Patricia's family lived, everyone who had been in the Harlem clinic on the day of Patricia's visit, and everyone who had set foot in Willard Parker between March 8th and March 27th or in the Bellevue dermatologic ward between March 5th and March 8th or between March 25th and March 27th, but they did not comprise all those who might conceivably have been infected. This was no reflection on the resourcefulness of the Bureau men. Dr. Weinstein and his associates had known from the outset that the city contained innumerable possible smallpox cases who were beyond the timely reach of any investigators. They were the people among whom La Bar, on March 5th, and Patricia, on March 21st, and Acosta on March 25th, had passed on their way to the hospital. It was largely Acosta's means of getting there that prompted Dr. Weinstein to try to stimulate in the public an orderly but general desire for vaccination. La Bar had travelled in the moderate seclusion of a cab, and Patricia had left the clinic in an ambulance. Acosta had taken the subway and a crosstown bus.

The immediate response to Dr. Weinstein's exhortation, which he quickly condensed for press and radio use into the slogan "Be Sure, Be Safe, Get Vaccinated!," was only mildly gratifying. Undismayed, he instructed the Bureau of Laboratories to at once set about converting its bulk supplies of vaccine into handy, one-dose units and to make these available without charge, through drugstores, to all physicians and, directly, to all hospitals and to the city's twenty-one district health centers. He issued a public statement emphasizing that the protection he recommended was free as well as simple and harmless. Over the weekend, his meaning appeared to have been caught only by the prudent and the panicky, but on Monday, April 7th, an encouragingly widened comprehension was perceptible. There was good reason. Two new cases of suspected smallpox had turned up and been proclaimed. Acosta's wife, who was twenty-six years old and in the seventh month of pregnancy, was one of them. She had become ill at her home on Saturday night. The following morning the inspector assigned to patrol the building took one alert look at her and summoned a Willard Parker ambulance. The other was a Cuban, who, as it later turned out, had nothing worse than chicken pox, but by the time his case was correctly diagnosed, another case of smallpox had come to light. This was on Thursday, April 10th. The patient was a forty-three-year-old wanderer named Herman G——, whose condition had come to the attention of a physician in the dermatologic ward at Bellevue where he had been confined for treatment of syphilis since March 10th. The next day, April 11th, still another victim was reported. He was a businessman of fifty-seven named Harry T——, and his case, too, was discovered in the Bellevue dermatologic ward. He had been admitted there, suffering from lymphoblastoma, on March 19th. His misfortune, as the newspapers loudly and uneasily pointed out, brought the number of smallpox cases to seven. It also had the effect of abruptly increasing to around a hundred thousand the number of people who had heeded Dr. Weinstein's admonition.

While dutifully notifying the United States Public Health Service of the outbreak and its transcontinental origin, Dr. Weinstein had expressed a normal interest in Mrs. La Bar's whereabouts and the state of her health. It was his understanding, he said, that she had continued on to Maine soon after her husband's funeral; nothing had been heard from her since, although the true cause of her husband's death had been widely publicized. As might be expected, Dr. Weinstein's curiosity concerning Mrs. La Bar was at least equalled by that of the Public Health Service. He was promised an early reply, and on Wednesday, April 9th, his day was enlivened by a report from the Service on its findings. They were numerous and in some respects reassuring, in others highly disturbing. Mrs. La Bar was at the home of a relative in East Winthrop, Maine, and in excellent health. Information obtained from her had enabled the Service to alert the health authorities in the towns at which the La Bars' bus had stopped—Laredo, San Antonio, Dallas, Tulsa, Joplin, St. Louis, Indianapolis, Cincinnati, and Pittsburgh. None had reported any local evidence of smallpox. La Bar's illness apparently hadn't reached a highly contagious stage during the journey. What distressed Dr. Weinstein was the disclosure that the La Bars had arrived in New York from Mexico City on Saturday afternoon, March 1st. This meant that they had been in the city five days before La Bar finally tottered into Bellevue. During that time, they had stayed at a hotel, which the Health Department has charitably never seen fit to identify. Fortunately, because of La Bar's unrelenting aches and pains, they seldom left their room. The only time they went outside the hotel, as far as Mrs. La Bar could recall, was on the Monday after their arrival here, when they took a stroll up Fifth Avenue and made a few trivial purchases at McCreery's, at a ten-cent store, and at the Knox hat shop. The report added that Mrs. La Bar's earlier reticence had been caused by a lifelong aversion to red tape.

A somewhat similar reticence was discovered in an assistant manager of the La Bars' hotel by a squad of Dr. Greenberg's agents who stopped by later that Wednesday. It was their intention to vaccinate all the hotel's employees and permanent residents and to gather the names and addresses of all transient guests registered there between March 1st and March 5th. The opposition that they encountered was rigid, but it was not prolonged. It vanished at a thawing murmur from Dr. Greenberg over the telephone to the effect that the full text of Mrs. La Bar's memoir could easily be substituted for the tactfully expurgated version, omitting the name of the hotel, that was then being prepared for the press. His words induced a cordiality of such intensity that the manager himself trotted out the records and asked to be the first to bare his arm. By bedtime Wednesday night, the inspectors had made a satisfying start on both their tasks, and they finished up the following day. Approximately three thousand people had spent one or more of the first five days of March under the same roof as La Bar. Nearly all were from out of town, and the names and addresses of these, who included residents of twenty-nine states, were transmitted to the health authorities of those states. Dr. Greenberg's men added what guests there had been from New York City to their already generous list of local suspects. In time, all the three thousand, except for a few dozen adventurers who had registered under spurious names, were hunted down and, as it happily turned out, given a clean bill of health.

Meanwhile, Dr. Weinstein and Dr. Greenberg had decided that there wasn't much they could do in the way of disinfecting the La Bars' month-old trail up Fifth Avenue. They tried to console themselves with the realization that private physicians and the district health centers were experiencing another substantial increase in the demand for safety and certainty. This followed the newspaper publication, on Thursday, of Mrs. La Bar's censored revelations, which contained a discomfortingly vague reference to "a midtown hotel," in and about which La Bar had passed five days at nearly the peak of his contagiousness. Practically all the hotels in Manhattan at which a transient would be likely to stop are in the midtown area.

Bright and early Saturday morning, April 12th, there was more unpleasant news. It was relayed to Dr. Weinstein by the New York State Department of Health, and it came from the village of Millbrook, in Dutchess County. A boy of four, Vernon L—, whose family lived in the Bronx, had been sick there for several days with what Dr. Smadel, in whom the state health authorities also had confidence, had just diagnosed as smallpox. The boy, an inmate of the Cardinal Hayes Convalescent Home, on the outskirts of town, was not, it appeared, critically ill. The source of the infection was no mystery. Before being admitted to the Home, on March 13th, Vernon had spent eighteen days, from February 21st to March 10th, at Willard Parker, under treatment for scarlet fever. He was one of a number of Willard Parker alumni no longer in the city whom the state investigators had been asked to trace. The news of the Millbrook case was conveyed to Dr. Weinstein by telephone. The morning brought him two more agitating calls. One was from Dr. Muckenfuss and the other from Dr. Tolle. Dr.

Muckenfuss reported that the municipal supply of vaccine was going fast. Two hundred thousand units had been distributed during the past week, and no more than that number were still on hand. Dr. Tolle called to say that Mrs. Acosta had just died.

At one-thirty that afternoon, Dr. Weinstein, accompanied by Dr. Bernecker and a couple of his other associates, hopped around to Gracie Mansion for a candid chat with Mayor O'Dwyer, whom they found enduring an instant of repose. It has been Dr. Weinstein's original and commendable determination to spare the Mayor any direct concern with the calamity. Dr. Muckenfuss's information, on top of everything else, had compelled him to change his mind. After Dr. Weinstein and his colleagues had successfully communicated their uneasiness to the Mayor, they divulged a more specific reason for their visit. They asked for an appropriation of five hundred thousand dollars. Most of this sum, which, after a little ritualistic sparring, the Mayor agreed to wheedle out of the Board of Estimate, would be expended for vaccine, Dr. Weinstein explained, and the rest for other extraordinary expenses of the Health and Hospital Departments, including the hiring of a thousand doctors and a couple of hundred clerks to man additional public vaccination centers in various parts of the city. Then, also at the request of Dr. Weinstein, the Mayor led the group down to City Hall, where at five o'clock he met in his office with the commissioners of all municipal departments and instructed them to see to it that no city employee delayed an instant in getting vaccinated. Before knocking off for the day, the Mayor called in the press, invited the photographers to unlimber their cameras, and allowed Dr. Weinstein to vaccinate him. This, he pointed out, was his fifth vaccination in six years, the others having been acquired during his service in the Army, but it was better to be safe than sorry.

Over the weekend, the words and insinuating example of Mayor O'Dwyer, which were supplemented, on the air at nine o'clock Sunday evening, by a sudden, inflammatory chirp from Walter Winchell, resulted in a powerful quickening of the instinct for self-preservation, and this was still further heightened by word from the convalescent home in Millbrook that three more smallpox cases—two of them child inmates and the other an elderly nun on the staff of the institution—had been discovered there. Eighty-four thousand people, including hundreds in the remotest wastes of Staten Island, were vaccinated on Monday. On Tuesday, following the announcement of yet another case of smallpox originating at Bellevue—that of a sixty-year-old man who had been in the hospital suffering from a serious skin ailment for many months—two hundred thousand more were vaccinated. So great was the drain on the municipal reserves of vaccine that the Mayor summoned before him representatives of all the big pharmaceutical firms that have plants or offices here and extracted from them a collective promise to make available to the city an abundant and immediate supply of the preparation. Pending the fulfillment of their pledge, he arranged, over the telephone, for an interim loan of vaccine from the Army and Navy. Wednesday night, in the course of announcing that emergency clinics would be opened the following morning in all of the city's eighty-four police stations, Dr. Weinstein found an opportunity to tacitly revise his earlier description of smallpox. It was, he now declared, "the most contagious of diseases." He was rewarded on Thursday evening with word that half a million vaccinations had been performed during the day.

There was no perceptible letup in the public's desire for immunization during the remainder of the week, and on Sunday, April 20th, some additional interest was created by an announcement from Brigadier General Wallace H. Graham, the White House physician, that President Truman's preparations for a three-hour visit to New York the next day had included a brand-new vaccination. During the next week, two hundred Health Department teams, each composed of a doctor and a nurse, moved through the public elementary and high schools, vaccinating some eight hundred and eighty-nine thousand children. Toward the end of the week, Dr. Weinstein was sufficiently satisfied with the way things were going to reveal that the six surviving smallpox patients at Willard Parker and the four in Millbrook appeared to be out of danger. On Saturday, at his direction, the vaccinators were withdrawn from the police stations.

Six days later, on Friday, May 2nd, Dr. Weinstein formally announced the end of the outbreak and the completion of the biggest and fastest mass-vaccination campaign in the history of the world. Within the space of only twenty-eight days, he said, a total of at least six million three hundred and fifty thousand people had been vaccinated in the city. Practically everyone in New York was now immune. Although Dr. Weinstein had the delicacy not to say so, it was about time.

[*1949*]

AUTHOR'S NOTE: Smallpox was one of the first diseases of international scope to come to the official concern of the World Health Organization. A worldwide program of eradication was initiated in 1948. At that time smallpox was considered to be endemic in thirty-three countries—in virtually the whole of Africa south of the Sahara; in Southeast Asia (Bangladesh, India, Nepal, Pakistan, and Afghanistan); in Indonesia; and in Brazil. There were at least ten million cases reported each year. The WHO program involved isolation of patients and vaccination of all persons having had any contact with them. By 1973, smallpox had been eradicated in every country but Ethiopia, Botswana, India, Bangladesh, Nepal, and Pakistan. The last case of smallpox in India was reported in 1975. The last case of smallpox in the world was reported in Ethiopia in 1977. A resolution adopted by the thirty-third World Health Assembly in Geneva, Switzerland, on May 8, 1980, read: "The world and all its peoples have won freedom from smallpox . . . an unprecedented achievement in public health."

CHAPTER 3

The Fog

———————————◆———————————

THE MONONGAHELA RIVER rises in the middle Alleghenies and seeps for a hundred and twenty-eight miles through the iron and bituminous-coal fields of northeastern West Virginia and southwestern Pennsylvania to Pittsburgh. There, joining the Allegheny River, it becomes the wild Ohio. It is the only river of any consequence in the United States that flows due north, and it is also the shortest. Its course is cramped and crooked, and flanked by bluffs and precipitous hills. Within living memory, its waters were quick and green, but they are murky now with pollution, and a series of locks and dams steady its once tumultuous descent, rendering it navigable from source to mouth. Traffic on the Monongahela is heavy. Its shipping, which consists almost wholly of coal barges pushed by wheezy, coal-burning stern-wheelers, exceeds in tonnage that of the Panama Canal. The river is densely industrialized. There are trucking highways along its narrow banks and interurban lines and branches of the Pennsylvania Railroad and the New York Central and smelters and steel plants and chemical works and glass factories and foundries and coke plants and machine shops and zinc mills, and its hills and bluffs are scaled by numerous blackened mill towns. The blackest of them is the borough of Donora, in Washington County, Pennsylvania.

Donora is twenty-eight miles south of Pittsburgh and covers the tip of a lumpy point formed by the most convulsive of the Monongahela's many horseshoe bends. Though accessible by road, rail, and river, it is an extraordinarily secluded place. The river and the bluffs that lift abruptly from the water's edge to a height of four hundred and fifty feet enclose it on the north and east and south, and just above it to the west is a range of rolling but even higher hills. On its outskirts are acres of sidings and rusting gondolas, abandoned mines, smoldering slag piles, and gulches filled with rubbish. Its limits are marked by sooty signs that read, "Donora. Next to Yours the Best Town in the U.S.A." It is a harsh, gritty town, founded in 1901 and old for its age, with a gaudy main street and a thousand identical gaunt gray houses. Some of its streets are paved with concrete and some are cobbled, but many are of dirt and crushed coal. At least half of them are as steep as roofs, and several have steps instead of sidewalks. It is treeless and all but grassless, and much of it is slowly sliding downhill. After a rain, it is a smear of mud. Its vacant lots and many of its yards are mortally gullied, and one of its three cemeteries is an eroded ruin of gravelly clay and toppled tombstones. Its population is 12,300. Two-thirds of its men, and a substantial number of its women, work in its mills. There are three of them—a steel plant, a wire plant, and a zinc-and-sulphuric-acid plant—all of which are operated by the American Steel & Wire Co., a subsidiary of the United States Steel Corporation, and they line its river front for three miles. They are huge mills. Some of the buildings are two blocks long, many are five or six stories high, and all of them bristle with hundred-foot stacks perpetually plumed with black or red or sulphurous yellow smoke.

Donora is abnormally smoky. Its mills are no bigger or smokier than many, but their smoke, and the smoke from the passing boats and trains, tends to linger there. Because of the crowding bluffs and sheltering hills, there is seldom a wind, and only occasionally a breeze, to dispel it. On still days, unless the skies are high and buoyantly clear, the lower streets are always dim and there is frequently a haze on the heights. Autumn is the smokiest season.

The weather is close and dull then, and there are persistent fogs as well. The densest ones generally come in October. They are greasy, gagging fogs, often intact even at high noon, and they sometimes last for two or three days. A few have lasted as long as four. One, toward the end of October, 1948, hung on for six. Unlike its predecessors, it turned out to be of considerably more than local interest. It was the second smoke-contaminated fog in history ever to reach a toxic density. The first such fog occurred in Belgium, in an industrialized stretch of the Meuse Valley, in 1930. During it several hundred people were prostrated, sixty of them fatally. The Donora fog struck down nearly six thousand. Twenty of them—five women and fifteen men—died. Nobody knows exactly what killed them, or why the others survived. At the time, not many of the stricken expected to.

The fog closed over Donora on the morning of Tuesday, October 26th. The weather was raw, cloudy, and dead calm, and it stayed that way as the fog piled up all that day and the next. By Thursday, it had stiffened adhesively into a motionless clot of smoke. That afternoon, it was just possible to see across the street, and, except for the stacks, the mills had vanished. The air began to have a sickening smell, almost a taste. It was the bittersweet reek of sulphur dioxide. Everyone who was out that day remarked on it, but no one was much concerned. The smell of sulphur dioxide, a scratchy gas given off by burning coal and melting ore, is a normal concomitant of any durable fog in Donora. This time, it merely seemed more penetrating than usual.

At about eight-thirty on Friday morning, one of Donora's eight physicians, Dr. Ralph W. Koehler, a tense, stocky man of forty-eight, stepped to his bathroom window for a look at the weather. It was, at best, unchanged. He could see nothing but a watery waste of rooftops islanded in fog. As he was turning away, a shimmer of movement in the distance caught his eye. It was a freight train creeping along the riverbank just south of town, and the sight of it shook him. He had never seen anything quite like it before. "It was the smoke," he says. "They were firing up for the grade and the smoke was belching out, but it didn't rise. I mean it didn't go up at all. It just spilled out over the lip of the stack like a black liquid, like ink or oil, and rolled down to the ground and lay there. My God, it just lay there! I thought, Well, God damn—and they talk about needing smoke control up in Pittsburgh! I've got a heart condition, and I was so disgusted my heart began to act up a little. I had to sit down on the edge of the tub and rest a minute."

Dr. Koehler and an associate, Dr. Edward Roth, who is big, heavyset, and in his middle forties, share an office on the second floor of a brownstone building one block up from the mills, on McKean Avenue, the town's main street. They have one employee, a young woman named Helen Stack, in whom are combined an attractive receptionist, an efficient secretary, and a capable nurse. Miss Stack was the first to reach the office that morning. Like Dr. Koehler and many other Donorans, she was in uncertain spirits. The fog was beginning to get on her nerves, and she had awakened with a sore throat and a cough and supposed that she was coming down with a cold. The appearance of the office deepened her depression. Everything in it was smeared with a kind of dust. "It wasn't just ordinary soot and grit," she says. "There was something white and scummy mixed up in it. It was just wet ash from the mills, but I didn't know that then. I almost hated to touch it, it was so nasty-looking. But it had to be cleaned up, so I got out a cloth and went to work." When Miss Stack had finished, she lighted a cigarette and sat down at her desk to go through the mail. It struck her that the cigarette had a very peculiar taste. She held it up and sniffed at the smoke. Then she raised it to her lips, took another puff, and doubled up in a paroxysm of coughing. For an instant, she thought she was going to be sick. "I'll never forget that taste," she says. "Oh, it was awful! It was sweet and horrible, like something rotten. It tasted the way the fog smelled, only ten times worse. I got rid of the cigarette as fast as I could and drank a glass of water, and then I felt better. What puzzled me was I'd smoked a cigarette at home after breakfast and it had tasted all right. I didn't know what to think, except that maybe it was because the fog wasn't quite as bad up the hill as here downstreet. I guess I thought my cold was probably partly to blame. I wasn't really uneasy. The big Halloween parade the Chamber of Commerce puts on every year was to be held that night, and I could hear the workmen down in the street putting up the decorations. I knew the committee wouldn't be going ahead with the parade if they thought anything was wrong. So I went on with my work, and pretty soon the Doctors came in from their early calls and it was just like any other morning."

The office hours of Dr. Koehler and Dr. Roth are the same, from one to three in the afternoon and from seven to nine at night. Whenever possible in the afternoon, Dr. Koehler leaves promptly at three. Because of his unsteady heart, he finds it desirable to rest for a time before dinner. That Friday afternoon, he was just getting into his coat when Miss Stack announced a patient. "He was wheezing and gasping for air," Dr. Koehler says, "but there wasn't anything very surprising about that. He was one of our regular asthmatics, and the fog gets them every time. The only surprising thing was that he hadn't come in sooner. The fact is, none of our asthmatics had been in all week. Well, I did what I could for him. I gave him a shot of adrenaline or aminophyllin— some anti-spasmodic—to dilate the bronchia, so he could breathe more easily, and sent him home. I followed him out. I didn't feel so good myself."

Half an hour after Dr. Koehler left, another gasping asthmatic, an elderly steelworker, tottered into the office. "He was pretty wobbly," Miss Stack says. "Dr. Roth was still in his office, and saw him right away. I guess he wasn't much better when he came out, because I remember thinking, Poor fellow. There's nothing sadder than an asthmatic when the fog is bad. Well, he had hardly gone out the door when I heard a terrible commotion. I thought, Oh, my gosh, he's fallen down the stairs! Then there was an awful yell. I jumped up and dashed out into the hall. There was a man I'd never seen before sort of draped over the banister. He was kicking at the wall and pulling at the banister and moaning and choking and yelling at the top of his voice. 'Help! Help me! I'm dying!' I just stood there. I was petrified. Then Dr. Brown, across the hall, came running out, and he and somebody else helped the man on up the stairs and into his office. Just then, my phone began to ring. I almost bumped into Dr. Roth. He was coming out to see what was going on. When I picked up the phone, it was just like hearing that man in the hall again. It was somebody saying somebody was dying. I said Dr. Roth would be right over, but before I could even tell him, the phone started ringing again. And the minute I hung up the receiver, it rang again. That was the beginning of a terrible night. From that minute on, the phone never stopped ringing. That's the honest truth. And they were all alike. Everybody who called up said the same thing. Pain in the abdomen. Splitting headache. Nausea and vomiting. Choking and couldn't get their breath. Coughing up blood. But as soon as I got over my surprise, I calmed down. Hysterical people always end up by making me feel calm. Anyway, I managed to make a list of the first few calls and gave it to Dr. Roth. He was standing there with his hat and coat on and his bag in his hand and chewing on his cigar, and he took the list and shook his head and went out. Then I called Dr. Koehler, but his line was busy. I don't remember much about the next hour. All I know is I kept trying to reach Dr. Koehler and my phone kept ringing and my list of calls kept getting longer and longer."

One of the calls that lengthened Miss Stack's list was a summons to the home of August Z. Chambon, the burgess, or mayor, of Donora. The patient was the Burgess's mother, a widow of seventy-four, who lives with her son and his wife. "Mother Chambon was home alone that afternoon," her daughter-in-law says. "August was in Pittsburgh on business and I'd gone downstreet to do some shopping. It took me forever, the fog was so bad. Even the inside of the stores was smoky. So I didn't get home until around five-thirty. Well, I opened the door and stepped into the hall, and there was Mother Chambon. She was lying on the floor, with her coat on and a bag of cookies spilled all over beside her. Her face was blue, and she was just gasping for breath and in terrible pain. She told me she'd gone around the corner to the bakery a few minutes before, and on the way back the fog had got her. She said she barely made it to the house. Mother Chambon has bronchial trouble, but I'd never seen her so bad before. Oh, I was frightened! I helped her up—I don't know how I ever did it—and got her into bed. Then I called the doctor. It took me a long time to reach his office, and then he wasn't in. He was out making calls. I was afraid to wait until he could get here—Mother

Chambon was so bad, and at her age and all—so I called another doctor. He was out, too. Finally, I got hold of Dr. Levin and he said he'd come right over, and he finally did. He gave her an injection that made her breathe easier and something to put her to sleep. She slept for sixteen solid hours. But before Dr. Levin left, I told him that there seemed to be an awful lot of sickness going on all of a sudden. I was coughing a little myself. I asked him what was happening. 'I don't know,' he said. 'Something's coming off, but I don't know what.' "

Dr. Roth returned to his office at a little past six to replenish his supply of drugs. By then, he, like Dr. Levin, was aware that something was coming off. "I knew that whatever it was we were up against was serious," he says. "I'd seen some very pitiful cases, and they weren't all asthmatics or chronics of any kind. Some were people who had never been bothered by fog before. I was worried, but I wasn't bewildered. It was no mystery. It was obvious—all the symptoms pointed to it—that the fog and smoke were to blame. I didn't think any further than that. As a matter of fact, I didn't have time to think or wonder. I was too damn busy. My biggest problem was just getting around. It was almost impossible to drive. I even had trouble finding the office. McKean Avenue was solid coal smoke. I could taste the soot when I got out of the car, and my chest felt tight. On the way up the stairs, I started coughing and I couldn't stop. I kept coughing and choking until my stomach turned over. Fortunately, Helen was out getting something to eat—I just made it to the office and into the lavatory in time. My God, I was sick! After a while, I dragged myself into my office and gave myself an injection of adrenaline and lay back in a chair. I began to feel better. I felt so much better I got out a cigar and lighted up. That practically finished me. I took one pull, and went into another paroxysm of coughing. I probably should have known better—cigars had tasted terrible all day—but I hadn't had that reaction before. Then I heard the phone ringing. I guess it must have been ringing off and on all along. I thought about answering it, but I didn't have the strength to move. I just lay there in my chair and let it ring."

When Miss Stack came into the office a few minutes later, the telephone was still ringing. She had answered it and added the call to her list before she realized that she was not alone. "I heard someone groaning," she says. "Dr. Roth's door was open and I looked in. I almost jumped, I was so startled. He was slumped down in his chair, and his face was brick red and dripping with perspiration. I wanted to help him, but he said there wasn't anything to do. He told me what had happened. 'I'm all right now,' he said. 'I'll get going again in a minute. You go ahead and answer the phone.' It was ringing again. The next thing I knew, the office was full of patients, all of them coughing and groaning. I was about ready to break down and cry. I had talked to Dr. Koehler by that time and he knew what was happening. He had been out on calls from home. 'I'm coughing and sick myself,' he said, 'but I'll go out again as soon as I can.' I tried to keep calm, but with both Doctors sick and the office full of patients and the phone ringing, I just didn't know which way to turn. Dr. Roth saw two or three of the worst patients. Oh, he looked ghastly! He really looked worse than some of the patients. Finally, he said he couldn't see any more, that the emergency house calls had to come first, and grabbed up his stuff and went out. The office was still full of patients, and I went around explaining things to them. It was awful. There wasn't anything to do but close up, but I've never felt so heartless. Some of them were so sick and miserable. And right in the middle of everything the parade came marching down the street. People were cheering and yelling, and the bands were playing. I could hardly believe my ears. It just didn't seem possible."

The sounds of revelry that reached Miss Stack were deceptive. The parade, though well attended, was not an unqualified success. "I went out for a few minutes and watched it," the younger Mrs. Chambon says. "It went right by our house. August wasn't home yet, and after what had happened to Mother Chambon, I thought it might cheer me up a little. It did and it didn't. Everybody was talking about the fog and wondering when it would end, and some of them had heard there was sickness, but nobody seemed at all worried. As far as I could tell, all the sick people were old. That made things look not too bad. The fog always affects the old people. But as far as the parade was concerned, it was a waste of time. You really couldn't see a thing. They were just like shadows marching by. It was kind of uncanny. Especially since most of the people in the crowd had handkerchiefs tied over their nose and mouth to keep out the smoke. All the children did. But, even so, everybody was coughing. I was glad to get back in the house. I guess everybody was. The minute it was over, everybody scattered. They just vanished. In two minutes there wasn't a soul left on the street. It was as quiet as midnight."

Among the several organizations that participated in the parade was the Donora Fire Department. The force consists of about thirty volunteers and two full-time men. The latter, who live at the firehouse, are the chief, John Volk, a wiry man in his fifties, and his assistant and driver, a hard, round-faced young man named Russell Davis. Immediately after the parade, they returned to the firehouse. "As a rule," Chief Volk says, "I like a parade. We've got some nice equipment here, and I don't mind showing it off. But I didn't get much pleasure out of that one. Nobody could see us, hardly, and we couldn't see them. That fog was black as a derby hat. It had us all coughing. It was a relief to head for home. We hadn't much more than got back to the station, though, and got the trucks put away and said good night to the fellows than the phone rang. Russ and I were just sitting down to drink some coffee. I dreaded to answer it. On a night like that, a fire could have been real mean. But it wasn't any fire. It was a fellow up the street, and the fog had got him. He said he was choking to death and couldn't get a doctor, and what he wanted was our inhalator. He needed air. Russ says I just stood there with my mouth hanging open. I don't remember what I thought. I guess I was trying to think what to do as much as anything else. I didn't disbelieve him —he sounded half dead already—but, naturally, we're not supposed to go running around treating the sick. But what the hell, you can't let a man die! So I told him O.K. I told Russ to take the car and go. The way it turned out, I figure we did the right thing. I've never heard anybody say different."

"That guy was only the first," Davis says. "From then on, it was one emergency call after another. I didn't get to bed until Sunday. Neither did John. I don't know how many calls we had, but I do know this: We had around eight hundred cubic feet of oxygen on hand when I started out Friday night, and we ended up by borrowing from McKeesport and Monessen and Monongahela and Charleroi and everywhere around here. I never want to go through a thing like that again. I was laid up for a week after. There never was such a fog. You couldn't see your hand in front of your face, day or night. Hell, even inside the station the air was blue. I drove on the left side of the street with my head out the window, steering by scraping the curb. We've had bad fogs here before. A guy lost his car in one. He'd come to a fork in the road and didn't know where he was, and got out to try and tell which way to go. When he turned back to his car, he couldn't find it. He had no idea where it was until, finally, he stopped and listened and heard the engine. That guided him back. Well, by God, this fog was so bad you couldn't even get a car to idle. I'd take my foot off the accelerator and—bango!—the engine would stall. There just wasn't any oxygen in the air. I don't know how I kept breathing. I don't know how anybody did. I found people laying in bed and laying on the floor. Some of them were laying there and they didn't give a damn whether they died or not. I found some down in the basement with the furnace draft open and their head stuck inside, trying to get air that way. What I did when I got to a place was throw a sheet or blanket over the patient and stick a cylinder of oxygen underneath and crack the valves for fifteen minutes or so. By God, that rallied them! I didn't take any myself. What I did every time I came back to the station was have a little shot of whiskey. That seemed to help. It eased my throat. There was one funny thing about the whole thing. Nobody seemed to realize what was going on. Everybody seemed to think he was the only sick man in town. I don't know what they figured was keeping the doctors so busy. I guess everybody was so miserable they just didn't think."

Toward midnight, Dr. Roth abandoned his car and continued his rounds on foot. He found not only that walking was less of a strain but that he made better time. He walked the streets all night, but he was seldom lonely. Often, as he entered or left a house, he encountered a colleague. "We all had practically the same calls," Dr. M. J. Hannigan, the president of the Donora Medical Association, says. "Some people called every doctor in town. It was pretty discouraging to finally get someplace and drag yourself up the steps and then be told that Dr. So-and-So had just been there. Not that I blame them, though. Far from it. There were a couple of times when I was about ready to call for help myself. Frankly, I don't know how any of us doctors managed to hold out and keep going that night."

Not all of them did. Dr. Koehler made his last call that night at one o'clock. "I had to go home," he says. "God knows I didn't want to. I'd hardly made a dent in my list. Every time I called home or the Physicians' Exchange, it doubled. But my heart gave out. I couldn't go on any longer without some rest. The last thing I heard as I got into bed was my wife answering the phone. And the phone was the first thing I heard in the morning. It was as though I hadn't been to sleep at all." While Dr. Koehler was bolting a cup of coffee, the telephone rang again. This time, it was Miss Stack. They conferred briefly about the patients he had seen during the night and those he planned to see that morning. Among the latter was a sixty-four-year-old steelworker named Ignatz Hollowitti. "One of the Hollowitti girls, Dorothy, is a good friend of mine," Miss Stack says. "So as soon as I finished talking to Dr. Koehler, I called her to tell her that Doctor would be right over. I wanted to relieve her mind. Dorothy was crying when she answered the phone. I'll never forget what she said. She said, 'Oh, Helen—my dad just died! He's dead!' I don't remember what I said. I was simply stunned. I suppose I said what people say. I must have. But all I could think was, My gosh, if people are dying —why, this is tragic! Nothing like this has ever happened before!"

Mr. Hollowitti was not the first victim of the fog. He was the sixth. The first was a retired steelworker of seventy named Ivan Ceh. According to the records of the undertaker who was called in—Rudolph Schwerha, whose establishment is the largest in Donora—Mr. Ceh died at one-thirty Saturday morning. "I was notified at two," Mr. Schwerha says. "There is a note to such effect in my book. I thought nothing, of course. The call awakened me from sleep, but in my profession anything is to be expected. I reassured the bereaved and called my driver and sent him for the body. He was gone forever. The fog that night was impossible. It was a neighborhood case—only two blocks to go, and my driver works quick—but it was thirty minutes by the clock before I heard the service car in the drive. At that moment, again the phone rang. Another case. Now I was surprised. Two different cases so soon together in this size town doesn't happen every day. But there was no time then for thinking. There was work to do. I must go with my driver for the second body. It was in the Sunnyside section, north of town, too far in such weather for one man alone. The fog, when we got down by the mills, was unbelievable. Nothing could be seen. It was like a blanket. Our fog lights were useless, and even with the fog spotlight on, the white line in the street was invisible. I began to worry. What if we should bump a parked car? What if we should fall off the road? Finally, I told my driver, 'Stop! I'll take the wheel. You walk in front and show the way.' So we did that for two miles. Then we were in the country. I know that section like my hand, but we had missed the house. So we had to turn around and go back. That was an awful time. We were on the side of a hill, with a terrible drop on one side and no fence. I was afraid every minute. But we made it, moving by inches, and pretty soon I found the house. The case was an old man and he had died all of a sudden. Acute cardiac dilation. When we were ready, we started back. Then I began to feel sick. The fog was getting me. There was an awful tickle in my throat. I was coughing and ready to vomit. I called to my driver that I had to stop and get out. He was ready to stop, I guess. Already he had walked four or five miles. But I envied him. He was well and I was awful sick. I leaned against the car, coughing and gagging, and at last I riffled a few times. Then I was much better. I could drive. So we went on, and finally we were home. My wife was standing at the door. Before she spoke, I knew what she would say. I thought, Oh, my God—another! I knew it by her face. And after that came another. Then another. There seemed to be no end. By ten o'clock in the morning, I had nine bodies waiting here. Then I heard that De-Rienzo and Lawson, the other morticians, each had one. Eleven people dead! My driver and I kept looking at each other. What was happening? We didn't know. I thought probably the fog was the reason. It had the smell of poison. But we didn't know."

Mr. Schwerha's bewilderment was not widely shared. Most Donorans were still unaware Saturday morning that anything was happening. They had no way of knowing. Donora has no radio station, and its one newspaper, the *Herald-American*, is published only five days a week, Monday through Friday. It was past noon before a rumor of widespread illness began to drift through the town. The news reached August Chambon at about two o'clock. In addition to being burgess, an office that is more an honor than a livelihood, Mr. Chambon operates a moving-and-storage business, and he had been out of town on a job all morning. "There was a message waiting for me when I got home," he says. "John Elco, of the Legion, had called and wanted me at the Borough Building right away. I wondered what the hell, but I went right over. It isn't like John to get excited over nothing. The fog didn't even enter my mind. Of course, I'd heard there were some people sick from it. My wife had told me that. But I hadn't paid it any special significance. I just thought they were like Mother—old people that were always bothered by fog. Jesus, in a town like this you've got to expect fog. It's natural. At least, that's what I thought then. So I was astonished when John told me that the fog was causing sickness all over town. I was just about floored. That's a fact. Because I felt fine myself. I was hardly even coughing much. Well, as soon as I'd talked to John and the other fellows he had rounded up, I started in to do what I could. Something had already been done. John and Cora Vernon, the Red Cross director, were setting up an emergency-aid station in the Community Center. We don't have a hospital here. The nearest one is at Charleroi. Mrs. Vernon was getting a doctor she knew there to come over and take charge of the station, and the Legion was arranging for cars and volunteer nurses. The idea was to get a little organization in things—everything was confused as hell—and also to give our doctors a rest. They'd been working steady for thirty-six hours or more. Mrs. Vernon was fixing it so when somebody called a doctor's number, they would be switched to the Center and everything would be handled from there. I've worked in the mills and I've dug coal, but I never worked any harder than I worked that day. Or was so worried. Mostly I was on the phone. I called every town around here to send supplies for the station and oxygen for the firemen. I even called Pittsburgh. Maybe I overdid it. There was stuff pouring in here for a week. But what I wanted to be was prepared for anything. The way that fog looked that day, it wasn't ever going to lift. And then the rumors started going around that now people were dying. Oh, Jesus! Then I was scared. I heard all kinds of reports. Four dead. Ten dead. Thirteen dead. I did the only thing I could think of. I notified the State Health Department, and I called a special meeting of the Council and our Board of Health and the mill officials for the first thing Sunday morning. I wanted to have it right then, but I couldn't get hold of everybody —it was Saturday night. Every time I looked up from the phone, I'd hear a new rumor. Usually a bigger one. I guess I heard everything but the truth. What I was really afraid of was that they might set off a panic. That's what I kept dreading. I needn't have worried, though. The way it turned out, half the town had hardly heard that there was anybody even sick until Sunday night, when Walter Winchell opened his big mouth on the radio. By then, thank God, it was all over."

The emergency-aid station, generously staffed and abundantly supplied with drugs and oxygen inhalators, opened at eight o'clock Saturday night. "We were ready for anything and prepared for the worst," Mrs. Vernon says. "We even had an ambulance at our disposal. Phillip DeRienzo, the undertaker, loaned it to us. But almost nothing happened. Altogether, we brought in just eight patients. Seven, to be exact. One was dead when the car arrived. Three were very bad and we sent them to the hospital in Charleroi. The others we just treated and sent home. It was really very queer. The fog was as black and nasty as ever that night, or worse, but all of a sudden the calls for a doctor just seemed to trickle out and stop. It was as though everybody was sick who was going to be sick. I don't believe we had a call after midnight. I knew then that we'd seen the worst of it."

Dr. Roth had reached that conclusion, though on more slender evidence, several hours before. "I'd had a call about noon from a woman who said two men roomers in her house were in bad shape," he says. "It was nine or nine-thirty by the time I finally got around to seeing them. Only, I never saw them. The landlady yelled up to them that I was there, and they yelled right back, 'Tell him never mind. We're O.K. now.' Well, that was good enough for me. I decided things must be letting up. I picked up my grip and walked home and fell into bed. I was dead-beat."

There was no visible indication that the fog was beginning to relax its smothering grip when the group summoned by Burgess Chambon assembled at the Borough Building the next morning to discuss the calamity. It was another soggy, silent, midnight day. "That morning was the worst," the Burgess says. "It wasn't just that the fog was still hanging on. We'd begun to get some true facts. We didn't have any real idea how many people were sick. That didn't come out for months. We thought a few hundred. But we did have the number of deaths. It took the heart out of you. The rumors hadn't come close to it. It was eighteen. I guess we talked about that first. Then the question of the mills came up. The smoke. L. J. Westhaver, who was general superintendent of the steel and wire works then, was there, and so was the head of the zinc plant, M. M. Neale. I asked them to shut down for the duration. They said they already had. They had started banking the fires at six that morning. They went on to say, though, that they were sure the mills had nothing to do with the trouble. We didn't know what to think. Everybody was at a loss to point the finger at anything in particular. There just didn't seem to be any explanation. We had another meeting that afternoon. It was the same thing all over again. We talked and we wondered and we worried. We couldn't think of anything to do that hadn't already been done. I think we heard about the nineteenth death before we broke up. We thought for a week that was the last. Then one more finally died. I don't remember exactly what all we did or said that afternoon. What I remember is after we broke up. When we came out of the building, it was raining. Maybe it was only drizzling then—I guess the real rain didn't set in until evening—but, even so, there was a hell of a difference. The air was different. It didn't get you any more. You could breathe."

The investigation of the disaster lasted almost a year. It was not only the world's first full-blooded examination of the general problem of air pollution but one of the most exhaustive inquiries of any kind ever made in the field of public health. Its course was directed jointly by Dr. Joseph Shilen, director of the Bureau of Industrial Hygiene of the Pennsylvania Department of Health, and Dr. J. G. Townsend, chief of the Division of Industrial Hygiene of the United States Public Health Service, and at times it involved the entire technical personnel of both agencies. The Public Health Service assigned to the case nine engineers, seven physicians, six nurses, five chemists, three statisticians, two meteorologists, two dentists, and a veterinarian. The force under the immediate direction of Dr. Shilen, though necessarily somewhat smaller, was similarly composed.

The investigation followed three main lines, embracing the clinical, the environmental, and the meteorological aspects of the occurrence. Of these, the meteorological inquiry was the most nearly conclusive. It was also the most reassuring. It indicated that while the situation of Donora is unwholesomely conducive to the accumulation of smoke and fog, the immediate cause of the October, 1948, visitation was a freak of nature known to meteorologists as a temperature inversion. This phenomenon is, as its name suggests, characterized by a temporary, and usually brief, reversal of the normal atmospheric conditions, in which the air near the earth is warmer than the air higher up. Its result is a more or less complete immobilization of the convection currents in the lower air by which gases and fumes are ordinarily carried upward, away from the earth.

The clinical findings, with one or two exceptions, were more confirmatory than illuminating. One of the revelations, which was gleaned from several months of tireless interviewing, was that thousands, rather than just hundreds, had been ill during the fog. For the most part, the findings demonstrated, to the surprise of neither the investigators nor the Donora physicians, that the affection was essentially an irritation of the respiratory tract, that its severity increased in proportion to the age of the victim and his predisposition to cardio-respiratory ailments, and that the ultimate cause of death was suffocation.

The environmental study, the major phase of which was an analysis of the multiplicity of gases emitted by the mills, boats, and trains, was, in a positive sense, almost wholly unrewarding. It failed to determine the direct causative agent. Still, its results, though negative, were not without value. They showed, contrary to expectation, that none of the several stack gases known to be irritant—among them fluoride, chloride, hydrogen sulphide, cadmium oxide, and sulphur dioxide—could have been present in the air in sufficient concentration to produce serious illness. "It seems reasonable to state," Dr. Helmuth H. Schrenk, chief of the Environmental Investigations Branch of the Public Health Service's Division of Industrial Hygiene, has written of this phase of the inquiry, "that while no single substance was responsible for the . . . episode, the syndrome could have been produced by a combination, or summation of the action, of two or more of the contaminants. Sulphur dioxide and its oxidation products, together with particular matter [soot and fly ash], are considered significant contaminants. However, the significance of the other irritants as important adjuvants to the biological effects cannot be finally estimated on the basis of present knowledge. It is important to emphasize that information available on the toxicological effects of mixed irritant gases is meagre and data on possible enhanced action due to adsorption of gases on particular matter is limited." To this, Dr. Leonard A. Scheele, Surgeon General of the Service, has added, "One of the most important results of the study is to show us what we do not know."

Funeral services for most of the victims of the fog were held on Tuesday, November 2nd. Monday had been a day of battering rain, but the weather cleared in the night, and Tuesday was fine. "It was like a day in spring," Mr. Schwerha says. "I think I have never seen such a beautiful blue sky or such a shining sun or such pretty white clouds. Even the trees in the cemetery seemed to have color. I kept looking up all day."

[*1950*]

CHAPTER 4

A Pinch of Dust

AMONG THE SEVERAL REPORTS and memoranda that came to the
attention of Dr. Morris Greenberg, then chief epidemiologist of
the Bureau of Preventable Diseases of the New York City Department of Health and now its director, on Wednesday, January 21,
1942, was a note initialled by the head of the Department's Bureau
of Records. It was on Dr. Greenberg's desk when he returned
from lunch. The message was short, explicit, and altogether flab-
bergasting. For a moment, Dr. Greenberg could only stare at it.
Then he shook himself, picked up the telephone, and called his
chief diagnostician, Dr. David A. Singer, who now heads the
Bureau's Manhattan division. He told Dr. Singer that he had
before him the names of six people whose deaths had recently been
reported to the Department, and asked to be provided as quickly
as possible with a full medical history of each. Five of the group
—four females and a male—had died in Roosevelt Hospital, at
Fifty-ninth Street and Ninth Avenue. Their names and death
dates were: Bab Miller, December 29th; Juanita Jackson, December 30th; Josephine Dozier, January 1st; Ida Metcalf, January 3rd;
and Charles Williams, January 8th. The sixth was a woman

50

named Ruby Bowers. She had died on January 19th, at Bellevue Hospital. All were Negroes, all were unmarried, all had lived in or near the San Juan Hill section west of Columbus Circle, and all were adults, their ages ranging from twenty-five to sixty-one. The cause of death was tetanus.

The abrupt thirst for knowledge that was excited in Dr. Greenberg by this generous set of coincidences was entirely understandable. So was his disconcertion, for tetanus is a disease of gothic ferocity. It has, however, one redeeming quality. It is not communicable. It is invariably the result of a wound into which a bacillus called *Clostridium tetani* has found its way. In the majority of cases, it is introduced by the instrument that inflicts the injury. Although the intestinal tracts of many animals provide a congenial habitat for *Clostridium tetani*, it is also commonly found in soil, especially that rich in manure. The adult organism, like many other bacilli, readily expires when exposed to air and sunlight, but the spores by which it perpetuates itself do not share this engaging trait. They are among the hardiest forms of life. Tetanus spores are impervious to most antiseptics, including the cruelest extremes of heat and cold, and, in the absence of the dark and airless environment that favors their maturation, practically immortal. They are also balefully abundant. Bacteriologists have encountered them on vegetables, in hay, hair, cobwebs, and clothing, in the dust of streets and houses, and even adrift in the air of hospital operating rooms. No wound is too small to admit a multitude of tetanus spores. In fact, the smallest wounds—abrasions and pricks and thready cuts—are sometimes warmly hospitable. There are two reasons for this apparent anomaly. One is that such wounds close rapidly and thus shield the mature or maturing organism from the withering touch of oxygen. The other is that they are nearly always ignored. The cause of tetanus is a toxin that possesses a shattering affinity for the central nervous system. Neither the chemistry of the toxin's generation nor the method by which it reaches its destination is fully understood, but its nature is no mystery. Five hundred times more explosive than strychnine, whose action it somewhat resembles, the toxin elaborated by *Clostridium tetani* is one of the most venomous poisons known to man.

Tetanus is the name generally preferred by physicians for lockjaw. They consider the latter more apt than adequate. The rigors of tetanus are by no means limited to an inability to move the jaw freely. Constriction of the masseter muscles is merely the characteristic symptom of onset. The physical manifestations of a full-fledged case of tetanus amply reflect the virulence of its cause. They are of such distinctive vigor and variety that the disease was among the first to be recognized as an entity. The accounts of clinical studies made by Hippocrates in the fourth century before Christ include one of a tetanus seizure that is still regarded as a model of acute observation. "The master of a large ship mashed the index finger of his right hand with the anchor," he wrote. "Seven days later a somewhat foul discharge appeared; then trouble with his tongue—he complained he could not speak properly. The presence of tetanus was diagnosed, his jaws became pressed together, his teeth were locked, then symptoms appeared in his neck; on the third day opisthotonos appeared, with sweating. Six days after the diagnosis was made he died."

Opisthotonos is a spine-cracking muscular spasm. Numerous physicians have been inspired to describe the appearance of a patient in opisthotonos, but a Cappadocian named Aretaeus, who conducted a wide and successful practice in Rome in the second century, is usually acknowledged to be its classic delineator. "Opisthotonos," he noted, "bends the patient backward, like a bow, so that the reflected head is lodged between the shoulder blades; the throat protrudes; the jaw sometimes gapes, but in some rare cases it is fixed in the upper one; respiration stertorous; the belly and chest prominent . . . the abdomen stretched, and resonant if tapped; the arms strongly bent back in a state of extension; the legs and thighs are bent together, for the legs are bent in the opposite direction to the hams." Not all victims of tetanus are called upon to experience the excruciation of opisthotonos. More commonly, though no less disastrously, the systematic paralysis that marks the disease is not accompanied by tonic convulsions. Sometimes, however, a spasm the reverse of opisthotonos occurs. Aretaeus's description of this form of tetanic attack is not only definitive but perhaps the most elegiac passage in medical literature. "But if [the sufferers] are bent forward," he wrote, "they are protuberant at the back, the loins being extruded in a line with the back, the whole of the spine being straight; the vertex prone, the head inclining toward the chest; the lower jaw fixed upon the breastbone; the hands clasped together, the lower extremities extended; pains intense; the voice altogether dolorous; they groan, making deep moaning. Should the mischief then seize the chest and the respiratory organs, it readily frees the patient from life; a blessing this, to himself, as being deliverance from pains, distortion, and deformity; and a contingency less than usual to be lamented by the spectators, were he a son or a father. But should the powers of life still stand out . . . the patient is not only bent up into an arch but rolled together like a ball. . . . An inhuman calamity! An unseemly sight! A spectacle painful even to the beholder! An incurable malady! . . . But neither can the physician, though present and looking on, furnish any assistance as regards life, relief from pain or from deformity. For if he should wish to straighten the limbs, he can only do so by cutting and breaking those of a living man. With them, then, who are overpowered by this disease, he can merely sympathize."

Aretaeus's melancholy view of tetanus has not been rendered seriously obsolete by the accomplishments of modern medicine. Tetanus, once its grip is fixed, is still an essentially incurable malady, with whose victims the physician can for the most part merely sympathize. A remedy effective at any but the earliest stages of the disease has yet to be devised; its treatment is largely confined to the prevention of complications and the moderation of pain, and surviving an attack precipitated by a large number or an undebilitated strain of *Clostridium tetani* is anything but likely. "The outlook in cases of generalized tetanus is always grave," Dr. Warfield M. Firor, visiting surgeon at Johns Hopkins Hospital, in Baltimore, has noted in a recent monograph. "Even in the best hospitals the death rate is frequently more than fifty per cent." In other than the best hospitals, and among those victims to whom no hospital care is speedily available, the death rate is seldom as low as fifty per cent.

Nevertheless, in most parts of the world, tetanus is no longer a very domineering menace. Not for some years has its avoidance been wholly a matter of chance. Since the late nineteenth century,

when an extensive inquiry into the mechanics of the disease cul-
minated, in 1889, in the isolation of *Clostridium tetani* by the
Japanese bacteriologist Shibasaburo Kitazato, a prophylactic antitoxin (and, more recently, a toxoid that will confer an absolute and
a reasonably durable immunity) has been within easy reach. Inoculation against tetanus is now compulsory in the armed forces of
all nations, many business concerns throughout the world emphatically commend it to their employees, and in an increasing
number of countries, among which the United States is outstanding, it is fast becoming an integral part of pediatric routine. For
these reasons, and because most physicians are in the habit of
administering a prophylactic charge of antitetanic serum whenever they are confronted by a suspicious-looking wound, the disease has been for nearly a generation—in this country, at least—
something of a rarity. Its current incidence in the United States
is hardly two thousand cases a year. Of these, on the average, only
around fifteen turn up in New York City, and they are usually
pretty well scattered among the five boroughs. Also, as might be
expected from the solitary nature of the disease, they are generally
far apart.

The clinical biographies commissioned by Dr. Greenberg on that
winter afternoon in 1942 were compiled with the dispatch to
which he is accustomed. They reached him the following morning,
Thursday, January 22nd, at about ten o'clock. The first of the six
on which he happened to fix his eyes was that of Charles Williams.
"I visited Roosevelt Hospital today," wrote the operative Dr.
Singer had assigned to the job, "and examined the records of
Charles Williams. . . . History reveals that he [was] an old colored
man, sixty-one years of age, and single. He was admitted to the
hospital on January 4, 1942, at 7:00 P.M., with complaints of pain
in the back of his neck for the past twenty-four hours and difficulty
in swallowing for the past forty-eight hours. History shows that
he was a [heroin] addict, having used injections into the skin for
the past two years. On examination, the neck was rigid and his
pupils reacted sluggishly to light. On January 4, 1942, he was
given 100,000 units of tetanus antitoxin. On January 5th, he developed opisthotonos. . . . " Dr. Greenberg didn't bother to read any

more of it. Instead, he turned to the next dossier. After a line or two, he let it drop, and glanced sharply at each of the others. A glance was all he needed. It was enough to convince him that he was indeed up against a series of related cases of tetanus. It was also enough to give him an excellent idea of how they must have originated. Like Williams, Bab Miller, Ida Metcalf, Juanita Jackson, Josephine Dozier, and Ruby Bowers had all been firmly addicted to heroin. Dr. Greenberg returned the reports to their folder with a somewhat muted sense of triumph. He was conscious that he had just made a vividly illuminating discovery but scarcely a reassuring one. If, as seemed probable, the six Negroes had contracted the disease from a common source, it might very well be one that was still accessible to others who happened to share their failing.

The task of determining the source of the infection fell to a field epidemiologist whose name, because he is now engaged in private practice and prefers anonymity, shall here be Ernest Clarke. He was not an arbitrary choice. Dr. Clarke was, and is, an investigator of some distinction in the field of tetanus, and it was Dr. Greenberg's expectation that the congeniality of the subject would supply him with an unusual and perhaps a rewarding zest for the task. He knew he would need it. Dr. Clarke accepted his attractive assignment with a rather clearer notion of what he was looking for than of where to find it. It could be anywhere in the warrens of San Juan Hill, and the only known people who might have been able to direct him were dead. On the other hand, he could conceive of just two possible vehicles that would be compatible with the evidence. A contaminated hypodermic needle was one. The other was a contaminated batch of heroin. At the moment, Dr. Clarke was inclined to favor the former. He was aware, however, that it really didn't much matter. One could hardly be less lethal, or elusive, than the other.

Before actively buckling down to the hunt, Dr. Clarke retired to his office and made a series of sedentary casts. At the end of an hour on the telephone, he was satisfied that nothing even suggestive of tetanus had been seen in the past few weeks at any Manhattan hospital except Bellevue and Roosevelt, and that if something, especially in a drug addict, did appear, he would be promptly informed. Then he dropped in at a restaurant around the corner and had a thoughtful lunch. From there, no livelier course having occurred to him, he headed first for Bellevue and then for Roosevelt. His retracing of the steps of Dr. Singer's agent did not imply a lack of confidence in the agent's ability as a medical historian. He merely hoped that his colleague, in a natural preoccupation with the clinical aspects of the outbreak, had overlooked some biographical detail that would give him a serviceable lead. If he had, Dr. Clarke was soon persuaded, it hadn't been at Bellevue. There was nothing whatever in the recorded history of Ruby Bowers that he did not already know. Still hopeful, though weighted by a new and discomfiting appreciation of his predecessor's thoroughness, Dr. Clarke moved on to Roosevelt. It was a little past two when he presented himself to the librarian of the record room there. He emerged from his studies at three, possessed of only one trifling nugget of additional knowledge. For what it was worth, he now knew that at least two of the six victims were linked by more than race, geography, and misfortune. Ida Metcalf and Josephine Dozier had been friends. During most of 1941, they had shared a room in a lodging house on West Fifty-second Street.

As Dr. Clarke rose to go, the librarian came hurrying over and asked if she could be of any further help. Dr. Clarke said he guessed not—unless, of course, he added wryly, she could conjure up another case of tetanus for him. The librarian gave him a reproachful smile. After all, she remarked, five cases in less than two weeks were— She stopped, looking stunned. As a matter of fact, she said in amazement, it was just possible, if sudden memory served, that she could. Then, sped by a stare from Dr. Clarke, she vanished into the stacks. When she returned, she had another folder in her hand. Dr. Clarke sank back into his chair, crossed his fingers, and opened the folder. Its subject was a woman named Lulu Garcia. She was colored, single, and fifty-three years of age. Her address was 530 West Forty-fifth Street. She had been admitted to the hospital on January 5th for observation, the findings of the examining physician having been provocative but inconclusive. They included headache, nausea, and a stiff jaw and neck. Also, the clinician noted in passing, she was plainly addicted to drugs. That night, the house physician took a look at her, and though what he saw failed to inspire even a tentative diagnosis, he prescribed a liberal dose of tetanus antitoxin. It was not repeated. There was no need. Nine days later, on January 14th, she was judged to be recovered from whatever had ailed her, and discharged. Dr. Clarke reached jubilantly for his hat.

At a quarter to four, Dr. Clarke bounded up the eroded stoop of 530 West Forty-fifth Street. At five, he slowly descended. He hadn't seen Lulu Garcia. She didn't live there any more. She had moved away a week earlier, and he could find nobody in the building who was able, or at any rate willing, to tell him where.

Dr. Clarke's withdrawal from 530 West Forty-fifth Street was only temporary. He was destined to become a familiar figure on the block. Two weeks later, he was still there and still stumped. He had by then had an endless monotony of conversation with every inhabitant of the building and with most of the people who lived next door or across the street. He had talked to the janitor and the rent collector and a dozen delivery boys. He had spent hours of inquisitive loitering among the loiterers in the corner stores and bars and lunchrooms. Twice, driven less by hope than by exasperation, he had made a long and garrulous tour of the other addresses on his list. But nothing had come of any of it. Lulu Garcia was not merely gone; she had vanished without a trace. Toward the end of the second week, Dr. Clarke sought out Dr. Greenberg for a word of counsel. Dr. Greenberg wasn't much help. He had nothing to recommend but persistence. The disappearance of Lulu Garcia, he admitted, was nettling, but, he added optimistically, matters could be a lot worse. The important thing, he reminded his colleague, was that she existed. Dr. Clarke began to wonder, as he glumly resumed his rounds, if she really did. A day or two later, on Saturday, February 7th, he received a telephone call that further tried his resilience. The call, which reached him at home and at breakfast, was from the medical superintendent of Harlem Hospital. He understood that Dr. Clarke had asked to be notified if a case of tetanus with evidence of drug addiction should happen to turn up at Harlem. Well, one had. The victim was a woman named Mildred Stewart. She was twenty-six years old, unmarried and colored. Her home was on West 140th Street, and she had lain there, ill and alone, for several days. An ambulance summoned by neighbors had brought her to the hospital about an hour before. Dr. Clarke cut in with an impatient volley of thanks. He said he would be right up for a talk with her. The medical superintendent cleared his throat. That, he was sorry to say, would be impossible. The patient was dead.

Monday morning, February 9th, found Dr. Clarke back on West Forty-fifth Street again. He had nowhere else to go. An active but uneventful weekend among Mildred Stewart's effects and neighbors had merely confirmed his belief that Lulu Garcia, in spite of her increasingly chimerical aspect, was probably still his only chance of success. It was about ten o'clock when he dropped off a crosstown trolley and made his way up Tenth Avenue to the familiar corner. As he stood there, trying to decide which of his usual haunts was the least hopeless, a man emerged from a nearby areaway, stared at him for a moment, and then raised a beckoning finger. He wanted to ask a question. Wasn't he the fellow who had been asking around for Lulu Garcia? Dr. Clarke took a deep breath and said he certainly was. Was he sure enough a doctor? Dr. Clarke produced his credentials. The man gave them an inscrutable glance. Most people on the block thought different, he said. They thought he was most likely a bill collector or a process server, or even a detective. He himself—he shrugged—he didn't know or care. But he saw no harm in doing a man a favor. It might come back to him someday. Bread on the waters. If Dr. Clarke was interested, Lulu Garcia had a friend or a relative or something named Mrs. Johnson. She lived at 417 West Fifty-second Street.

The house at 417 West Fifty-second Street turned out to be a battered brownstone a few doors west of Ninth Avenue. Mrs. Johnson's apartment was on the fifth floor. A tall, robust woman of indeterminate age opened the door. Dr. Clarke introduced himself and, after explaining that his mission was both urgent and innocuous, said he was seeking a woman named Lulu Garcia. Mrs. Johnson, he understood, was acquainted with her. The woman gazed at him. Then she nodded, and stepped aside to let him enter. "Mrs. Johnson won't be back till later," she said. "But take a seat. I'm Lulu Garcia. What did you want to see me about?"

Dr. Clarke walked into Dr. Greenberg's office at dusk. Dr. Greenberg was just leaving, but at a provocative murmur from Dr. Clarke he discarded his hat, hung up his overcoat, and sat cheerfully down. "Congratulations," he said, and indicated a chair. "Which was it?"

"I don't know," Dr. Clarke said. "I've got a pretty good idea, though. Everything points to the heroin. For one thing, I'm satisfied that it wasn't a contaminated needle. It couldn't have been. Not if we believe Lulu, and I do. She has her own outfit. And so, she says, did Juanita Jackson and Ida Metcalf and Charles Williams. Charles Garcia, I should say. According to Lulu, that was his real name, and she ought to know. It seems they used to be married. And they were still friends. He and Lulu and Juanita and Ida generally took their shots together. The last time was at Lulu's place, somewhere around Christmas, just before they all got sick. And there's another reason for ruling out the needle theory. Lulu flatly denies knowing any of the others. And I believe her. Why should she lie? Why should she admit knowing Ida Metcalf, say, and deny knowing Ruby Bowers unless it was the truth? There'd be no point in it. But they're all linked up. Lulu didn't know Ruby Bowers or Bab Miller or Josephine Dozier or Mildred Stewart, but she had heard of them—from Juanita Jackson. Juanita knew them all. She was what Lulu calls the runaround. They all got their heroin through her."

"And tetanus?" asked Dr. Greenberg.

"Yes, I know," Dr. Clarke said. "Juanita wasn't a real peddler. She just bought a little batch every so often, and resold it—what she could spare of it—to her friends. Well, one of those little batches was contaminated. I'm not entirely guessing. Lulu has an idea that the stuff they had at Christmastime looked different. Dirtier than usual, I gather. So it was probably cut. It was probably cut a good many other times, but I mean by Juanita. Hers was the one that did the damage. Otherwise, we wouldn't have had eight cases of tetanus. We'd have had dozens. I don't know what she cut it with, but you know how those addicts operate. They'll use anything that's handy. My guess is she mixed in a pinch of dust."

"I suppose that's as good a guess as any," Dr. Greenberg said.

"Except for one thing. It doesn't explain why Lulu is still alive."

"I was coming to that," Dr. Clarke said. "As a matter of fact, it does. It's about the only explanation that seems to stand up. The last few times Lulu and her friends met, Lulu didn't get a regular shot. She didn't have any money for drugs. All she got, she says, was what she could cadge from the others. And they weren't overly generous. They only gave her just enough to keep her going."

[*1951*]

CHAPTER 5

A Lonely Road

———————◆•◀▶•————————

AROUND TEN O'CLOCK one September evening in 1934, a native of Puerto Rico, whose name shall here be Roberto Ramirez, was sitting at ease in the kitchen of his three-room flat on West 114th Street, a cigarette in his hand and a bottle of beer at his elbow, when he became aware of an odd and pungent odor. Ramirez, a married man of forty-one, with a nine-year-old son and a daughter of eleven, was alone in the room. His wife was out, at a movie with a neighbor, and the children were in bed and asleep. For an instant, Ramirez thought of fire. He cocked his head and sniffed. But the smell was not the smell of smoke and smoldering wood. It was more like the smell of something cooking. It smelled like meat, like roasting meat—and it was. As he pushed back his chair to investigate, he saw it. It was his hand. His cigarette had burned away to a ruddy coal between the first and second fingers of his left hand, and the flesh for half an inch around was cracked and curling and darkly red. He dislodged the remains of the cigarette with a convulsive jerk, and stared at his wound. The sight of it made him shudder, but it might have been the hand of another man. It didn't hurt at all. Ramirez got up and went to the cupboard and smeared his fingers with lard. Then, in a panic of bewilderment, he sat down again and waited for his wife. Her consternation was anything but reassuring.

The next morning, still dazed with dismay, Ramirez presented himself at the general clinic of Harlem Hospital for a word of explanation. His confidence in medical science was not misplaced. The examining physician was neither greatly perplexed nor much perturbed. Loss of sensation, he explained, after inspecting the burn and modernizing its dressing, was not an unheard of phenomenon. It could hardly be called even rare. It bespoke a neuritis —an inflammation of the nerves—and was more or less symptomatic of numerous ailments. They included tumors, certain deficiency diseases, and several bacterial infections. At the moment, the doctor went on, the evidence, though far from abundant, seemed to indicate that Ramirez's complaint was nutritional in origin. He suspected, he said, a chronic deficiency of vitamin B_1. If such was the case, the trouble was readily reparable. He then turned his attention from theory to therapy. He wrote out a prescription for thiamine hydrochloride, recommended a diet rich in milk and liver and whole-grain cereals, and advised a minimum of exercise. In addition, and as a matter of course, he exacted from Ramirez a firm promise to return in a couple of weeks for review and further instructions.

Ramirez was more than punctual. He was back at the clinic the following week. His burn was healing, but he had made an unsettling discovery. He thought the doctor ought to know. That morning, while washing, he had come upon a new, or at least another, patch of insensitivity. Like the first, it was on his left arm, but higher up, just above the wrist. He rolled back his sleeve and pointed it out. The spot he indicated was the color of parchment and slightly depressed. It was about the size of a quarter. The doctor gave it a long, reflective, and increasingly uneasy look. It didn't, he had to admit, much resemble the lesions characteristic of any deficiency disease. Nor was it strongly suggestive of any of the more familiar infections that had earlier crossed his mind. What it did resemble, he found hard to believe. He was astonished that the idea had even occurred to him. After a time, he stood up and stepped across the office to a tier of cabinets. He returned with a scalpel, a glass slide, and a carefully disarming smile. His explanation of his purpose was also shaped by discretion. There was a possibility, he said, that his original diagnosis had not been entirely correct. In order to make sure, he was going to extract a drop of material from the lesion for a bacteriological examination. It was a simple, bloodless operation, and took only a moment. Now, if Ramirez would just . . . exactly! He discarded the scalpel and held out a friendly hand. Analysis, of course, took somewhat longer. But Ramirez would be notified of the result in a day or two. Meanwhile, he was to continue as before.

When the door had closed, the doctor picked up the telephone and put in a call to the laboratory. He told the bacteriologist on duty there that he was sending along a skin scraping on which he wanted a prompt report. It was to be examined for acid-fast bacilli by the Ziehl-Neelsen method. Half an hour later, as he was preparing to duck out for a hurried lunch, the laboratory called back. They had received the scraping and it had been stained as requested. The reaction was positive. For a moment, the doctor was silent. Then he uttered a grunt of thanks, hung up, and reached for his pen and a piece of writing paper. The message he wrote was addressed to the director of the Bureau of Preventable Diseases of the New York City Department of Health. It informed him that Roberto Ramirez, male, of — West 114th Street, had been examined by the undersigned and found to be suffering from leprosy.

Of all the diseases that beset the human race, leprosy is by far the hardest to bear. It is usually disfiguring, it is often crippling, and it not uncommonly results in death. It is also chronic and contagious. In addition, it is incurable. What distinguishes leprosy from all other ailments, however, is not the progressive physiological dissolution that its victims must frequently endure. It is the fear and horror and violent loathing that it ordinarily excites in others.

The belief that leprosy unfits its victims for either the sympathy or the society of other men is supported by more than mere aversion. It has the sanction of Holy Writ. Both the Bible and the writings of Mohammed endorse it. "Run away from an Arabian leper as you run away from a tiger," the prophet advised his disciples at the beginning of the seventh century. Mohammed's inspiration, in this instance, was more derivative than divine. His attitude toward leprosy had been molded by an earlier prophet. The architect of lepraphobia was Moses. In the opinion of most medical historians, the universal abhorrence of leprosy is largely attributable to the heaven-sent dread of the disease that Moses communicated to the children of Israel. "And the Lord spake unto Moses and Aaron," the anonymous author of the Book of Leviticus records, "saying, When a man shall have in the skin of his flesh a rising, a scab, or bright spot, and it be in the skin of his flesh like the plague of leprosy; then he shall be brought unto . . . the priest. . . . Then the priest shall look upon it: and, behold, if the rising of the sore be white reddish . . . he is a leprous man, he is unclean: the priest shall pronounce him utterly unclean. . . . And the leper in whom the plague is, his clothes shall be rent, and his head bare, and he shall put a covering upon his upper lip, and shall cry, Unclean, unclean. All the days wherein the plague shall be in him he shall be defiled; he is unclean: he shall dwell alone; without the camp shall his habitation be." Moses received these explicit instructions some twelve or thirteen hundred years before the birth of Christ. Until then, lepers had been only informally shunned. Their good fortune vanished in the wake of the wandering Jews. Within a century or two, the intolerable impurity of the leprous had been sensed throughout the civilized world. The first full-dress demonstration of lepraphobia occurred around 1250 B.C., in Egypt. At the order of Ramses II, the monarch of the moment, eighty thousand lepers were wrested from their homes and resettled in a compound on the edge of the Sahara Desert. There is no record of how long they survived. The most recent display took place in China, in June of 1952, when the sub-prefect of a back-country province ordered approximately one hundred inmates of the local leprosarium burned to death. Three escaped the holocaust.

Leprosy probably originated in Egypt. It is possible that the Jews first encountered it there. There are allusions to an adhesive skin disease of catastrophic ferocity in many of the oldest Egyptian religio-medical writings, including the encyclopediac "Papyrus Ebers," which was assembled nearly four thousand years ago and is the most venerable manual of medicine in existence. "Papyrus Ebers" also suggests a remedy. "To drive away leprous spots on the skin," it reads, "cook onions in sea salt and urine, and apply as a poultice." The spread of leprosy from Egypt is indistinctly charted. It is certain only that it was among her earliest exports and that its advance in the beginning was rapid and easterly. By 1000 B.C., it was endemic in all of Asia. Its westward sweep, though eventually equally thorough, was somewhat less galvanic. It failed to get a foothold in Europe until almost the time of Christ. Leprosy was unknown to the ancient Greeks. It is, in fact, one of the few diseases of indisputable antiquity that Hippocrates neglected to describe. The introduction of leprosy into Europe is usually attributed to the legions of Pompey the Great. They acquired it, along with the treasures of Mithridates, during their triumphant tour of Asia Minor, and in 62 B.C. it accompanied them back to Rome. From there, in line of duty and in the course of time, they carried it on to Spain and France and Germany, and across the Channel into Britain. They also distributed it among the Greeks. To the Romans, the disease was known as *"elephas."* The Greeks gave it its present name. "Leprosy" derives from *"lepros,"* an adjective meaning "scaly." The first reasonably recognizable clinical account of leprosy was composed by an Augustan aristocrat of scientific leanings named Aulus Cornelius Celsus. "In this [leprosy] the whole body becomes so affected that even the bones are said to be diseased," he noted, about the year 30 A.D., for the illumination of his friends. "The surface of the body presents a multiplicity of spots and of swellings, which, at first red, are gradually changed to be black in color. The skin is thickened and thinned in an irregular way, hardened and softened, roughened in some places with a kind of scales; the trunk wastes, the face, calves, and feet swell. When the disease is of long standing, the fingers and toes are sunk under the swelling: feverishness supervenes, which may easily destroy a patient overwhelmed by such troubles."

Celsus, though otherwise a sharp observer, seems not to have grasped the brutalizing quality of the new disease. His contemporaries were similarly obtuse. The Romans, like the aborigines of Egypt, were slow to develop an immoderate horror of leprosy. Its uniqueness had to be explained to them. Among the missionaries who contributed to their ultimate enlightenment, three are out-standing. One of these was the celebrated physician and teacher Aretaeus of Cappadocia. Aretaeus, who established himself in Rome toward the latter half of the second century, possessed a gift for portraying the serious side of disease that has almost never been equalled. His likeness of leprosy is generally considered his masterpiece. "The disease named 'elephas' and the animal named elephant have many properties in common," he wrote. "Formerly, this affection was called 'leontiasis,' on account of the resemblance between the disease and the lion, produced by the appearance of the lower part of the forehead . . . 'Satyriasis,' on account of the redness of the cheeks . . . 'Herculean,' because there is no disease which is graver and more violent. Its power is indeed formidable, for of all diseases it is the one which possesses the most murderous energy . . . also, it is filthy and dreadful to behold, in all respects like the wild animal, the elephant. Lurking among the bowels, like a concealed fire, it smolders there . . . [then] blazes forth . . . the respiration is fetid . . . Tumors prominent . . . The hairs on the whole body die prematurely . . . The skin of the head [becomes] deeply cracked . . . nose elongated . . . ears red, black, contracted, resembling the elephant . . . Sometimes, too, certain of the mem-bers of the patient will die, so as to drop off, such as the nose, the fingers, the feet, the privy parts and the whole hands; for the ailment does not prove fatal, so as to relieve the patient from a foul life and dreadful sufferings, until he has been divided limb from limb . . . libidinous desires [are] of a rabid nature . . . Sleep slight, worse than insomnolency . . . neither food nor drink affords pleas-ure." Aretaeus concluded his study with a word of warning and advice. "There is also the fear that the disease may be com-municated," he pointed out. "Many, for this reason, remove their dearest ones to solitude or to the mountains. Some preserve them from hunger for a time, others not at all, desiring their death." The other leading, if less overt, disseminators of the Oriental concep-tion of leprosy were the apostles Peter and Paul. The Church of their founding was not based altogether on the compassionate gospel of Jesus. It also embodied the fierier teachings of Moses.

Lepraphobia and Christianity are closely linked. Both emerged from the ruins of Rome to sweep almost unimpeded through the

Western world in the deeps of the Dark Ages, and both achieved their richest maturity during the long medieval twilight. The convulsive acceptance of the Trinity was everywhere in Europe followed by an equally convulsive aversion to the leprous. In 583, the delegates to the Council of Lyon, the first ecclesiastical convention held in France, unanimously approved a decree that prohibited lepers, under penalty of death, from fraternizing with any but their own kind. Their pious example soon fired the imagination of all wide-awake temporal authorities. Among the first to respond was an early ruler of Lombardy named Rothari. At his command, in 644, all leprous Lombards were seized and permanently sequestered in an abandoned building on the outskirts of Milan. Their support was left to the inclination of their friends. Pepin the Short, who was the father of Charlemagne and mounted the throne of the Frankish kingdom in 751, carried the Levitical ideas of his predecessors a step further. In addition to discarding his leprous subjects, he forbade them to marry, and declared that those already married could be divorced by their mates. Around 1000, during the reign of Olaf II, of Norway, who was subsequently canonized for his good works, the lepers of that country were simultaneously excommunicated, disenfranchised, and banished from all towns and villages. They were also pledged to celibacy. Olaf, a recent convert, was in one respect a trifle behind the times. By then, in the more civilized centers of Europe, it had become the custom to drive a leper into the wilderness only if he had the misfortune to be poor. Well-to-do victims of the disease were permitted, upon dividing their possessions between the Church and the Crown, to retire to a cell in a public asylum. At the beginning of the thirteenth century, according to Matthew Paris, a contemporary English historian, there were nineteen thousand lazarettos, as such retreats came to be called, in Europe alone. The term is of Biblical origin. It derives from a passage in St. Luke: "And there was a certain beggar named Lazarus, which was laid at his gate full of sores." One of the first English lazarettos was established in 1096, at St. Albans. A book of rules drawn up for the guidance of its inmates has been preserved. "Amongst the infirmities," the opening injunction reads, "the disease of leprosy may be considered the most loathsome, and those who are smitten with it ought at all times, and in all places, and as well in their conduct as in their dress, to bear themselves as more to be despised and as more humble than all other men."

In 1179, the Church introduced an additional mortification. It informed its deputies, by way of an ecumenical decree, that the banishment of lepers, while wholesome, was being carried out with offensive haste and informality. In the future, it continued, their separation from human society, instead of following immediately upon positive diagnosis by a physician (or, as was the custom in some places, by a magistrate), was to be preceded by a seemly religious service. The decree was accompanied by several sample ceremonials. "On [the] day [of exile], the leper must be clad according to his station, very simply," one of these, as elaborated by a twelfth-century French cleric, stipulates. "He must have on his head a white shroud, falling low behind, and a grave cloth over [his garments] and carry in both his hands a little wooden cross; and so move from his house accompanied by the church cross and by his friends mourning over him until he reaches the church. And when he has come to the entrance, the priest and clergy shall meet him and sprinkle holy water over him and take him by the hand and bring him into the cemetery and sing *Libera me Domine.* When they have come to the church, the priest shall begin the Vigils and the Commedaces, and when these are finished, the priest shall pray for him and say the Requiem Mass as for a dead man, with lights and candles. The leper, attired in his shroud and grave cloth, with his little wooden cross, shall kneel and lean on a low stool, his head bowed toward the altar—there where they are accustomed to place the bodies of the dead. And when the service is finished, the priest shall go to the leper, and read what is read to the dead, and then give him the holy water. Then the priest takes him by the hand, and when they are come to the cemetery, the priest makes him kneel, and throws earth over him three times, saying, 'Be dead to the world, and again living to God.' The priest shall then bless and present to the leper a hooded robe, a pair of gloves, and a bell to warn others of his approach, called the Lazarus Bell. He shall then admonish him: 'I forbid you ever to enter into church, abbey, fair, mill, or market, or into the company of others. I forbid you to go without your habit. I forbid you to wash your hands or anything about you at the stream or fountain, or to drink there, and if you need water to drink, take it in your cup. I forbid you to touch anything that you bargain for, or buy, until it is yours. I forbid you to go into any tavern, and if you want wine, whether you buy it or men give it to you, have it put in your cup. I forbid you to touch children or to give them anything. I forbid you to eat or drink from any vessel but your own. I forbid you to drink or eat in company, unless with lepers. If you go on the roads and meet another person who speaks to you, I forbid you to answer until you place yourself against the wind.' "

The wisdom of the Church in thus definitively demonstrating to the leprous their difference from ordinary pariahs was promptly and enthusiastically acknowledged by most medieval Christians. There were, however, in the course of the next hundred years or so, a few spasms of dissent. Several highly placed lepraphobes, including Henry II of England, his great-grandson Edward I, and Philip V of France, took the position that the recommended ritual was unnecessarily symbolical. The revisions instituted by Henry and Philip were similar. Both chose to replace the religious service with a simple civil ceremony. It consisted of strapping the leper to a post and setting him afire. Edward adhered a trifle more closely to the letter of the ecumenical decree. Lepers, during his reign, were permitted the comforts of a Christian funeral. Then they were led down to the cemetery and buried alive.

As a plague of pandemic proportions, leprosy reached its zenith in Europe in the thirteenth and fourteenth centuries. Its grip then suddenly slackened. It began to vanish around the middle of the fifteenth century. By the middle of the sixteenth, it was almost extinct. Numerous reasons have been advanced to account for its abrupt disappearance. Three are generally accepted. The unflagging zeal with which its victims were hounded and harried is, of course, one. Another is the several successive explosions of the Black Death, which, between 1347 and 1568, very nearly depopulated Europe. The third is the timely development of a diagnostic technique flexible enough to frequently distinguish from leprosy such other defacing afflictions as acne and scabies and scurvy. Of these reasons, the last is now widely considered the most persuasive. It is the current conviction of most authorities that only a fraction of the innumerable victims of medieval lepraphobia were actually suffering from leprosy.

Modern leprologists are capable to some extent of understanding the extraordinary horror of leprosy that haunted ancient and medieval man, but they find its present-day persistence peculiar. Any resemblance it may bear to reality is entirely coincidental. Leprosy is no longer obtrusively prevalent much of anywhere. Nor is it by any means the mystery it once was. Its source, its nature, and its clinical manifestations have all been pretty well fathomed. Nothing about it contains any unusual inducements to panic.

The cause of leprosy, which was determined by Gerhard Armauer Hansen, a pioneer Norwegian bacteriologist, in 1874, is a funguslike microbe of unparalleled sluggishness known as *Mycobacterium leprae*. Its lethargy approaches the comatose. Most pathogenic organisms make their presence felt within a week or two of arrival. A month is almost the limit. The incubation period in leprosy is rarely less than two years and it has run as high as thirty. Ordinarily, it is close to seven. The organism is also highly selective in its choice of habitat. Many parasites are able to adapt themselves to practically any physiological environment in a wide variety of animal hosts. *Mycobacterium leprae* can exist in no creature but man (all attempts to cultivate it in laboratory animals have failed), it much prefers men to women (the ratio is two to one), and it finds just two sites fully congenial. They are the under surface of the skin and the peripheral nervous system. When it lodges in the skin, the resulting infection is called lepromatous leprosy. Nerve involvement results in a type known as tuberculoid leprosy. Although the two types of leprosy may appear in conjunction, their characteristics are clinically distinct.

Lepromatous leprosy is the form usually envisioned by lepraphobes. It is marked by the gradual eruption on the face and hands and feet of a multitude of small, lumpy lesions that tend in cases of classic severity to grotesquely merge and ulcerate, and though its progress is slow, it ends nearly always in death. The life expectancy of a victim of lepromatous leprosy is approximately fifteen years. Tuberculoid leprosy is less conspicuously formidable. The lesions by which it manifests itself are macular, anesthetic, and somewhat resemble scar tissue. They vary enormously in size (from an inch in diameter to eight or ten) and they may appear on almost any part of the body. In a considerable number of cases, a few small blemishes remain from beginning to end the only perceptible evidence of the disease. In a majority, however, the destruction of nerve fibres is accompanied by some impairment of certain muscles, most often those in the fingers and toes. A few victims, in time, become helpless cripples. But, at worst, tuberculoid leprosy is merely disabling. It is very infrequently attended by pain, and it has never been known to be fatal.

Just how *Mycobacterium leprae* gains admittance to the body is uncertain. Both the respiratory passage and the gastrointestinal tract have been suggested as likely portals. A third, and to many epidemiologists a likelier, possibility is that it enters by way of a bruise or laceration. But whatever the path to which it is partial, one thing is unequivocally clear. It can transfer itself from one host to another with only the utmost difficulty. Contrary to popular persuasion, leprosy is among the least contagious of all contagious diseases. In fact, under ordinary conditions its contraction is next to impossible. The disease is almost invariably, but by no means inevitably, a result of prolonged and intimate association with a lepromatous leper. Tuberculoid leprosy, to the best of medical opinion, is rarely, if ever, in any way communicable.

Although medical science has yet to find a cure for leprosy, the debilitating advance of the disease can often be hindered and sometimes even halted. There are several drugs to which it is more or less vulnerable. The oldest is chaulmoogra oil. Chaulmoogra oil, which may be administered orally, intramuscularly, or intravenously, is extracted from the seeds of a tree native to Burma. Its discoverer and first beneficiary, according to legend, was a leprous Burmese prince who happened upon it in time to return from banishment and claim his rightful throne. Chaulmoogra oil has been used in the Orient for a thousand years or so and in the West since the late nineteenth century, but because it is cruelly toxic and erratically effective, its popularity now is everywhere waning. The pharmacopoeia in current favor includes streptomycin, cortisone, and the sulfones. The last, which are distant derivatives of the sulfonamide group, are by far the most masterful. They were developed for general germicidal use by a team of British chemists in the middle thirties, but an American, the late Guy H. Faget, for many years medical officer in charge of the National Leprosarium at Carville, Louisiana, was the first to detect their value in the treatment of leprosy. Sulfone therapy was initiated at Carville in 1940. In 1947, after seven years of careful observation, Dr. Faget was able to report, "Experience has shown that the relation of improvement to duration of treatment [with the sul-fones] can be approximately estimated. After six months of treat-ment almost twenty-five per cent of the patients show some im-provement. After one year this percentage is increased to sixty, after two years to seventy-five, after three years to almost one hundred." Subsequent investigators have more than confirmed his findings. A large majority are fully satisfied that sulfone therapy, if continued for a minimum of three years, will result in at least some improvement in all but the most forlorn and far-gone cases.

There are approximately four million lepers in the world. Around three million are concentrated in southeastern Asia, cen-tral Africa, and tropical Latin America. Most of the rest are widely scattered. The only considerable areas almost wholly free of leprosy are Canada and Siberia. It is endemic even in Iceland. In Europe, it is now largely confined to Spain, Portugal, Greece, Norway, Italy, and parts of the Soviet Union. Leprosy reached the United States, by way of the West Indies and the African slave trade, in the mid-eighteenth century, but it has never made much headway here. The American Leprosy Foundation estimates that there are at present not more than two thousand lepers in the entire country. Fully two-thirds of them, the Foundation esti-mates, acquired the disease elsewhere. Leprosy is endemic in just four of the forty-eight states—Florida, Louisiana, Texas, and, but only in its southern tip, California. Why this should be so has yet to be adequately explained. It is, however, demonstrably a fact. From time to time, cases of leprosy turn up in other states, but nearly all of them can be traced, directly or indirectly, to some foreign source. Four or five lepers, on the average, are discovered in New York City every year. In the fall of 1934, when Roberto Ramirez suffered his unsettlingly painless burn, the names of twenty-three local lepers were on file at the Department of Health. He brought the total to twenty-four.

The note from Harlem Hospital was handed to Dr. Samuel Frant, then director of the Bureau of Preventable Diseases and now Deputy Commissioner of Health, on Friday morning, September 25th. He gave it a long, unhappy look, added a few well-chosen words of instruction, and, as is usual in such matters, passed it promptly along to the Department's chief diagnostician, Dr. David A. Singer, for thorough investigation. Dr. Singer's reaction to Ramirez's plight was equally brisk and methodical. He tossed the report, the note, and a word or two of his own across to his secretary, and she typed out the customary letter. It read, "Will you please call on me at my office on Monday, October 1st, at 4 P.M. If you cannot appear at that time, kindly telephone my secretary and she will arrange another appointment." Dr. Singer signed the letter before he left for lunch, and it went out in the afternoon mail.

"Ramirez performed as expected," Dr. Singer says. "He didn't telephone and he didn't fail me. They very seldom do. They're afraid to. Our letter reads like a summons. They don't dare ignore it. It's too official. On the other hand, it very carefully says nothing that could possibly scare them away. Leprosy is a nightmare word. One hint of what we want to see them about, and they might simply pack a bag and run. That's happened. And, of course, you can't really blame them. They don't know any better. Most people are still living in the Middle Ages as far as their understanding of leprosy is concerned. Particularly of how we handle it. They still think in terms of quarantine and segregation—life imprisonment in a leper colony. In other words, a fate worse than death. Nothing could be farther from the truth. At least, in most parts of the country. Two-thirds of the lepers in the United States live pretty much like everybody else. Carville is for the very unfortunate few. And it's hardly a prison. It's a hospital—one of the finest in the world. The fact is only ten states—most of them, as might be expected, in or near the endemic areas—still insist on some form of isolation. Notification of the health authorities is the most required by law in any of the others. Most of us still feel that notification is desirable. But our reasons have changed a good deal. Up to a generation or so ago, the main idea was to protect society from the leper. That's only part of it these days, even in the Deep South. We're more interested now in the leper—in doing what we can to make his trouble more tolerable. Which includes protecting him from the ignorance and cruelty of society.

"Well, as I say, Ramirez showed up. He came in on Thursday at four on the dot. Obviously worried to death. I gave him a cigarette and we talked a bit and I got what I needed in the way of history. Born, raised, and married in San Juan, Puerto Rico. Moved to New York in 1929. A painter by trade. All very much as usual. At least forty per cent of our cases originate in the Caribbean area. Then I had a look at his arm. It was leprosy, all right—tuberculoid leprosy. Not that I'd had any serious doubts. A positive Ziehl-Neelsen doesn't leave much room for argument. But, naturally, I like to see for myself. And I didn't merely look. I went over him from top to toe. Also, if only for the record, I took another skin scraping and some material for a nasal smear. Then I sat down and broke the news. I made it as easy as I could, but I told him the truth. All of it. There's no other way. I began with the report from Harlem, and went on from there. I told him what the test had showed, what leprosy is and what it isn't, and what we do about it—or, rather, what we don't do. I made that plainer than plain. That we had no intention of sending him away. That his life was no more over than mine. That he could continue to live and work and do pretty much as he pleased—for years, probably. And that no one would ever know but him and his family and us. All we asked was that he follow a few simple instructions, the first of which was to return the following week—same day, same time—for a talk about treatment. Then I went back and explained it all again. I won't say he took it with a smile. There were, as always, several very bad moments. But he took it. He finally came around. At any rate, he wasn't going to do anything rash. I was sure of that. You can generally tell. So we were over the hump. The rest, I had every reason to hope, was just a matter of time.

"I don't know when Ramirez broke the news to his family. Or how. That part of the business, thank heaven, doesn't often devolve on me. The job of telling the patient is painful enough. I waited a couple of days, until I could assume they had heard and thrashed it out. Then, on Monday, I sent a medical inspector up to the home for a good look at Mrs. Ramirez and the children.

We don't very often find more than one case of tuberculoid leprosy in the same family. But it happens. Offhand, I can think of five or six cases. So we always make certain. That goes without saying. Moreover, we like to see how our people live. It's only common sense to insist on the fundamentals of hygiene. Adequate toilet facilities, for example, and a separate bed for the children. By Thursday, when Ramirez came down for his second session, everything was well in hand. Nobody had sprung any surprises. As expected, our laboratory was in full agreement with Harlem. Both of my samples were unequivocally positive. The inspector's report was also unequivocal. Ramirez was our only problem.

"My second meeting with Ramirez was a good deal happier than the first. A week had done wonders for him. He had a good grip on himself and he couldn't have been more coöperative. Maybe his wife had helped. I met her some years later—a very sensible woman. But, however it happened, it was a big relief. They sometimes come back worse than ever. It all depends upon how much nonsense they've managed to absorb. Nevertheless, I didn't take any chances. Leprosy is a lonely road. Even the best of them need plenty of encouragement. So I went over all the facts again and repeated all my promises. From there, I moved on to what we expected of him. It wasn't much. Certainly nothing very onerous. We wanted to see him at least once a year—my secretary would call or write—to evaluate his progress and make the usual tests. That was the major requirement. Of the others, the only one worth mentioning is this. He wasn't to sleep with or kiss or fondle his children. I don't mean to imply that they were in any real danger. Still, since children seem to be rather more susceptible than adults, it's just as well to play safe. I then took up the question of treatment. In those days, that meant chaulmoogra oil —an injection twice a week, administered by a doctor. He could get his shots from a private physician or at one of the several big public dermatological clinics. Just as he liked. My advice was the latter. As a matter of fact, I told him, I had talked to a man I knew at New York Skin and Cancer Hospital and arranged a tentative appointment for nine o'clock Saturday morning. He nodded. Whatever I said. And he meant it. He went. Around noon on Saturday, I called the hospital and checked. It wasn't necessary.

I just thought I would. He'd been there, they said, and would be back on Wednesday. Well, that was that. He was on his way.

"During the next few years, I got to know Ramirez pretty well. I was seeing him twice a year here at the office, and every now and then I'd run into him up at Skin and Cancer and we'd stop for a minute and talk. We finally came to be something like friends. That's where I met his wife—at the clinic. As far as I know, he never missed a treatment. He must have had well over a thousand shots. I wish I could say they did him some good. But I doubt it. In fact, I doubt if chaulmoogra oil ever did anybody any good. The arrests we used to brag about were probably pure coincidence. Leprosy is very peculiar. It sometimes just plain peters out. Ramirez had no such luck. He was a better than average patient, but his case was fairly typical. Almost every time I saw him, I'd find a new lesion. By the end of 1942, or thereabouts, he had at least a dozen—all sizes—on his arms and legs and back. It could, of course, have been worse. Considerably so. For one thing, it didn't, as can easily happen, develop into an infection of the lepromatous type. Also, nobody ever knew—except, I suppose, his son-in-law. His daughter married—with our blessing—in 1944. She lives in Boston now. And his only disability was his left hand. Eventually, the first and second fingers—the site of the original lesion—become badly clawed. New lesions kept turning up, though. Six months or a year would go by and we'd begin to hope. And then there it would be—another. Until 1949. Two years before, in 1947, we started using the sulfones, and Ramirez, like all of our cases, was switched to that. At the end of a year, we couldn't be sure. There were no new lesions, but that had happened before. In 1949, however, we really had reason to hope. By 1950, we were sure. He was more than holding his own. There was actually some objective improvement. Don't misunderstand me. He wasn't cured. A cure for leprosy is still in the future. He wasn't even arrested. The samples I took at his second 1950 visit were still very definitely positive. But something had changed. Things were slowing down.

"There's no way of knowing what might have happened. No two cases are the same. Our 1950 meeting was the last time I ever saw him. Early in 1951, a few days before he was due to come in again, I had a call from Mrs. Ramirez. Her husband wouldn't be down. He was sick. He'd had a heart attack of some kind—it sounded like coronary sclerosis—and was up at Harlem Hospital. Apparently in very bad shape. The next thing I heard, he was dead."

[*1953*]

CHAPTER 6

Lost

———————◆◆◆———————

I'LL CALL HIM UHLAN—Walter Uhlan. The date was August 29, 1950, the day was a Tuesday, and the time was a little past noon. That, to the best of his subsequent recollection, was the moment of emergence. It was then that consciousness stirred and quickened, and he found himself—a tall, stooped, bespectacled man of thirty-nine, in a blue polo jersey and tan gabardine trousers, with a rumpled tweed jacket slung over his arm—standing in front of the Doubleday bookstore on the Long Island level of Pennsylvania Station. For several minutes, Uhlan had been cloudily aware of a mounting sense of strangeness and confusion. Now, with an almost jarring suddenness, he realized why. He didn't know who he was or where he was or what he was doing there.

Loss of memory is the familiar phenomenon familiarly known as amnesia. It invariably manifests itself as a disturbance in the essential processes that form the library of the mind. These include the prompt reception, the orderly conversation, and the accurate reproduction of mental impressions. Like those of most cerebral aberrations, its possible causes are almost astronomically numerous. All amnesias, however, stem from one or another of two distinctly different sources. They have their roots in either an organic or a functional debility. Of these, amnesia of organic origin is by far the more common. It is also less extensive, and less difficult to trace to its seat. The immediate cause of organic amnesia is a neural languor that renders the brain temporarily incapable of retaining and recalling stimuli. Organic amnesia is not in itself a disease, though, or even, in the usual sense, a symptom of one. It is merely a more or less insignificant corollary of some physiological dishevelment (an acute infection, an epileptic seizure, a metabolic convulsion) or an addling blow on the head.

The range of functional amnesia is protean (it may obscure little or much or even the whole of memory), its term is unpredictable (it may lift in a day, in a week, or only after many months). It is precipitated not by a mechanical breakdown but by the descent of an emotional block. Its gravest form, which science has come to call fugue, embraces three classically dramatic phases. The first of these is a brief interval of complete dissociation, closely resembling somnambulism. This is eventually followed by a period of lightened oblivion, in which only certain facts and events remain beyond the reach of the victim. The final stage, which may occur spontaneously or as a result of psychiatric manipulation, is a return to full-functioning consciousness. But, whatever its pattern, an attack of functional amnesia of the fugue type is seldom susceptible to either a ready or a reassuring explanation. In almost every instance, including, as it turned out, that of Walter Uhlan, it reflects the presence of a racking psychoneurosis—a constitutional inability to withstand the rigors of reality—whose beginnings lie deep in the encysted complex of the past.

Uhlan was an only child. He was born to Rufus Uhlan, a bookkeeper employed by a wholesale hardware company, and Grace Thompson Uhlan, the youngest of six daughters of a Manchester, New Hampshire, veterinary, in a railroad flat in South Boston on June 18, 1911. Ten months later, in the spring of 1912, Mrs. Uhlan developed acute leukemia, and in five or six weeks she was dead. During her illness, Walter had been taken in and cared for by his eldest maternal aunt, a childless widow with a comfortable pension, who lived just down the street. His mother's death prolonged his stay considerably. He remained there, cherished by his aunt and largely ignored by his father, until shortly after his fourth birthday. Rufus Uhlan had by then remarried, and in July, 1915, having persuaded his bride to be a stepmother as well as a wife, he brought the boy home again. Walter endured a month of home-sickness so keen that he still recalls it with anguish. Then, one afternoon, he slipped out of the flat, down the block, and into the arms of his aunt. After an hour of tears and kisses and cookies, she led him back up the street. That was his first attempt. By the time he was six, he had fled to his aunt at least a dozen times. Finally, a family council was called. Facts were faced, convenience was consulted, and eventually the problem was solved. Early in 1918, Uhlan was returned once more to his aunt. For several years, he spent every Sunday with his father, and they sometimes had an outing together. Then, as time went on, their meetings became less frequent. Toward the end of 1930, Rufus Uhlan was transferred by his firm to Chicago. The son never saw him again.

Uhlan was then nineteen. He had graduated from his neighbor-hood high school, he had passed a random year at Boston University, and he was restlessly in search of a job. He found one the following spring, as a shipping clerk in the local retail branch of a mammoth mail-order house. It was the best he could do, and he made the best of it. In the course of the next ten years, he rose from clerk to salesman to assistant manager of the work-clothes department. But, with responsibility, his restlessness returned. After two years of executive tension, he resigned, talked things over with his aunt, and decided to study law. In the fall of 1941, he reënrolled at Boston University. His second appearance on the campus lasted just six months. In February of 1942, his aunt suffered a coronary thrombosis, and he dropped out of school to take care of her. She died in the middle of May. Two months later, he was inducted into the Army.

Uhlan applied himself to the Army as he had to business, and with much the same result. At the end of the basic-training period, he was recognized as a potential officer, and, because of his experi-ence as a merchandiser, dispatched to the Quartermaster School at Camp Lee, Virginia. For the first ten weeks of a three-month course there, he was an apt and ardent pupil. Then an accident occurred. One afternoon, while he was demonstrating his ability to conduct close-order drill, a rumor reached him that a general recently returned from North Africa had joined the usual observers in the stand. Uhlan's reaction was sudden and shattering. He called out an order, tried to call it back, tried to give another, and then stood frozen with panic. His men shambled into a fence. Uhlan turned and ran from the field. An officer, investigating, discovered him a few minutes later, collapsed on his cot in an agony of tears. That was in February of 1943. The following October, after a regimen of rest and psychiatric rehabilitation at Walter Reed Army Hospital, in Washington, he was honorably separated from the service with a certificate-of-disability discharge.

Uhlan returned to civilian life in good health but low spirits. He had no plans, no prospects, and very little money. Also, now that his aunt was dead, he had no ties anywhere. During the next few months, he drifted from place to place—Philadelphia, Baltimore, New York—and from one aimless job to another. April found him back in Boston. There, one night in a bar on Scollay Square, he ran into a boyhood friend. It soon developed that he, too, was idle and restless and alone, and the two young men settled down to a long evening of beer and talk. They parted, toward morning, fired with a desire to go into business together. The notion survived a second meeting. All that remained was to turn up a promising project. By the first of June, they had one—a personnel service designed to supply wartime industry with competent maintenance men. It was a modest idea, but timely, and, to the best of their knowledge, unique. They opened an office, made the rounds of the local factories, and waited. The response was overwhelming. Before the year was out, they had satisfied clients from Maine to Maryland, and were scouring the countryside for recruits. But as time went on and the business steadied, Uhlan's enthusiasm waned. Finally, late in 1945, he was seized once more by the familiar longing for change. He sold out his interest, pocketed the proceeds, and began to drift again.

Uhlan chose, this time, to stay in Boston. The spell lasted almost a year. It ended, abruptly, at a cocktail party one afternoon in December of 1946. The reason was a girl. She lived in South

Boston, where her father, a widower, kept a corner haberdashery shop; she had a job with an advertising agency on Tremont Street; and her name, I'll say, was Mildred Morris. Uhlan fell in love at a glance. His courtship was swift and triumphant. He and Miss Morris announced their engagement in February, 1947, and on the nineteenth of May they were married. Ten days later, after a honeymoon week in New York at the St. Moritz Hotel, on Central Park South, they were comfortably settled in a pleasant apartment near Franklin Field. Meanwhile, inspired by love or necessity, Uhlan had ceased his drift from job to job and was again in business for himself. In March, he had conceived and set in motion a monogram-embroidering service. Like the employment agency, it got off to a most encouraging start. Throughout the spring of 1947, the orders poured in. Then, with summer, they began to dwindle. Uhlan told himself that it was merely a seasonal slump. But it wasn't. Fall was, if anything, worse. With the last of his savings, he managed to hold out through Christmas. The creditors then closed in. Uhlan made his final appearance at his office on January 28, 1948. The following morning, he refused to get up. He said he couldn't. He said he had a paralyzing headache, he said he was a born failure, he burst into tears. A doctor, summoned by his frightened wife, arrived around noon and found him buried in the bedclothes, sobbing and moaning and shaking. Having taken his temperature and his history, the doctor gave him a sedative and suggested a consultation with a psychiatrist. He named a reliable colleague. Early in April, on the psychiatrist's recommendation, Uhlan was admitted to a suburban sanitarium for observation and treatment. Mrs. Uhlan went back to work and back to live with her father.

Uhlan's second immersion in psychotherapy lasted a little over six weeks. He was discharged, reasonably restored to normality, at the end of the third week in May. He returned to his wife, who continued to work, and a new apartment, and at once set out in search of a suitable job. He didn't immediately find one. The trouble was he didn't quite know what he wanted. His efforts were hampered by two contradictory desires. He was determined to somehow distinguish himself, but he lacked the nerve to risk another failure. He was still looking for an acceptable compromise when chance settled the problem for him. Shortly after Thanksgiving, his father-in-law was struck down by a hypertensive cardiovascular stroke. It was neither fatal nor crippling, but it left him dangerously prostrated. What he needed, the family doctor reported, was several months of rest, preferably in a milder climate. Mrs. Uhlan did what she could. She gave up all thought of quitting her job, and arranged for her father to spend the winter with a cousin in Dover, Delaware. Meanwhile, she suggested, Uhlan could take over the haberdashery store. Uhlan heard her proposal with dismay. It was the mail-order house all over again, only worse. It was even more harrowing than the Army. It offered him responsibility, and no chance whatever to satisfy his ambition. But he couldn't very well refuse. Besides, it was only temporary. In the end, he reluctantly agreed to keep the business going.

In his new position, Uhlan opened the shop at nine in the morning. Five days a week, Monday through Friday, he locked up for the night at eight. On Saturdays, he stayed open until eleven. That had been Mr. Morris's custom. Uhlan was expected to follow it. During the first few weeks, in the intervals between customers, he kept busy by familiarizing himself with the stock. After that, in the intervals, he leaned on the counter and waited —for spring, for Mr. Morris, for his release. In June, Mrs. Uhlan had a letter from her father's doctor in Dover. Mr. Morris had suffered a mild relapse. It was advisable that he remain in Delaware through the summer. Uhlan took a deep breath. In September, the doctor wrote again. He felt it would still be risky for Mr. Morris to return to work. Perhaps a few more months of rest would put him back on his feet. Two weeks later, on October 7, 1949, there was another letter from Dover. Mr. Morris had just had a second stroke. There was, however, no particular cause for alarm. In fact, except for some difficulty in articulation and a partial paralysis of his left arm, he had made a strong recovery. But it would be understood, of course, that this new development meant that in all probability . . . Uhlan put down the letter, and swallowed. He understood exactly what it meant. His stomach tightened with panic. He was trapped.

When Uhlan emerged to an awareness of his surroundings that August afternoon in 1950 and found himself lost and nameless in the depths of Pennsylvania Station, his first reaction again was one of panic. He stood for a moment transfixed. Then, as he moved on, an overhead sign caught his eye. It read, "8TH AVE. SUBWAY STRAIGHT AHEAD." His panic at once subsided. "I knew where I was," he says. "Eighth Avenue and a subway could only mean New York. Well, New York was a place I knew. So I wasn't completely helpless. The next thing I remember was walking—and the heat. I've never been so hot. My shirt was soaking wet. Maybe I'd been running. I was on some street, and I had a vague kind of feeling that I was trying to get away from something. Or, rather, that I had got away. Because I didn't feel nervous or frightened, or anything like that. What I felt was relieved. Then I was looking at a telephone book. It was a classified directory, and I had it open to the section on hotels. I was tired and I wanted to take a bath and rest. The hotel I picked was in the West Forties, just off Broadway. At least, that was the one I tried first. But I only stayed a minute. The room they gave me was filthy. It had a ragged old rug on the floor and the bed was falling apart—that's my impression, anyway. I went down to the desk and asked for my money back. I didn't have any luggage, so I'd had to pay in advance. The clerk said no. I didn't argue. It didn't really matter. I just left, and went a couple of blocks up to the Taft. The room I got there must have been all right. At any rate, I took it. I remember looking at myself in the bathroom mirror. In a way, I guess, I was curious. All I remember, though, is thinking that whoever I was and wherever I came from, I hadn't been gone long. From the look of my beard, I had shaved that morning, and my pants were pressed and my shirt was reasonably clean. But, actually, I wasn't much interested. I was too tired. I flopped down on the bed and went to sleep."

Uhlan's deductions, as far as they went, were correct. He hadn't been gone very long. His wanderings had begun only that morning. "Walter left the house about eight," Mrs. Uhlan says. "That was a little early, but I wasn't surprised. We had agreed the night before that he would get breakfast on his way to the store. I was on vacation that week, and wanted to sleep late. Well, I heard him leave, and then I dozed off again, and it was after nine when I finally got up. Everything seemed perfectly normal. His shaving things were all over the bathroom, as usual, and I found his pajamas where I always did—on the floor beside the bed. I dressed and had breakfast and tidied up the house. Then I went down the street and did some marketing. When I got back, I thought it would be nice to call the store and say good morning. That must have been around ten-thirty. I called, but the phone just rang. There was no answer. I decided he'd probably stepped out for a minute. Either that, or he was busy with a customer. I tried again at eleven. Again no answer. I waited a few minutes, and tried once more. Still no answer. Well, that *was* peculiar. I checked with the operator. There was nothing the matter with the phone. They just didn't answer, she said. But why? I'm not the nervous type, but I began to feel very uneasy. Something had happened. I was sure of it. It was nearly eleven-thirty by then. He couldn't be waiting on a customer for almost an hour. Or out. It wasn't possible. I tried to think what to do. Then I had an inspiration. I called the store next door. It was a little bakery, and the man who ran it was an old friend of Daddy's. I told him the story. He didn't know what to make of it, either. But he told me to hang on—he'd go take a look and see if there was anything wrong. He came back completely bewildered. Walter wasn't there. The front door was locked, the mail slot was full of letters, and the night light in the rear was still burning.

"I thanked him and hung up. I was too stunned to say another word. I was simply paralyzed. For a minute, I just sat there. The only thing I could think of was an accident. He was always in such a hurry. It always gave him the fidgets to have to wait for the light to change. I could almost see him darting across the street, and the brakes screaming, and the people running up—and the ambulance. But then I began to calm down. I told myself that you always imagine the worst. There was probably some perfectly ordinary explanation. Maybe he'd had to see one of the jobbers. Or our lawyer. There might even be some sort of trouble with the bank. He could have mentioned it the night before, and I could have just forgotten. That had happened more than once. So I tried to be sensible. I called the bank and the jobbers and the lawyer —everybody and every place I could think of. Even a few of his business friends. But none of them knew a thing. That left the hospitals and the police. I tried the hospitals first. I started with those near the store. Then I called the big ones, like City Hospital and Massachusetts General. After that, I went straight down the list. It took me all afternoon, and I learned absolutely nothing. Except, of course, that he hadn't been hit by a car or suddenly taken sick. If he had, there would almost certainly have been some kind of record at one of the hospitals. At least, they'd have his name. Because his wallet was always stuffed with personal papers and all kinds of identification. I suppose that should have been some comfort, but it wasn't. I was frantic. In a way, I think, I'd almost hoped that a hospital would say yes. Nothing is worse than not knowing.

"My only hope then was the police. Even if they didn't know anything, they might at least be able to help. But I didn't have the strength to face them alone. I'd always been used to fending for myself, but somehow this was different. It was too much for me. I needed—well, moral support. So I called up a girl I knew and told her what had happened. If she wasn't my best friend then, she is now. She was simply wonderful. I couldn't have managed without her. She threw some things in a bag and jumped in her car and came straight over, and she stayed right through to the end. The first thing we did was drive to the store. I knew Walter wasn't there—I'd kept calling off and on all afternoon—but I wanted to see for myself. It looked the way it always does at night. I had a key, and we went in, and something made me open the cash register. It was empty. That meant Walter hadn't been in the store since he closed up the evening before. He never left money overnight at the store. He always brought it home with him. And he always put it back in the register the very first thing in the morning. It also meant that, whatever had happened, he was well supplied with money. He probably had over a hundred dollars. I looked around to make sure everything was all right, and then locked up again. Then we drove down to Police Headquarters. We ended up in the Missing Persons Bureau. The sergeant there wasn't much impressed at first. When I told him that Walter had only been missing since morning, he gave me an awfully funny look. I think he thought that we'd quarrelled, or something, and Walter had simply walked out. But when he heard the whole story —about Walter's nervous breakdown, and so on—he couldn't have been nicer. Or more sympathetic. He said they'd send out a bulletin with a full description and recheck all the hospitals and do everything else that was possible. The minute they had some news, he would let me know."

It was a little past three when Uhlan flopped down on his bed in the Taft. He awakened at four, streaming with sweat but re-freshed. Almost at once, a wave of restlessness rolled over him. It swept him off the bed and through the door and down the stairs to the street. "I had to get going," he says. "It didn't matter where. All I wanted was out. I felt hemmed in. Otherwise, though, I felt all right. And as soon as I started walking, I was fine. I completely relaxed. I cut over to Ninth Avenue, I remember, and headed south. I wasn't going anywhere and there wasn't any hurry. I just walked along looking in the windows and watching the people and enjoying the sights. It was an Italian neighborhood, and there were fruit-and-vegetable stands out in front of the stores. They were piled with wonderful food—all kinds of squash, and big yellow tomatoes, and a lot of things I'd never even seen before. I stopped at one place and bought a couple of beautiful bananas. Everything seemed new and different. Even the people. It was very interesting. But I kept on walking, and pretty soon I was in the Village. That was interesting, too. I was fascinated. I'd never been there before. There was one street of old red brick houses with shiny doorknobs and knockers, and I have a kind of memory of a bookstore window full of big pictures that looked carved out of wood. I don't really remember much about what I did, though. Mostly, I think, I just wandered around. I don't even know if I had any dinner. Maybe I had a hamburger or something. I did have a few beers. But that was later on, after it got dark. It was still hot and I had a terrible thirst. When I couldn't stand it any longer, I'd find a bar and go in and drink a glass of beer. Then I'd start walking again. After one time, I remember sitting on a bench in Washington Square. I was smoking a cigarette, and it must have

been late. It had that feel. The next thing I remember, I was back
at the hotel.

"I hardly slept at all that night. It was too hot and I was too
tired and I couldn't seem to get comfortable. Finally, about seven-
thirty, I stopped trying and got up. That was Wednesday morning.
I took a shower and got dressed as fast as I could, and left. It was
like the day before. I couldn't stay still. I had to keep moving. As
long as I was going somewhere or doing something, I kept feeling
all right. I must have headed straight for the Village. At any rate,
I was back there by ten o'clock. My first recollection is one of
those streets around Wanamaker's. There was a walkup hotel in
the middle of the block. I went in and got a room, but it was so
dark and dirty I came right out. Then I tried another. It was even
worse. I don't think it was even a real hotel. It was some kind of
dive. The clerk asked me how many hours I planned to stay. So
I walked out of that one, too. I kept walking until I found a place
that at least looked clean. It was on Eighth Street, I think, not far
from Fifth Avenue. I sat in my room there for a while, just looking
out the window. It was hot and sticky and beginning to rain. All
of a sudden, I felt something crawling on my legs. It was a terrible
feeling. I kicked off my pants and got under a good light and
examined myself. My legs were alive with little animals. I don't
know what they were. They weren't bedbugs or lice, or anything
like that. I can't even describe them. They were sort of red and
clammy and all tangled up in my hair—it was horrible. The only
thing I could think to do was shave my legs. I pulled on my pants
and ran down to the street. There was a drugstore a couple of
doors away. I went in and bought a razor and some blades and
a tube of shaving cream. While I was at it, I bought a toothbrush.
I felt filthy all over. Then I ran back to the hotel, and stripped,
and got in the bathtub and started in. It took a long time. I really
had to scrape to dig them out. They were practically embedded.
By the time I got the last one off, my legs were bleeding in a dozen
places. But I didn't care about that. The awful mess was down the
drain, and I was clean. Then I scrubbed the razor and put in a new
blade and had a regular shave, and brushed my teeth. Then I took
a long hot bath. Then I got dressed and went out. I started walking
again.

"I walked until it began to get dark. I don't know where I went. I was still in the Village, though, and so hungry my head was spinning. Except for a cup of coffee, I hadn't had a bite to eat all day. The part of the Village I was in was down below Washington Square. It was full of restaurants. The one I picked was an Italian place in a basement, with a menu in the window. I had a big plate of spaghetti and a bottle of beer. Then I felt better. After that, I walked back up to Eighth Street. I didn't have any plans, but when I came to a movie theatre, I decided to go in. They were showing one of those Italian pictures—like 'Paisan' or 'Open City.' Also, I remember, there was a sort of lounge where they served coffee. I guess I saw about half the picture. But I couldn't get interested. I couldn't concentrate. Something kept kind of nagging at me. So I finally left and found a bar and had a beer. But that wasn't what I wanted, either. While I was standing there at the bar, it suddenly hit me that I didn't know who I was. I mean, it hit me in a new way. I'd been aware all along that there was something wrong, and every now and then I'd stop and wonder, but it hadn't really made any impression on me. This was different. I don't know how to explain it, but all of a sudden I was scared. It was as if I'd looked in a mirror and there wasn't any reflection. I remember standing there and trying to think. I thought of the hotel registers I'd signed, and tried to remember the name I'd written down. It was something Ward, I think, or Walsh. But I was sure that wasn't my name. It didn't sound right. I got to shaking so I could hardly hold my glass. Then I was out on the street, almost running. It was like something was chasing me. The next thing I remember, I was up in my hotel room. I started turning out my pockets. I knew I had a wallet. I remembered seeing it in the drugstore. If I could find it, there was sure to be something inside it that at least would give me a clue. But there wasn't any wallet. All I found was half a pack of cigarettes and some matches and money—all kinds of money. Every pocket was stuffed with bills. I don't know how much I had. I didn't count it. That didn't interest me. Instead, I took off my clothes and examined them. But they didn't tell me anything, either. My jersey had only an Arrow label, and all the label in my jacket said was Hart, Schaffner & Marx. Then I had an idea. I don't know how

or why, but suddenly I decided I wanted to go to Philadelphia. I
got dressed as fast as I could and ran down the street and headed
for Penn Station. It must have been around three o'clock in the
morning when I got there. Only I didn't go to Penn Station. I went
to a bus depot near there. There was a bus just leaving, and I
wasn't sure about the trains and I wanted to be in Philadelphia
by morning. So I took the bus."

Uhlan arrived in Philadelphia, at the Broad Street Station, just
after daybreak on Thursday, August 31st. He found an all-night
lunchroom near City Hall and had a bowl of cereal and a cup of
coffee. After breakfast, he walked down Broad Street until he
came to a hotel. "It was the John Bartram," he says. "They gave
me a nice room, and I went to bed and slept for a couple of hours.
I'd had a miserable night on the bus—hardly even dozed. When
I woke up, it was gray and gloomy, and I felt terribly depressed.
And bewildered. I didn't know what I was doing in Philadelphia.
If I'd had a reason, it was gone now. I took a bath and got dressed.
I needed a shave, but I'd lost my shaving things. Maybe I'd left
them in New York, or on the bus. I didn't really care, though. I
was too discouraged, and I was beginning to get jumpy and restless again. As soon as I got dressed, I went out and started walking. It was raining, but that didn't bother me, either. I walked the
streets until I got tired. Then I went back to the hotel and tried
to rest. After that, I walked some more. Every now and then, I
had the feeling I was looking for something. I don't know what.
Mostly, though, I just walked because I couldn't stay still. Pretty
soon, it was dark. I was on Locust Street, I remember, carrying
a little kit bag with a razor in it and some other things I'd bought,
and I decided I'd had enough of Philadelphia. I had to get back
to New York. So I walked over to Broad Street and up to the
station and got a ticket on the next bus. I don't know when it left,
but it must have been very late, because when I came out of the
depot in New York, it was broad daylight.

"I had some breakfast in a cafeteria on Thirty-fourth Street.
Then I headed back to the Village. It was another hot day, and
something kept hurrying me, and by the time I got there I was
dripping wet and half dead. The first place I went was that hotel

on Eighth Street where I'd stayed before. But they were full up. Or so they said. Maybe it was the way I looked. I was filthy. I'd slept and sweated and walked through the rain in the same clothes for almost four days. Also, I had a two-day growth of beard. The only place that would take me in was a hole-in-the-wall down on Bleecker Street. Meanwhile, before I got there, I'd stopped and bought myself some underwear and a pair of socks and a regular shirt and a necktie. I still had the kit bag and the things I'd bought in Philadelphia. I showered and shaved and put on my new clothes. The old stuff I just threw in the wastebasket. Then I left. For a while, I felt better. At least I was clean. But then my mind started working. I got to worrying about who I was and what had happened. And what was going to happen. The only way I could keep halfway calm was to keep walking. Whenever I stopped, I'd begin to get panicky, and have to move on again. About two o'clock, I was in Times Square and I came to an out-of-town-newspaper stand. That gave me an idea. I was certain that I came from somewhere near New York. I had that feeling. And I was pretty sure it was a big city—because the traffic didn't bother me. That narrowed things down quite a bit. It was possible, I figured, if I got some papers from all the likeliest places, maybe one of them would look familiar. It might ring a bell. At any rate, it was worth trying. So I did. I bought a whole armful and carried them up Forty-second Street to Bryant Park and found a bench. I sat down and started reading. I began with Philadelphia—the *Bulletin* and the *Inquirer*. Then I went through the Baltimore *Sun* and *News-Post*, the Washington *Post* and *Times-Herald*, the Wilmington *News*, the Providence *Journal*, the Newark *News*, and the Hartford *Courant*. I ended up with the Pittsburgh *Post-Gazette*. But nothing happened. They all looked exactly the same. It was all I could do to keep from crying. It wasn't just disappointment. That was only part of it. It was mainly—I don't know. I just felt so helpless, and alone.

"I don't remember leaving the park. The next thing I remember is some boys playing ball in a big field up on Riverside Drive. I sat on the grass and watched them for quite a while. Then I got restless, and started walking again. Around eight o'clock, I was back in the Village. I had a sandwich somewhere. It was a Greek place, I think. After that, I walked down to Bleecker Street. I realized that I'd left my kit bag in that hotel there and I had to get it. I couldn't afford to keep buying razors. My money was going too fast. By the time I found the hotel and got my bag, it was dark. It was hot, too, and I was thirsty. I walked around until I found a bar, and went in and had a beer. Only, it wasn't just a bar. It turned out to be some kind of a night club. There was a band playing and people dancing, and pretty soon a floor show started up. One of the entertainers was a strip-tease girl. I stood at the bar and watched her. She wasn't pretty. As a matter of fact, she was kind of homely. But she had a beautiful body. It was really sensational. I guess she saw me watching her. When the show ended, she came over to the bar and said hello, and we started talking. I could hardly believe it. That was the first time in four days that anybody had even noticed me. It made me feel almost real. Her name was Arlene, she said, and then she asked me if I'd like to buy her a drink. That was the whole idea, of course, but I didn't mind. It was worth it. We sat down at a table and I ordered another beer and she asked for some whiskey. When the waiter left, she sat there for a minute, just looking at me. It was as if she hadn't really seen me before. Finally, she said, 'There's something wrong, isn't there? You're in some kind of trouble.' I was startled, but I told her no. I said I was fine. 'No,' she said. 'You're in trouble. I can tell.' Well, there didn't seem to be any point in arguing. So I told her. I told her the whole story—what there was to tell. I don't know whether I expected her to believe me or not, but she did. She kept shaking her head, and saying, 'Oh, you poor thing.' She couldn't have been sweeter, or more understanding. She was wonderful. Then she jumped up and went over to the bar for a minute, and when the waiter brought our drinks, it was two beers. She'd cancelled her whiskey. I had to save my money, she said.

"We sat there and talked until it was time for her next show. I waited, and after that we talked some more. She asked me all sorts of questions. She really tried to help. One question, I remember, was did I think I was married? I said yes. That hadn't really occurred to me before, but now I was sure of it. I had that feeling. Also, she wanted to know where I'd been staying. When I told her down on Bleecker Street, she threw up her hands. I ought to be in someplace clean and decent, she thought. If I'd meet her when she got off work, she said, maybe I could get a room where she lived. That was a sort of apartment hotel up near Columbus Circle, and we agreed to meet there at around four. It must have been about one o'clock by then, but I'd had all the sitting and talking I could stand. I spent the next three hours just walking, and when I got to Arlene's place, she was in the lobby, waiting for me. But they didn't have any rooms. The clerk suggested the Alvin, on Fifty-second Street, so we tried that, and I got a room there. Arlene handled everything. We sat in the lobby for a while and talked. Then we said good night. I think if I'd said the word, she would have come up to the room with me. She wanted to, I'm pretty sure. But I didn't. I couldn't. That was the last thing in the world I felt like. Not with anybody."

It was morning, on Saturday, when Uhlan fell asleep, but he was up and out by nine. After a cup of coffee at a drugstore, he walked down to the out-of-town-newspaper stand on Times Square. He bought another Baltimore *Sun* and, on an impulse, a Cleveland *Plain Dealer*, and then hurried back to the Alvin. The telephone was ringing as he let himself into his room. "It was Arlene," he says. "She wanted to know how I was. She also suggested that we have breakfast together. I didn't particularly want to—I felt more like reading—but I said all right. We met at a Childs, on Columbus Circle, and it turned out she had a plan. She thought I ought to see her doctor. He would know what to do. She gave me his address, and asked me to meet her there at three. I said all right to that, too. Maybe I meant it. But the minute I left her, I knew I wouldn't. Instead, I found a drugstore and bought a little bottle of toilet water and had it wrapped as a gift. I took it over to Arlene's place and left it, with a card thanking her for everything. I was grateful to her, but I'd had enough. She was beginning to make me uncomfortable.

"I bought some clean clothes and went back to the Alvin and changed. Then I took my kit bag and checked out. I'd been there long enough. I headed for the Village again. But it wasn't the way it had been. There were too many people and the streets were too narrow. Everything was different. I began to get panicky. That's the last thing I remember for I don't know how long. Then I was all alone on a path at the south end of Central Park, and across the street was the St. Moritz Hotel. I went over and walked past the entrance, and there was something about it. It meant something. When I reached the corner, I turned around and came back. There were people going in and out, and I stood there and watched them. I kept walking back and forth and hanging around the entrance and watching them for about an hour—until the doorman noticed me. He gave me a very suspicious look. I didn't want to leave. I hated to leave. There was something there that made me feel sort of sad and peaceful and almost happy. But I couldn't stay there with him watching me. I was afraid something might happen. The next time I reached the corner, I kept going. I kept on going until I came to a bus depot. It was around Times Square somewhere. There was a bus loading up. I asked where it was going and they said to Newark, and I don't know why, but I got on. It was something to do. One place was as good as another, I guess. We got to Newark at about eight-thirty in the evening. I found a bar and went in and had a beer. Then I walked around a little, and pretty soon I passed a burlesque house. That appealed to me. It sounded new and interesting. But it wasn't. The show was awful and the audience was worse. It was Saturday night, and everybody was drunk and yelling. I couldn't stand it. Besides, my feet were killing me. I left, and asked the ticket girl where I could find a decent hotel. She directed me to one called the Douglas. I got a room and went right to bed.

"It was too hot to sleep. Newark was even worse than Manhattan. I just lay there and looked at the ceiling and waited for it to get light. Finally, around seven, I got up. My feet were in terrible shape. They were so swollen I could hardly get my shoes on, and I had a big blister on my right heel. I squeezed into them, though, and got my things together and went downstairs. The coffee shop wasn't open yet. I sat in the lobby and looked at the Sunday papers and waited. When it opened, I went in and ordered a big breakfast —everything I could think of. My stomach was so empty it hurt. But when my order came, I couldn't eat. I was too tired and restless. After a few bites, I gave up. I had to get back to New

York. It was as if I was missing something. They told me at the desk that the quickest way was the Hudson Tube. I guess I took it. I remember a tunnel and climbing a long flight of steps, and an empty street. It was almost ten o'clock in the morning, but it felt like the dead of night. It felt dark. There wasn't a soul in sight. There wasn't even a car or a truck going by. There was nothing but empty streets and closed doors and old warehouses. I felt like the last man on earth. There wasn't a sound, even—nothing. I didn't know which way to turn. Every street I tried looked just like all the rest. But I kept walking, and one of them came out at a ferry shed. It was the Erie ferry to New Jersey. I didn't want to take it, but I was afraid not to. I couldn't face those empty streets again. On the way over, I talked to a man and he told me I could get another Manhattan ferry on the Jersey side. It went to Christopher Street, he said. He even showed me the way. Maybe he was wrong. Either that or I didn't pay enough attention. Whatever happened, I never found it. The next thing I knew, I was in the middle of a railroad yard. There was nothing but tracks and freight cars as far as I could see. I started walking between two strings of cars. I walked for about a mile, and then the tracks ended at a high wire fence. On the other side of the fence were more cars. I tried to follow the fence, but there were old boxcars and piles of junk blocking the way, and I lost it. Then I was back in the middle of the yard again. I started climbing under the cars and over the couplings, trying to get out that way. But there wasn't any way out. I remember trying to run and I couldn't. I didn't have the strength. It began to rain. I crawled underneath a car and lay there. Then I heard somebody coming. It was a watchman. He saw me and started yelling, but I was already coming out. He was pretty tough for a minute. After I'd talked to him, though, he was all right. He led me down the tracks a few hundred yards to his shack. Beyond it was an open gate, and a street.

"I went out the gate and down the street, until I came to some buses. One of them was half full and ready to leave. I jumped on. That's the last thing I remember for about an hour. I must have gone right to sleep. When I woke up, it was the end of the line. I asked somebody where I was. North Bergen, he said. I looked around for another bus, and saw one marked 'BROADWAY.' But it was the wrong Broadway. I ended up in Hoboken. I knew there was a ferry there, and I tried to find it. All I could find was bars. There was nothing but bars and drunks and hills. I tried to ask people the way, but I was too tired and groggy and miserable, and they wouldn't listen. They just walked on. Finally, it was raining so hard I couldn't keep going. I got on some bus. Then somebody was shaking me. I got up and got off, and I was back in North Bergen. I don't know how I ever got out of that place. I don't know whether I took a bus or a train or what. I don't remember anything more until I was standing on the corner of Forty-second Street and Seventh Avenue. That was about dusk. Then I was in Brooklyn, at the Hotel Pierrepont, on Pierrepont Street. I was sitting on a sofa in the lobby. There was a wedding reception going on in one of the banquet rooms. I could see the people talking and laughing. I sat there and watched them enjoying themselves, and I felt so lonely. It was worse than walking those empty streets. And all of a sudden I couldn't stand it. I broke down and started to cry.

"I woke up the next morning in a room at the Pierrepont. All my things were there—my bag, and my clothes, and a copy of *U.S. News & World Report* I'd bought—so it was my room. I must have checked in whenever it was I got there. I still felt groggy—everything seemed out of focus. It was as if I'd lost my glasses. And I hurt all over. It wasn't just my feet. Even my bones ached. Every move was agony, but I managed to get up and get dressed. I had to get out of there. I couldn't stay in Brooklyn. It was all wrong. I went down and checked out, and started up Pierrepont Street toward Borough Hall. It was close to eight by then, but the streets were deserted. There was hardly anybody even on Fulton Street. It didn't feel like Monday. Everything had that Sunday look. Then I realized it was Labor Day, and I don't know why, but an awful, helpless, terrified feeling came over me. I felt hunted. The only thing I could think of was to get back to Manhattan as quickly as possible. That meant the subway. I wandered around until I saw an entrance. It was the I.R.T., and I ran down the stairs and got on the first train that came along. But as soon as they closed the doors, I began to get uneasy. I was alone in the car, and

I was afraid I'd made a mistake, and I couldn't stand it. Then the train stopped. I didn't know where I was, but I got off. I remember going up the stairs to the street. Only, it didn't seem like a street. There was a wall—a long, high wall. I started looking for a door or a gate or some other way out. There wasn't any. There was just the wall. I began to run. I ran as long as I could, and then I walked until I had to stop and rest. But the wall was still there. I started walking again. It was like a nightmare. I don't know how far I walked. It must have been miles. But finally I came to a saloon. It was on a corner in a block of factories. I went in and sat down and had a beer. The bartender was a big, smiling fellow, and I remember talking to him. He told me how to find the subway.

"I must have got off around Chatham Square. It was some-where on the Bowery, anyway. The sidewalks were full of all kinds of bums and drunks, and there was an old woman lying in a doorway. She got up and came after me. I gave her a dime. It wasn't just to get rid of her. In a way, I knew how she felt. I knew how they all felt. The only difference was I still had some money. But I had to get out of there, too. So I started hurrying. At Houston Street, I cut over to Broadway, and then headed north again until I reached Times Square. After the Bowery, I felt dirty and contaminated, and I started looking for a hotel. I found one around three o'clock. It was the Century, on Forty-sixth Street, near the Luxor Baths. I showered and shaved, and rested a little. Then I soaked my feet in cold water so I could get my shoes back on, and went out. It was all I could do to walk, but I had to. I don't know how to explain it. There was something driving me. It was getting closer and closer every minute, and I had to keep moving. I had to get somewhere. But everywhere I went was the wrong place. I remember walking down Madison Avenue, and how empty it was. Another time, I was way over east—around Beekman Place. Maybe that was earlier, though. Because I re-member going through Union Square, and after that I was back in the Village, on Eighth Street. I didn't know which way to turn. Then I thought of the St. Moritz. I started back up Fifth Avenue. It was getting dark, and I tried to hurry, but I was too weak. I kept weaving and stumbling. Nothing had ever been more impor-tant. It was vital. I had to get there. But it didn't seem possible

I could make it. I was too tired and sick and crippled—I'd never make it. It was too much, and I started to cry. There were people going by, but I didn't care. I couldn't help it. I couldn't stop.

"I don't know how I ever got to the St. Moritz. Or when— except that it was late. But I got there. I made it. I stood on the other side of Central Park South, where I could see the entrance, and watched. I kept looking at the faces of the women going in and out. It was as if there might be one I knew. I must have stood there a long time. Because finally I couldn't hold out any longer. I was too exhausted even to cry. I had to lie down. So I left and started back to my hotel. But I didn't know where to go. I'd forgotten the name of it, and where it was, and everything. There had been so many hotels. I turned back and went into the Park. I sat down on a bench and tried to think. And I couldn't. My mind was dead. I was too miserable. It was cold and damp, and I began to get the shakes. Pretty soon, looking through the trees, I saw a policeman standing on the corner. I dragged myself off the bench and went over to him. He was very polite. I guess he thought I was drunk and was trying to humor me. At first, anyway. But after we'd talked a few minutes, I knew he believed me. He got inter-ested. He suggested we go along to the precinct station on West Fifty-fourth Street. That scared me. I thought he was going to call the patrol wagon. I said I wouldn't be treated like a criminal. I said I'd go, but I wouldn't go that way. I pulled out a handful of money, and told him we'd go like respectable citizens. We'd take a cab."

Uhlan and the patrolman reached the Fifty-fourth Street station at about two o'clock in the morning. He told his story again, to the desk sergeant and to several detectives. They questioned him until nearly three. By that time, it was apparent that, whatever his trouble, he needed medical attention. He was taken first to St. Clare's Hospital, on West Fifty-first Street. The examining physi-cian, noting that his symptoms were predominantly emotional, dispatched him promptly to Bellevue Hospital. There, after a crisp examination and a few questions, he was admitted for observation, and led away to bed in a psychiatric ward. "I spent an awful night," he says. "I'd heard about Bellevue, and when I realized that's where I was, all I wanted was out. I could hear people moaning and mumbling. I was terrified. But mostly I was in such pain. They'd almost had to cut my shoes to get them off, and my feet were like boils. They hurt so I hardly cared if I lived or died. Somehow, though, I fell asleep. Maybe they gave me something. I woke up crying, but there was a nice nurse standing there. She brought me some breakfast. She had a wonderful quiet voice, and after a while, I guess, I just lay there and rested. The next thing, the nurse was helping me down the hall, and I was in an office and a doctor was asking me questions. I tried to answer them, but my mind kept jumping around. I can't describe the way it felt. Then, suddenly, it was as if a door opened. All of a sudden, I knew. I remembered. I jumped up and shouted. I yelled, 'I know—I can remember! I remember my wife's name. It's Mildred. We live in Boston. I can even tell you the address. And my name is Uhlan —Walter Uhlan.' "

[1954]

CHAPTER 7

One of the Lucky Ones

AMONG THE MORE obviously ailing suppliants who appeared at Mount Sinai Hospital, on upper Fifth Avenue, on the afternoon of Tuesday, February 15, 1949, was a man I'll call Arnold Schneider. Schneider was only thirty-seven years old, but that day he could have passed for sixty-five or seventy. His back was bent, his gait was slow and shuffling, and his hands, his face, and the whites of his eyes were a ghastly lemon yellow. He felt as wretched as he looked. He had a blinding headache, he told the examining physician, there was a burning pain in the pit of his stomach, and he was dizzy, diarrheic, and nauseated—violently nauseated. He hadn't had a bite to eat since Sunday. The very thought of food was enough to double him up. To the best of his recollection, it was Sunday night, at supper, that his trouble had begun. Nothing had tasted right. Also, he had felt tired and his bones had ached. His wife suggested that he probably had a touch of the flu. He thought so, too. So, to be on the safe side, as soon as they had cleared the table and done the dishes he went straight to bed. A few hours later, around midnight, he had an attack of cramps, and vomited. That seemed to help, and Monday morning he felt a trifle better. Enough, at least, to get up. But on the way to work—he owned a half interest in a cleaning-and-pressing shop on West Ninety-sixth Street, just down the street from his flat—he had another seizure, and it was all he could do to get back home. Since then, he had been in almost constant misery. What really worried him, though, was his urine. It was dark brown, almost black. He had never heard of such a thing. This morning was the first time he had noticed it, and it had sent him, as rapidly as he could drag himself into his clothes and around the corner, to the nearest doctor. The doctor had sent him to the hospital. Schneider reached in his pocket and brought out an envelope. Here was a note from the doctor. The examining physician smiled a reassuring smile, glanced at the note, and clipped it to an admittance form. Apart from identifying its author as a man of conventional prudence, the message told him nothing that he hadn't known since the patient entered the room. Schneider, as his color alone made pitifully plain, had jaundice.

The following morning, after a fitful night in an observation ward, Schneider was roused, raised, and rolled away for a barrage of diagnostic tests and soundings. That was routine but imperative. Jaundice is a morbid condition, and often a serious one, but it is not in itself a disease. Like chills and fever and malaise, it is merely a sign of disease. The immediate cause of jaundice is an excess of bile pigment in the blood. Since the manufacture, the storage, and the discharge of bile (a citreous fluid essential to the digestive process) are functions of some of the body's most highly specialized organs, a bilious complexion is rather more than disfiguring. It inevitably signals one or another of three largely distinct debilities. One of these is a derangement of the cells of the liver. A second is an obstruction in the bile duct. The third is a catastrophic destruction of red corpuscles. By the time Schneider was back in bed again it was clear to the resident in charge of the study that both a blocked duct and a blood breakdown could safely be eliminated as possible sources of trouble. That narrowed it down to the liver. A little past noon, the final returns came in from the laboratory, and they narrowed it down still further. Schneider's liver was ravaged in a manner that could have been accomplished only by some sudden, shattering assault. The resident took a brief turn among the now comfortably limited alternatives and un-capped his pen. He entered on the record a tentative diagnosis of acute infectious—or virus—hepatitis.

Some four or five hours later, on his evening tour of inspection, the attending physician was brought at first sight to much the same conclusion. The clinical findings, as enumerated on the chart in the ward nurse's office, were all in excellent harmony with a reading of hepatogenous jaundice. So, he soon satisfied himself, was the general appearance of the patient. Schneider lay as limp as a string—oblivious, apparently, to everything but pain. After a moment of silence and sympathy, the doctor turned away, to-ward the next of his scheduled stops. But halfway, he halted, arrested by a freak of perception. He then swung around and walked thoughtfully back up the ward to the office. Unless his memory was completely confused, there was an entry in the rec-ord that rendered it less than likely that Schneider's hepatitis stemmed from a virus infection. The record had been returned to the file, but he found it without any trouble and drew out the opening page. He hadn't been mistaken. The notation was there, just below the patient's name, age and address. It read, "Occupa-tion: dry cleaner." The doctor sat down at the desk and picked up the telephone and called the administration office. He asked the clerk who took his call to notify, the first thing in the morning, the Division of Industrial Hygiene and Safety Standards of the New York State Department of Labor—an agency, at 80 Centre Street, whose functions include the prompt and thorough investi-gation of any illness anywhere in the state that appears to be occupational in origin—that the hospital had under treatment a case of what looked very much like carbon-tetrachloride poison-ing.

Some sixty million people in the United States, or a trifle over half the total adult population, are regularly employed in industry, business, agriculture, and the professions. Their presence on the job, however, is somewhat less than regular. Every day in the year, at least a million and a half of them are absent from work because of sickness. Of this number, a considerable minority—perhaps two hundred thousand—are victims of more than the common run of aches and pains and contagions that harry mankind. Their ailments are a natural, if not an unavoidable, result of the nature of their work. Occupational disease is a peculiarly sinister source of human misery. It is also an inexhaustible one. None of the astronomically various methods by which man makes his living is wholly without some hazard to physical or mental health. The fisherman's rheumatism, the waiter's fallen arches, the surgeon's hypertension, the miner's silicosis, the boilermaker's deafness, the bus driver's peptic ulcer, and the housemaid's bursitic knee are all, like a thousand other complaints, more or less directly attributable to the environmental conditions under which their victims work. The scope of occupational disease is vast almost beyond calculation. In one or another of its several entities, it sounds practically the full scale of physiologic, biochemic, and metabolic disharmonies known to modern medicine. It comes, in fact, unpleasantly close to being the major public-health problem of our time, and is probably the most permanent.

Like most diseases, those of occupational origin are distinguished not by their manifestations but by their causes. They differ, however, from those of general incidence in two important respects. One is that their causes all are pretty well known. The other is that they are all—potentially, at least—preventable. That they continue to occur with formidable frequency can be laid only partly to greed or need or carelessness. Nor is their awesome abundance and variety much of a factor. Their persistence is due largely to the fact that there are few such diseases whose presenting signs and symptoms unmistakably reflect their cause. In most, the clinical evidence can be anything but etiologically illuminating. It is often even misleading. For, in one way or another, most occupational diseases resemble with striking exactness one or another of the rather more familiar disorders. As a result, except among physicians trained in industrial medicine they are seldom recognized—and hence seldom reported and investigated—for what they are.

Despite its encyclopedic reach, most authorities recognize just four basic sources of occupational disease. Their roots, though occasionally entwined, are perceptibly distinct. One is emotional stress. Physical stress (heat, cold, damp, noise, glare, vibration, radiant energy) is, of course, another. A third is infection—anthrax, tularemia, undulant fever. Of these three fundamental hazards, only the first (inasmuch as it can spring with equal ease from fear, anxiety, or brain-washing boredom) is of compellingly wide significance, and together they probably account for little more than fifty per cent of all cases. The other source of occupational disease is poison. A poison may enter the body by way of the mouth, the lungs, or the skin. Its usual conduit in outbreaks among the general population is the gastrointestinal tract. In industrial poisoning, it follows a different itinerary. The mouth is seldom the portal of entry, the passage through the skin is only a trifle less rare. It almost always makes its entrance through the respiratory system.

There are literally thousands of substances whose dusts or vapors are toxic. They include most heavy metals, many coal-tar distillates and hydrocarbon derivatives, and certain natural or combustion gases. Some of them have menaced man for centuries. From the earliest hours of civilization, the asphyxiating powers, if not the nature, of such products of decomposing vegetable matter as carbon dioxide and hydrogen sulphide have been painfully familiar to miners, well diggers, and other burrowers underground. Both these gases are sluggish, inconspicuous, and tend to accumulate in pockets. Carbon dioxide, whose generation depletes the oxygen in the air, is known to mineworkers as black (or choke) damp, and their use of mice, canaries, or lighted candles to detect its presence is among the most venerable techniques of industrial-disease control. Hydrogen sulphide, in the popular vocabulary, is sewer gas. Unlike carbon dioxide, which has only a faint and scratchy odor, it emits a warning stench (the rotten-egg smell common to all sulphur compounds), but this forthright characteristic is more than offset by its nearly instantaneous action. In Texas, in 1929, a whim of the wind drew a cloud of hydrogen sulphide from an oil well and blew it into a nearby herd of mules. The animals were dead before they could wheel and bolt.

Carbon monoxide has at least as long a history. It is formed by the incomplete combustion of some carbonaceous material (wood, coal, petroleum) and has been a hazard to man since the domestication of fire. It is violently toxic (ten times more so than carbon dioxide), it is uniquely versatile (no other gas is so capable of inducing both chronic and acute reactions), and it is by far the most insidious of all asphyxiants. For all practical purposes, carbon monoxide is indistinguishable from air. It has almost exactly the same free-flowing buoyancy, and it is equally colorless, odorless, and tasteless. Moreover, its inhalation, its passage through the lungs to the blood stream, and its accumulation there, where it displaces oxygen in the hemoglobin molecule, are seldom accompanied by any reliably alerting discomfort. Its action is less equivocal. An exposure of even five minutes to air containing as little as one per cent of carbon monoxide is almost always fatal. Chronic poisoning (marked by persistent headache, frequent vertigo, and, sometimes, a progressive anemia) can result from prolonged daily exposure to concentrations of less than one-fifth of one per cent. The gas is also ferociously plentiful. Its sources, though they have always been abundant, are now rapidly approaching the ubiquitous. Carbon monoxide is generously present in the effluvia of all internal-combustion engines, most industrial plants, and many mines, mills, and workshops. In automobile-exhaust fumes, for example, it averages about seven per cent. Because of the widespread installation of safety devices (fans, baffles, alarm meters), most cases of carbon-monoxide poisoning in industry these days are chronic, rather than acute, and even these are generally attributable to accidents. Industrial toxicologists are persuaded that thousands of workers—particularly automobile mechanics and storage-garage jockeys—suffer some degree of intoxication every day. Traffic policemen have lately been added to the list. A recent survey in Philadelphia demonstrated the presence of carbon monoxide in the blood of fourteen members of a downtown traffic squad. In six of these men, the amount ranged from twenty to thirty per cent. Anything much over ten per cent is usually considered dangerous.

Metal poisoning is almost entirely an occupational phenomenon. Except for an occasional freakish accident, its appearances outside industry are invariably either homicidal or suicidal in origin. They are just as invariably sudden and shattering and, unless the poison, which always enters the body through the mouth, is eliminated by immediate vomiting, invariably end in

death. In industry, metal poisoning is rarely, if ever, fatal. This is
not, however, much cause for jubilation since, on the other hand,
it is chronic, systemic, and, sometimes, incurable. Among the
many metals whose fumes (or dusts) can seldom be inhaled with
impunity, lead and mercury are notorious. White phosphorus
(which, though not a metal, toxicologists find it convenient to
classify as one) has much the same reputation. It shares with lead
and mercury an inimitable capacity for highly specialized destruction. Phosphorus has a predilection for the jawbones, the gums,
and the teeth. Long exposure to its fumes produces a necrotic
condition known as "phossy jaw." This is characterized by a
grotesque enlargement of the lower face and a slow, agonizing
dissolution of the teeth. In severe cases, its spread throughout the
body often can be checked only by the surgical removal of the
entire jaw. Phossy jaw was once a common consequence of steady
employment in a match factory. Since shortly before the First
World War, when the manufacture of white-phosphorus matches
was universally prohibited, its victims have been largely confined
to workers in chemical, fertilizer, and ore-reduction plants.

Mercury has the distinction of inspiring the first attempt on
record to control occupational disease by legislation. That was the
passage of a law limiting the work of men employed in mercury
mines at Idrija, in what is now Yugoslavia, to a maximum of six
hours a day. It became effective in April of 1665. Chronic mercury
poisoning, or mercurialism, was well known long before that time,
certainly since the first Christian century. (The writings of Plu-
tarch contain a rebuke to a mine-owner for using slaves who were
not also criminals in his mercury mines.) It could hardly have
failed to be. Like phosphorus poisoning, the damage it inflicts is
only too apparent. Mercury strikes at the central nervous system.
With one exception (a pyorrheal inflammation of the mouth), the
dominant signs of mercurialism all have a neural cast. Two are
sufficiently singular to require specific listing in most medical
dictionaries. One of them is a progressive intention tremor called
hatter's shakes. The other is a personality derangement for which
an eighteenth-century English investigator coined the term "erethism." Erethism is marked by constant anxiety, black depression,
and alternating spells of infantile timidity and savage irritability.

Sometimes, in advanced cases, its victims are racked by nightmare hallucinations, and even near-epileptic convulsions have been reported. The tremor of mercurialism takes its name from the trade that has always been a major source of the disease. Until about a generation ago, when several less toxic substitutes were devised, mercury was an essential ingredient in the processing of felt for hats. The use of mercury in hat-making is now illegal in many European countries and in most American states. In less enlightened parts of the world, about the only defense available to hatters is chewing tobacco. Many hatters believe, though without much justification, that constant spitting will eliminate the poisonous fumes. Hatter's shakes first affects the muscles of the eyelids, the fingers, and the tongue. It then moves on to the arms and legs. In time, its victims may become wholly incapacitated—unable to eat, dress, or walk without assistance. The saying "mad as a hatter" and the Mad Hatter of "Alice in Wonderland" both derive from the lurching gait, the tangled tongue, and the addled wits of mercurialism.

Lead poisoning, or plumbism (the term derives from *plumbum*, the Latin word for "lead"), has also enriched our literature, though rather less conspicuously. Its clinical manifestations are celebrated in "Alexipharmaca," one of the two surviving works of the pre-Christian Greek poet Nicander. The poem reads in part:

> The mouth it [lead] inflames and makes cold from within,
> The gums dry and wrinkled are parch'd like the skin,
> The rough tongue feels harsher, the neck muscles grip,
> He soon cannot swallow, foam runs from his lip,
> A feeble cough tries it in vain to expel,
> He belches so much, and his belly does swell. . . .
> Meanwhile there comes a stuporous chill,
> His feeble limbs droop and all motion is still.

As Nicander intimated, and numerous cooler clinicians have subsequently confirmed, muscular atrophy, abdominal distention, and a curious stippling of the gums are classically suggestive of plumbism. The first of these (it usually takes the form of a limp, or "dropped," wrist) and the last (a dark-blue line, somewhat resembling a tattoo) always point to the presence of lead in the body. They are not, however, always, or even often, present. The usual seat of plumbism is the gastrointestinal labyrinth, and its usual indications are bloat and prolonged paroxysms of almost unendurable pain. This deranging colic can be subdued by prompt medication, but since it stems from a massive accumulation of lead in the body, usually absorbed (as dust or fumes) over a long period of time, such treatment is essentially only palliative. Unless the lead can be dissolved (by means of a most complex procedure) and excreted, the gassy pains tend to recur. The gum discoloration is permanent. So, if firmly established, is the characteristic palsy. During the past twenty-five years, largely as a result of educating workers, the incidence of plumbism has perceptibly declined, but the disease is still far from conquered. It still seizes hundreds, if not thousands, of victims every year. Its persistence, though hardly inevitable, is understandable enough. No metal is more widely used than lead. It is encountered in most of the traditional trades (painting, printing, plumbing, mining, pottery-making) and in many of recent origin. Altogether, according to the United States Department of Labor, some exposure to lead occurs in a hundred and fifty different occupations.

The exact number of occupations that involve the use of one or another of the coal-tar distillates and hydrocarbon derivatives is not known. New ones turn up too fast for ready computation. The only certainty is that these cabalistically complicated substances dominate modern industry. At least two hundred of them are now in general use. The most broadly serviceable compounds include benzol (or coal-tar benzene), beta-naphthylamine, carbon disulphide, carbon tetrachloride, and dinitrophenol. Most of this group figure importantly in the manufacture of numerous essentials of twentieth-century culture (mechanical refrigerators, lubricating oils, rubber cement, aniline dyes, plastics, explosives, and artificial silk), and all are incomparable solvents. They possess to perfection all the qualities that make a dry cleanser efficient. Their cost is low, their volatility (or speed of evaporation) is high, and their avidity for fats and greases is insatiable. They are also, however, almost incomparably toxic. The fumes of carbon disulphide derange the nervous system. Exposure to benzol vapor may produce the lethally wasting condition known as aplastic anemia. A possible result of beta-naphthylamine poisoning is cancer of the bladder. Dinitrophenol, which was once the effective essence of a popular reducing drug, has the power to race the metabolism to the point of irreparable collapse. Carbon tetrachloride is less narrowly selective. The areas to which it is drawn include the heart, the bowels, the lungs, the kidneys, and the liver.

The kaleidoscopic range of carbon tetrachloride is not its only distinction. It has, unfortunately, others. It is particularly partial to the overfed, the undernourished, and the alcoholic (the presence of even a small amount of alcohol in the blood will enormously intensify its action), and, with the possible exception of benzol, it is the most reliably ravaging of all familiar solvents. It is in addition, as the attending physician at Mount Sinai Hospital was nicely aware that February evening in 1949, the one most highly esteemed by a majority of American dry cleaners. The reason for its popularity is anything but arbitrary. It could hardly be more practical. Unlike benzol, beta-naphthylamine, carbon disulphide, and dinitrophenol, all of which will burst into flame at a spark, carbon tetrachloride is as incombustible as soapy water.

The report on Arnold Schneider was telephoned to the Division of Industrial Hygiene and Safety Standards of the New York State Department of Labor on Thursday morning, February 17th. As is customary, it was received and promptly recorded there by a clerk in the Medical Unit. That was around eight o'clock. When a physician on the staff of the unit—whose name, at his request, shall here be Paul Temple—reached the office some twenty minutes later, a memorandum containing the facts of the case (the name, address, and occupation of the patient, and the nature of his trouble and its suspected source) was lying on his desk. He read it with interest, and a kind of satisfaction.

"I don't mean to sound inhuman," Dr. Temple says. "Actually, my reaction was quite the reverse of heartless. I was simply gratified, as we always are down here, to learn that somebody in general medicine was thinking in terms of occupational disease. Most doctors in ordinary practice don't. That's only natural, of course. It's outside their field of training and experience. The possibility that the kind of work the patient does may be a vital factor in the problem just doesn't occur to them. Not very often, anyway. They tend to concentrate entirely on the clinical picture. That can be very misleading. It can even be fatal. The industrial diseases are pretty tricky. And not only because their symptoms are rarely pathognomonic. A clinically accurate diagnosis isn't enough. Neither is the best of treatment. Unless the fundamental cause is known, it's little better than nothing. It hardly suffices to save a man's life and then, because it never dawned on anybody to relate his job to his illness, let him go right back to the environment that sent him to the hospital in the first place. That isn't very successful therapeutics. It isn't very good preventive medicine, either.

"But in this case, apparently, the truth had dawned. Somebody had made a differential diagnosis on the basis of all the available facts. That was most refreshing. So I was pleased, and relieved. Not, of course, that I accepted the diagnosis as fact. Carbon-tetrachloride poisoning was merely the most reasonable assumption. It still had to be proved. But one thing, at least, was certain. Arnold Schneider was one of the lucky ones. From our standpoint, anyway. When and if he recovered, it would be permanent. He wouldn't come tottering back to the hospital in a couple of weeks with the same thing all over again. No matter what the cause of his trouble turned out to be. An attack of infectious hepatitis confers a fairly lasting immunity, and physical agents can be controlled. He would be safe. Moreover, and no less importantly, if the hospital was right, so would everyone else who worked in his cleaning establishment. We would see to that. And at once. Prevention is our first concern. Well, in this case that presented no problem. We knew where to begin. We had the suspected source. A look around the shop should answer a good many questions. That phase of our work is handled by the Chemical Unit. I called William J. Burke, the chief of the unit, and gave him the information I had. The rest was a matter of routine. One of his men would take it from there. I'd have the results as soon as he made his report.

"For the moment, that was that. There was nothing to do right now but wait. Our next move would depend on what we found at the shop. An investigation of the kind that was indicated here takes time. I didn't expect to hear from Burke for several hours, and I didn't. It was almost two when he called. He sounded puzzled. I must say he had his reasons. The findings at the shop were hardly what I'd led him to expect. Quite the contrary. The chemist assigned to the job had camped in the shop all morning. He had watched the work and examined the apparatus and made every possible test, and ended up in a glow. His report was practically a testimonial. Schneider and his partner—Thompson was his name—were one among many. Their shop was everything most dry-cleaning shops aren't. It was a model. The equipment was the best and the safest on the market. It was a single-vat machine, airtight and fully automatic. All the operator himself did was put in the clothes and take them out. Everything else—the introduction of the solvent, the cleaning-and-drying operations, and the extraction and disposal of the solvent—was controlled by buttons and levers. Also, the machine was almost new. They had been in business only a little over a year. There was just one point at all in line with expectations. The solvent they used was carbon tetrachloride. Under the circumstances, however, that didn't really signify. The chemist had run a test on the air in the shop. It showed a ratio of something like twenty parts of carbon tet to a million parts of air. The accepted maximum in New York State is thirty-five. In some states, anything under a hundred is considered safe enough. Well, that took care of that. I thanked Burke and hung up. The shop was out.

"I can't truthfully say I was sorry. As an industrial hygienist, I was bound to feel encouraged. A good shop is always good news. Still, I wasn't exactly elated. It didn't go very far toward explaining Schneider's trouble. Unless, of course, I took it to mean that his illness and his occupation were totally unrelated. In that event, as far as we were concerned, the case was closed. But I couldn't. I simply wasn't willing to dismiss the fact that he worked in a place where carbon tetrachloride was used as merely an odd coincidence. Not yet, at any rate. Besides, there was that diagnostician at Mount Sinai. He had made a very sensible deduction. It would be nice to justify his alertness. And then I was curious. I just plain wanted to know. But the trouble was there was nothing I myself could do about it. I was involved in a couple of other things that would keep me in the office all afternoon. I checked the schedule, and one of the other medical investigators was free. He's in private practice now, so I'll say his name was Boone. I called him in and he was interested, and we talked it over. That didn't take us long. There was only one real question. If Schneider did have toxic hepatitis—if it really was a case of carbon-tetrachloride poisoning —how and where was he exposed? Or, rather, if the shop was eliminated, where did we start? Boone didn't agree that the shop was definitely out. He wanted to see for himself. A talk with Thompson might put him on to something that a chemist could very easily overlook.

"But the shop *was* out. Thompson settled that. Boone called back in about an hour and gave me the story. It couldn't have been more conclusive. It would have finished the shop as a possible source even without the chemical report. Schneider had nothing to do with the mechanical end of the business. That was Thompson's department. Schneider worked up front. He kept the books and made deliveries and waited on the trade. So if there had been some kind of accident in the workroom—I gathered that's what Boone had had in mind—our victim wouldn't be Schneider. It would be Thompson. But Thompson was the picture of health. And there hadn't been any accident.

"Boone was still at the shop when he phoned. His next step, of course, was the hospital. Schneider himself seemed the only lead we had left. If, that is, he was still alive and could talk. Well, it turned out that he was and could, and did. Just barely—although he had managed to round the corner and was off the critical list —but enough. However, I didn't know that for some little time —not until almost six o'clock. I'd finally cleared my desk and was ready to call it a day when the phone rang. It was Boone. It was all over. He had it all tied up. The tone of his voice told me that. I sat down and waited for him to tell me the rest. He was calling from the Schneider apartment. Mrs. Schneider, whom he had met at the hospital, was with him. So was the source. I saw it the next day, on a shelf in the chemical lab. It was a gallon jug about two-thirds full of carbon tetrachloride. Schneider had filled it from a drum at the shop on Saturday and brought it home that night. The living-room rug needed cleaning. On Sunday afternoon, around three o'clock, he emptied part of the jug into a pail, dug up a scrubbing brush, and went to work. It was a wall-to-wall carpet, and what with shifting the furniture around and stopping every now and then to rest, the job took a couple of hours. I must say Boone gave me the picture. An open pail of carbon tet, a dripping brush, and Schneider down on his hands and knees with his face about a foot from the rug—it made my hair stand on end. It also made me wonder. It settled the question of Schneider, all right. But it raised another question.

" 'What about Mrs. Schneider?' I asked.

" 'Oh,' Boone said. 'She's fine. She wasn't at home that afternoon. She was up in the Bronx, or somewhere, visiting her mother. But it probably wouldn't have mattered either way. It's a good-sized room, with doors opening into the rest of the flat. Also, Schneider knew enough to open a couple of windows. What he didn't know was something else. While he was working, he had a bottle of beer, maybe two. He isn't sure which.'

" 'One could be plenty,' I said.

" 'Yes,' said Boone. 'And when he began to feel rotten and got into bed, his wife fixed him a nice hot toddy.' "

[*1955*]

CHAPTER 8

Birds of a Feather

ONE MORNING TOWARD THE END of April, in 1945, Dr. Karl F.
Meyer, Director of the George Williams Hooper Foundation for
Medical Research, at the University of California, received a
somewhat breathless letter from a doctor who introduced himself
as an attending physician at the Southampton Hospital, in Suffolk
County, Long Island. His name, I'll say, was Cornelius Barton,
and his letter was a request for help and counsel. Dr. Barton had
a hunch. A few days earlier, he informed Dr. Meyer, he had
encountered a case that struck him as uncomfortably provocative.
The patient was a handyman on one of the numerous duck farms
in that part of the Island, forty-four years old, and white. He had
been admitted to the hospital on April 6th, suffering from chills,
headache, and abdominal distention, and with a temperature of a
hundred and three. Auscultation revealed a slight respiratory rat-
tle. This was presently traced, by a chest X-ray, to a patchy
inflammation of the lower right lung. There was, however, no
cough, and, as it turned out, no further pulmonary involvement.
After three days, during which treatment was confined to bed rest
and small doses of sulfadiazine, his temperature dropped, his chest

cleared, and he was discharged to convalesce at home. He was now pretty well recovered. Having thus delivered himself of the pertinent facts, Dr. Barton moved on to speculation. The general nature of the case, of course, presented no great diagnostic challenge. It was almost certainly an atypical, or virus, pneumonia. Ordinarily, he would have been inclined to let it go at that. But this, he felt, was not an ordinary case. He had been inspired to attempt a more definitive reading. The trouble was he lacked the experience and the laboratory facilities to put it to a test. Dr. Meyer, he knew, possessed an abundance of both. Dr. Barton had on hand a sample of blood extracted from his patient on the third day of illness. Might he send it to him? He would like to have it examined by the complement-fixation method for evidence of ornithotic pneumonitis. Unless he was badly mistaken, he had just discovered a case of psittacosis acquired from a barnyard duck.

Dr. Barton's choice of a collaborator, though awkwardly transcontinental, was anything but arbitrary. It was practically unavoidable. Dr. Meyer is not merely the outstanding authority in this country on the ecology and epidemiology of psittacosis but back in 1945 he was almost the only one. The excitement that animated Dr. Barton's appeal was also natural enough. Psittacosis is parrot fever. At that time, its transmission was thought to be largely, if not altogether, confined to birds of the psittacine group. This includes such parrots as Amazons, African grays, cockatoos, macaws, parakeets, lovebirds, and lories. Although all psittacines are potential reservoirs of psittacosis, most outbreaks of the disease in man have been caused by either parrots or parakeets. Psittacosis was recognized as an entity of avian origin by Jacob Ritter, a perceptive Swiss pathologist, in 1879. His portrait of its clinical manifestations, which he observed in a family of seven whose misfortune it had been to acquire an infected parrot, is still considered a generally excellent likeness. Ritter called his discovery "pneumotyphus." Its present name, which derives from *psittakos*, the Greek for "parrot," was suggested in 1895 by a French physician named Antonin Morange.

Until 1929, psittacosis was universally regarded as among the rarest of rare diseases. In that year, a pandemic of almost global proportions rendered this agreeable assumption abruptly and permanently infirm. The last outbreak usually included in the pandemic occurred in October, 1930, in Hawaii. Exactly how many people were stricken in the course of those fifteen months has never been determined, and estimates vary widely. The most conservative put the number at approximately eight hundred. Probably, considering the unfamiliarity of the disease and the ambiguity of its symptoms, it was at least twice that. The number of fatal cases is less uncertain. There were, roughly, a hundred and fifty.

The pandemic had two immediate results. One, as might be expected, was a salubrious quickening of interest among medical scientists in the anatomy of psittacosis. Their efforts were richly and rapidly productive. By the end of 1931, its cause had been found, its mechanics charted, and Ritter's description of its salient signs revised for modern readers. Since then, though at a somewhat less headlong pace, many of its remaining riddles have been fathomed with equal thoroughness. The agent responsible for psittacosis is a filterable organism intermediate in size between a virus and a bacillus, but most authorities find it convenient to call it a virus. Fortunately, it has all the few redeeming weaknesses of both of its nearest relatives. It is vulnerable to most antibiotics, it confers on its surviving victims a more or less prolonged resistance to reinfection, and it is incapable of growth and reproduction outside the body of a living animal host. The communicability of psittacosis is also providentially peculiar. Although the organism is readily airborne and enters the body by way of the upper respiratory tract, its passage from one human being to another is almost unheard of; it has been reported just thirty times. To the best of medical knowledge, the only significant source of infection to man is dust heavily and freshly contaminated with the droppings of a psittacotic bird.

The other immediate result of the 1929–30 pandemic was the establishment by the affected nations of public-health regulations designed to prevent its recurrence. Those set up in the United States were among the most stringent. They included a federal embargo on all alien psittacines for commercial resale, restrictions largely prohibiting the interstate transportation of any members of the family, and an elaborate network of supplementary defenses devised by the various states. The majority of the regulations became effective early in 1930. Early in 1952, the embargo on imports was substantially modified and practically all the other regulations were rescinded. This action, though abrupt, was in no sense impulsive. It was, if anything, deliberate to the point of procrastination. Since the end of 1945, it had been abundantly plain that as a means of ridding the country of psittacosis the regulations were totally ineffectual. The disease is ineradicably here, and probably has been for years.

Dr. Meyer's reply to Dr. Barton's request was composed on Thursday, April 26th. It was delivered the following Monday. Dr. Barton found it on his desk when he came in at about five from a round of afternoon calls. "This is in reply to your letter of April 16th," Dr. Meyer wrote. "I want to tell you first that I will be only too glad to examine the blood serum of the patient who is now suffering from an atypical pneumonia which you suspect to be connected epidemiologically with Pekin ducks. In case we prove this pneumonia to be caused by the ornithosis or psittacosis agents, some steps should then be taken to test the blood serum of the Pekin ducks. Until relatively recently, only the representatives of the parrot family were suspected of being the hosts of ornithosis or psittacosis virus. With the discovery that the infection occurs quite extensively in pigeons . . . and also in seagulls, I see no reasons why the Pekin ducks should not be the hosts of a similar or identical virus. Recently, I had a letter from Philadelphia with a history of a man who was exposed to wild ducks. This serum gave a strongly positive reaction for the ornithosis virus. Therefore, the reasonableness that he became infected by handling ducks is great. . . . Any time you wish to send the sera, please do so. . . . Preferably, two samples should be sent—one collected during the first few days of the illness and another one between the fifteenth and twentieth days of convalescence. We have shown that penicillin is quite effective in the treatment of these infections. Ordinarily, we use a dosage of 20,000 units every three hours during the first forty-eight hours, and then reduce the dosage to ten. . . ."

"I don't know what kind of an answer I expected," Dr. Barton says. "But you may be sure it was nothing like that. Not even in my most hopeful moments. About all I really asked at that point was to be taken seriously. I didn't see how Dr. Meyer could turn me down. Not completely. Still, I can't deny that the possibility had occurred to me. And I knew if he did I was sunk. Just another general practitioner who had made a fool of himself. I was pretty sure I hadn't, but I could have, of course. Very easily. I knew next to nothing about ornithology, and not much more about psittacosis. I'd seen only one confirmed case in my life. That was back in 1930, at medical school, and he was dead. I sat in on a postmortem. Apart from a little reading, that was the extent of my knowledge. So far as I can recall, I never even thought of psittacosis again until that day in 1945. There was no occasion to. Why I happened to think of it then is hard to say. Psittacosis is a form of pneumonitis, and I was quite certain that my patient—Haupt was his name—had a pneumonitis, but pneumonitis doesn't necessarily mean psittacosis. Hardly. All I knew was that in Haupt's case I thought it did. And when I began to look around for a possible source of infection, the only birds in sight were ducks. There are some things you just can't explain. Something happens and your mind begins to percolate, and sometimes something comes out. Well, I thought this was one of those times. And Dr. Meyer agreed. At least, that was the impression I got. He isn't the type to get excited over trivialities. But his letter was a good deal more than encouraging. It was also most instructive. I think I knew that the virus had been demonstrated in pigeons and gulls. Vaguely. I had no idea how extensively, though, and, of course, the wild-duck angle was something altogether new. So was the tip on penicillin. Penicillin was still a good deal of an unknown quantity back in those days. Nobody was exactly sure what it could and couldn't do. When I came to that passage, I stopped and stared. Nothing could have been more opportune. Because over the weekend I'd come across what looked like two more cases of the same. They were a white man and a colored woman, both duck-farm people, and both sicker than Haupt ever was. And neither one had shown the slightest response to sulfadiazine.

"Well, Dr. Meyer's word was good enough for me. I trotted up to the wards and went right to work. To make up for lost time,

I started out with twenty-five thousand units for each. If that didn't do the job, I was prepared to go even higher. I won't say I was really worried. Neither one of them appeared to be in serious trouble. But you never know. I also took the precaution of arranging for a couple of samples of blood. However, Haupt was first on the list. I got a second specimen of his blood in the morning. He was a little past the twentieth day of convalescence, but I couldn't help that. At any rate, my package was on its way to Dr. Meyer by noon, air-mail special delivery. That was on Tuesday, May 1st. Then I waited. Or tried to. Until Sunday. On Sunday morning, as I sat down to breakfast, the telephone rang. It was Western Union with a wire from Dr. Meyer. The message read: 'SERUM PATIENT HAUPT FIXES COMPLEMENT WITH PSITTACOSIS ANTIGEN IN DILUTION ONE TO THIRTY-TWO. REACTION DIAGNOSTICALLY POSITIVE. PLEASE SEND SERA FROM SICK DUCKS.'

"So I was right. Or perhaps it would be more accurate to say I wasn't wrong. A ratio of one to thirty-two is unequivocal. In view of the other clinical findings, it meant that Haupt had very definitely suffered an attack of psittacosis. Which was extremely gratifying. But, of course, that's all it did mean. It merely confirmed the existence of a psittacosis problem. It didn't tell us where he got his infection. The real point at issue remained to be proved. My idea that the ducks were the source of the trouble was still just a notion. Unless we could show that the ducks were infected, I obviously hadn't accomplished very much. Well, there are two procedures by which the presence of psittacosis virus can be demonstrated in a bird. One is the blood-serum, or complement-fixation, test. The other is rather more complicated. It works something like this. A group of laboratory mice are inoculated with material obtained from the vital organs of the suspected host. Presently, if all goes well, the mice become sick and die. An autopsy is then performed and the spleen removed for microscopic examination. The result, when successful, is isolation of the organism. But it isn't always that simple. It's often necessary to make another passage to a second group of mice. In any event, it takes from two weeks to a month. Dr. Meyer preferred to start with the blood test. That was understandable. It isn't quite as satisfactory as the other—or at least not with birds. Nevertheless, as a preliminary check, it could save a lot of time and effort. It also made things a bit easier for me. I didn't have to cut up any ducks. Although even getting a few cc.s of duck serum wasn't exactly easy. I had to do a little persuading before the owner of the farm where Haupt had worked finally gave in and let me proceed. He didn't like the implications. In the end, I managed to bleed three birds. The samples reached Dr. Meyer on May 11th. Ten days later, on May 21st, I got his report. He had tested all three samples with every available antigen. The results were uniformly negative.

"That was pretty bitter. I won't say I was surprised. In a way, I'd even expected it. But you know how it is—you can't help hoping. The only consolation was that the findings were essentially inconclusive. A positive reaction—even one—would have been immensely significant. On the other hand, a negative report meant almost nothing. Approximately six million Pekin ducks are grown on Long Island every year. Haupt's employer alone raises several hundred thousand. And we'd examined three. As Dr. Meyer remarked in his report, that hardly constituted a fair test of my hypothesis. He had never supposed that a majority of the ducks might be infected. Possibly, he said, no more than five or ten per cent. A much larger sampling would have to be tested and proved negative before he would be willing to accept the present findings. Of course, all that more or less went without saying, but it helped to hear him say it. I needed all the encouragement I could get. Not just because I'd had high hopes of those samples. I had other worries. My two new patients had responded beautifully to penicillin. In fact, the woman had already gone back home. But the day she left, another case came in. A few days later, another arrived. And he was followed by a third. They were all exactly alike. Sex: Male. Occupation: Duck farmer. Diagnosis: Atypical pneumonia. As it happened, they weren't my cases. I only saw them. But that was enough to take all the joy out of life. In other words, unless Haupt had completely led me astray, we were up against something that looked unpleasantly like an epidemic.

"He hadn't. Dr. Meyer disposed of that possibility, if it was one, very promptly. All he needed was five specimens of blood. I didn't wait to be asked. As a matter of fact, I'd sent them off along with a full history of each patient, even before I got his report on the ducks. His answer came through on the twenty-eighth. Haupt had plenty of company. Of the five, two—cases 1 and 2—were definitely positive for psittacosis. No. 3 was probable. The two most recent cases—4 and 5—were uncertain. It was simply too early to tell. He suggested I bleed them again. He also asked for another sampling of duck sera. Then he gave me rather a start, for he added that he was sending a copy of his letter to Dr. Robert F. Korns, the acting director of the Division of Communicable Diseases of the New York State Department of Health, at Albany, with a recommendation that the state institute a thorough epidemiological investigation of the matter. I don't know why that should have surprised me—it was certainly the logical next step —but it did. It just hadn't occurred to me, I guess, that I had stumbled onto anything quite that big. It was a little hard to believe."

Dr. Meyer's letter had much the same effect on Dr. Korns. "To tell the truth, I had my doubts about the ducks," he said. "With all due respect for Dr. Meyer's opinion, I couldn't see that they were necessarily the focus of infection. He seemed to consider it probable. His letter to me contained an explanatory note saying, 'There is every likelihood that an ornithosis problem exists on the duck farms.' That struck me as a trifle strong. The evidence, as far as I could make out, was altogether circumstantial. It could be the ducks. Or it could be something else—gulls, perhaps, or pigeons. Chickens, even. If parrots were out, as they unquestionably were, almost anything was possible. The field was wide open. One thing, however, was sure. Something very strange was happening down on eastern Long Island, and it was up to the state health authorities to do something about it.

"Most of the work in the field was handled by an epidemiologist named Donald Tulloch—he's dead now, poor fellow. An extremely able man. He had to be for this particular job. About the only person whose help he could consistently count on was Dr. Barton. The rest of us came and went. Before Tulloch took off for Suffolk County, we had a little conference. It wasn't a very cheerful meeting. The longer we looked at the problem, the bigger it got. Bigger and broader and more complicated. I'd had a peculiar feeling about it ever since I got back from Long Island. But it wasn't until then that I began to understand why. Most epidemiological problems involve just one basic question. This one was different. It involved two. Six people in Suffolk County—they had all been confirmed by then—had psittacosis. Where did they get it? That was one question. The other was this: It was also a fact that those people lived and worked miles away from each other. That meant that the focus of infection was pretty widespread. So why were there only six cases? Six were plenty. But sixty would have been easier to explain.

"I didn't hear from Tulloch for more than a week. Then, on July 18th, he sent in a rough preliminary report. He had been to the hospital, he had talked to half the doctors in the county, and he had done a lot of digging on his own. The result was twelve more cases. All, like the first ones, were more or less mild. There was no question about the diagnosis. In each case, Dr. Meyer had confirmed it by the complement-fixation test. That brought the total up to eighteen. As it happened, not all of that was news to me. I'd had some inkling that the count was rising. I forget from whom—Dr. Barton, probably. He'd called me a couple of times. What *was* news, though, was that only ten of the new cases were duck-farm people. The other two had no connection with ducks at all. One was a section hand on the Long Island Railroad and the other a man who ran a butcher shop in Riverhead. But they both kept chickens, and the section hand's next-door neighbor owned a large flock of pigeons. That added to the confusion with a vengeance. It not only weakened the chain of circumstantial evidence that seemed to implicate the ducks but it also gave us a prominent new suspect. The butcher and the railroad man weren't the only chicken raisers among the whole eighteen victims. Ten of the others were, too. Moreover, just to snarl things up a little more, one of the new patients and one of the original six told Tulloch that they sometimes amused themselves by feeding wild pigeons. A nice mess.

"The rest of the report was an account of work in progress. In spite of the butcher and the railroad man and the chickens, the bulk of the evidence still pointed to the ducks—or, rather, it appeared to. Most of the patients were duck people. But then, so

was almost everybody else in that part of Long Island. Any disease
in that area would be bound to show a high incidence among
people who had something to do with ducks. In other words, was
there a real relationship between the farms and the outbreak? Or
was it merely fortuitous? Well, Tulloch was doing what he could
to find out. His approach was conventional. Exposure to the psittacosis virus may not always cause illness. That's true, of course,
of all communicable diseases. It does, however, almost always
cause certain relatively permanent changes in the blood—the development of immunizing substances called antibodies—and they
can be detected by the complement-fixation test. Tulloch reasoned
that if the ducks were the source of the trouble, the blood of all
—or at any rate many—of the other farmers would contain evidence of past infection. And the blood of people having no contact
with ducks would be normal. He had already bled twelve apparently healthy men and women who worked on one or another of
the implicated farms. He was now in the process of selecting a
dozen people from the general populaton in the epidemic area to
serve as controls. Both sets of specimens would be in Dr. Meyer's
hands by the middle of the following week. Our next move in that
phase of the investigation depended entirely upon the laboratory.

"Toward the end of the month, Tulloch came in from the field
for a couple of days to attend to some personal matter. He was
still around when Dr. Meyer's reports arrived. That was Monday
morning, July 30th. The results were not exactly what we had
expected. Or hoped for. Seven out of the twelve farmers gave
positive reactions. But so did three of the controls. Tulloch was
at a loss. It seemed to confirm our idea that the focus was pretty
widespread. Beyond that, he didn't know what to think. Neither
did I. Except that a new and larger sampling was very much in
order. Large enough to eliminate any possible distortion. I suggested another series from the implicated farms, one from farms
where no cases had occurred, one from a farm where only chickens were raised, and, naturally, a much larger group of controls.
Then we might be able to draw some definite conclusions. I also
suggested that he hop right to it. Tulloch didn't need any urging.
He left immediately after lunch.

"Tuesday morning, with one of the local doctors for a guide,

Tulloch started in. They began with the farms. Their first stop was a big establishment near Center Moriches, in the heart of the duck-growing area. I don't believe any of us were quite prepared for what happened next. We should have been, perhaps, but we weren't. What happened was the owner stopped them at the gate. He was pleasant enough, Tulloch told me later, but very firm. There wasn't going to be any bleeding on his place. Or on any other, he hoped. What were we trying to do—put them all out of business? Everybody in the neighborhood was talking about what they called duck fever. The workers were getting scared. A little more investigating and they'd all up and quit. And not only that. If the duck-fever gossip ever reached the market, there wouldn't be any more market. Nobody would even dream of eating another Long Island duck. That, of course, was plain silly. The psittacosis organism enters the body through the respiratory system, not the alimentary canal. Besides, the virus is extremely delicate and couldn't possibly survive the processing that a duck goes through before it reaches the market. Well, Tulloch told him all that and a good deal more, but the answer was still no. It was also no at the next farm. And the next.

"With the help of Dr. Barton and a couple of others, Tulloch rounded up eight or ten of the leaders and they agreed to meet him that night at somebody's house in Eastport. It was a ticklish situation. The growers were dead wrong. Still, you couldn't help but sympathize with them. They were in a tough spot. Tulloch handled it beautifully. He didn't try to argue, he simply stated the problem. Did they want the truth? Or did they prefer gossip and guesses and rumors? Then he left the room and let them decide for themselves. He must have bewitched them. When they called him back, the battle was more than won. They hadn't just withdrawn the complaint and agreed to coöperate. They had even voted to invite him to address the fall meeting of the Long Island Duck Growers Association. From then on, with the growers all behind him, Tulloch made good time. He ended up, on August 10th, with a total of sixty-six new samples. Thirty-three were taken from duck people in various parts of the area. The rest, including two chicken raisers, were all controls. If that didn't clarify the picture a bit, it was hard to say what would.

"Meanwhile, during the past few weeks, I'd had several letters from Dr. Meyer. His confidence in the ducks was still unshaken, but he had finally given up hope of ever proving anything by testing samples of their sera. None of the numerous samples that Dr. Barton had sent him had shown even a faintly positive reaction. So the time had come to try to isolate the organism from tissue. Would we please supply him with the necessary specimens for laboratory testing on mice? Well, we already had—a few, at any rate. Whenever Tulloch or Dr. Barton could, either of them, find the time. But now that Tulloch had wound up his serological survey, we could settle down in earnest. Dr. Barton let his practice practically drop. The only thing that really interested him any more was psittacosis, and by then the active phase of the outbreak was over. Long over. The last case was No. 12 in the group that Tulloch reported in July. Which was a great relief. Keeping Dr. Meyer supplied with material turned out to be a very big job. He wanted plenty and he wanted everything. Not just ducks—although, of course, they were his main concern—but also chickens, pigeons, gulls, crows, and even starlings. His results were negative, one and all. Toward the end of the month, Dr. Meyer sent one of this technicians, Dr. Bernice Eddie, on from the Coast to lend us a hand, and a few days later wrote that he himself was coming East sometime in September, and planned to pay us a visit. Those were about the only pleasant things I remember about the whole of August. Everything else was hard work and hard luck. And then, just after Labor Day, the report on Tulloch's bloods came through. It didn't bear much resemblance to the report on his first survey. Of the thirty-three controls, only two were definitely positive. The balance, or well over ninety per cent of the group, were either completely negative or inconclusive. Among the duck farmers, on the other hand, eight, or twenty-five per cent, were positive. And unmistakably so. Of course, that wasn't final proof. Not by any means. Those two positive controls—to say nothing of the three in the other series—meant that we still had a long way to go. But it was no longer possible to seriously doubt that the ducks were in the picture. They almost had to be.

"They were. Only, it turned out to be quite a sizable picture. And it took a good many weeks to piece it all together. Dr. Meyer had been to New York and out to Riverhead to see our plant and back in California for some little while before his laboratory tests turned up the first organism. The date was Tuesday, October 2nd. It came, very suitably, from the liver of a bird that was born and raised on the farm where Haupt had worked—a three-week-old drake. That cemented the duck as a carrier. But he was just the beginning. By the time we heard about him, there were more. And the news got bigger and bigger. On October 8th, two pigeons came through. Beautifully. Then a lot more ducks and a couple of gulls and a crow. In the end, around the first of November, when we closed up shop, the only bird that hadn't yielded was the starling. Which proved nothing. We hadn't made a really serious effort with starlings. I've forgotten the final score—we got forty or fifty positives from ducks alone—but I remember the estimates we eventually worked out on incidence. They tell the story well enough. Pigeons, we concluded, are the worst. Fifty per cent of them are infected. Gulls come next—forty per cent. Then ducks —thirty-three per cent. The others—chickens and crows—average about twenty. I say estimates. That's what they were at first. Now they're practically facts. Since 1945, there have been a number of other surveys. Every one of them has fully confirmed our conclusions. Psittacosis isn't peculiar to the ducks and gulls and pigeons and chickens and crows of Long Island. It's an endemic disease that may well appear in any bird anywhere.

"For us, isolation of the virus was the grand finale. But it didn't completely wrap things up. There were still a couple of problems. Diagnosis isn't a remedy. What, for example, were we going to do about the situation? Or, rather, what could we do? Well, the answer to that turned out to be wonderfully simple. Nothing. There wasn't anything we could do. Unless, of course, we killed off all the birds on Long Island. And kept them killed off. That may sound more like a rationalization than a solution. Actually, though, there was no great need to do anything. Then or since. The Long Island experience didn't merely broaden our understanding of the potential sources of psittacosis. It also broadened our understanding of the disease itself. We used to think of psittacosis as a pretty serious affair. That was natural. The serious cases were about the only ones we ever saw. Now, I think, it's generally agreed that severe attacks are really rather uncommon. The average victim, as Tulloch's survey very clearly suggested, doesn't even know he's sick. The other problem wasn't really a problem. It was just a loose end—something we wondered about. The cause of the trouble was obviously deeply rooted. Then why did the outbreak happen when it did? Why 1945? Instead of 1944, say, or 1943? We got the answer to that the following year, when there was another little flurry on the farms. So the chances are that 1945 wasn't the first year that part of Long Island had an outbreak of psittacosis. It's probably been going on for generations. Except that in 1945 there was Dr. Barton. And he opened his eyes and saw it."

[*1953*]

CHAPTER 9

Placebo

———————◆·◆———————

THE MOST WIDELY USED DRUGS in the modern medicine cabinet are not really drugs at all. They are mere accommodations. This is not to say that they are ineffective. Their use is often followed by incontestably salubrious results. They are, however, chemotherapeutically inert. They either possess no curative powers whatever or have none that are contextually relevant. The remedial vigor that they seem to manifest is as insubstantial as thought. Like that of the witch doctor's mask, the potentate's touch, and the food faddist's yeast and yoghurt, it exists only in the receptive mind of the beholder.

Such drugs are called placebos. The term is an unaltered acquisition from the Latin, which precisely describes their function. It is the first-person singular of the future indicative of the verb "*placere*," and means "I shall please." Nevertheless, despite its classic aptness, the word comes to medicine not from Latin but from English. "Placebo" has been an English idiom of varied meaning for nearly a thousand years. It entered the English language as an ecclesiastical colloquialism for vespers for the dead (from the Vulgate psalm recited in that service, which begins, "*Placebo Domino in regione vivorum*") around the twelfth century. Toward the end of the fourteenth century, while retaining (as it still does) its ecclesiastical meaning, it began to acquire a secular connotation. It was first so used, to judge from an allusion in "The Canterbury Tales" ("Flatereres been the deueles Chapelleyns that syngen euere Placebo"), as a metaphor suggesting supine sycophancy. By the middle of the fifteenth century, "placebo" was in general use as a simple synonym for "flattery" and "flatterer," and it continued to serve that purpose through the sixteenth and seventeenth centuries. It then came to mean a courtesy designed to soothe or gratify. Its inclusion in the vocabulary of medicine is rather more recent. It made its first clearly recorded appearance there (as "an epithet given to any medicine adapted more to please than benefit the patient") in the 1811 edition of *Hooper's Medical Dictionary*. It could hardly have been included much earlier. For until around the early part of the nineteenth century, when chemistry began to develop into a science capable of discerning the true nature and action of drugs, all medicines, as far as anyone could tell, were equally worthy or worthless.

The definition of a placebo has broadened since Hooper's time. His epithet is no longer confined to drugs that are prescribed solely to satisfy the patient's craving for medicine. It now embraces any form of therapy that is inappropriate to the complaint under treatment. All medical procedures may thus on occasion be placebos. (So, for that matter, may almost anything—a religious medal, a toilet ritual, the avoidance of drafts, a gold ring applied to a sty.) Most placebos, however, are drugs. They include true drugs, purported drugs, and deliberate counterfeits. A true drug becomes a placebo when its specific therapeutic properties are misapplied. The use of penicillin in the treatment of the common cold, the administration of cortisone to victims of osteoarthritis, and the casual prescription of tranquillizers, stimulants, and vitamins, though currently much in fashion, are among the many examples of true drugs so abused. The purported drugs are mainly patent medicines—blood refreshers, backache nostrums, acne cures, nerve tonics, virility restorers. Although most patent medicines contain some active chemical agent (alcohol, aspirin, caffeine), it is seldom one that has an active bearing on the need. A counterfeit drug is a pure placebo. It looks like a drug and tastes like a drug. It may even, if administered by injection, feel like a drug. But it is pharmacologically a drone. It is made of some inactive substance (starch, lactose, or salt), and so has no inherent power either to help or to harm. And yet, for all their great variety, all placebos—drugs or devices or charms—are essentially alike. The power they exert is not their own. It derives from the infinite capacity of the human mind for self-deception.

The pure placebo, it need hardly be said, is the only placebo that has a reputable place in modern medical science. But its place is a curious one. Contrary to common supposition, the placebo is no more than peripherally accepted in general clinical medicine. Many physicians, in fact, are magisterially opposed to any therapeutic use of placebos, considering it little better than quackery, and even those who condone the practice do so with many reservations. "A placebo should never be given on demand," Arthur K. Shapiro, professor of psychiatry and neurology at the New York University College of Medicine, points out in a recent study in the *Journal of Nervous and Mental Disease*. "It should never be continued for a long time, at least without regular reëxamination . . . or given unless the indications are more carefully examined than if a specific therapy were ordered. A placebo should never be given if the diagnosis is in doubt, if the doctor-patient relationship is in jeopardy, for retaining the confidence of those expecting but not requiring treatment, and unless the doctor believes it will help. A placebo should not be prescribed for neurotic patients whose complaints are based on anxiety and fear of disease. It should never, in any circumstances, be used as a substitute for psychotherapy. . . ." The circumstances in which a placebo may be given are equally well defined. "A placebo," A. Barham Carter, a staff physician at the Ashford Hospital, in London, has noted in a report to the *Lancet*, "may be the correct treatment for a patient who needs a material sign that we are trying to help him, and who (from a scientific point of view, at any rate) is past our help." The niche that the placebo chiefly occupies is in pharmacological research. Its usefulness there is undisputed. As a control in the clinical evaluation of drugs—screening out false or feeble claimants, verifying the true—it has, and can have, no substitute. And with every exposure of a sham or shallow drug, it has added to the formidable documentation of its own peculiar powers.

That the placebo effect exists is clear beyond dispute. It owes nothing to the imagination but its origin. Its reality has been abundantly demonstrated by the many control experiments whose results are now on record. So, almost as abundantly, has its range. The palliative powers with which suggestion can invest the placebo are extraordinarily broad. Their reach surpasses that of the powers inherent in the great majority of genuinely robust drugs. It extends (at least potentially) throughout the spectrum of psychophysiological distress.

The placebo can powerfully mimic the tranquillizing touch of certain ataractics. "There is no good evidence that meprobamate [the chemical name of Equanil and Miltown] can be distinguished from a placebo in treating anxiety in psychiatric outpatients," two clinical pharmacologists at the Johns Hopkins University School of Medicine—Victor G. Laties and Bernard Weiss—reported to the *Journal of Chronic Diseases* in a recent review of the subject. Their conclusion was largely derived from two well-controlled studies carried out in 1957. One of these, the work of Herbert Koteen, assistant professor of internal medicine at Cornell University Medical College, involved twenty-five patients, whose symptoms included anxiety, muscle tension, restlessness, and irritability. In the course of this trial, each patient consumed thirty-seven bottles of meprobamate capsules and thirty-six bottles of matching lactose placebo capsules. All were told simply that they were taking something that would help them. "The results," Koteen noted, "reveal that meprobamate in the currently recommended dose had no greater effect in relieving symptoms than did the placebo." If anything, the placebo was the more effective. An analysis of reports on the patients showed that twenty-three of the thirty-six bottles of placebo capsules produced marked improvement. For meprobamate the count was twenty-one out of thirty-seven. A team of English investigators—M. J. Raymond, C. J. Lucas, M. L. Beesley, B. A. O'Connell, and S. A. F. Roberts—

conducted the other study reviewed by Laties and Weiss. Fifty-one psychoneurotic patients took part in the test, and each was given five different ataractic drugs and a placebo. In addition to meprobamate, the drugs were amobarbital (Amytal), chlorpromazine (Thorazine), benactyzine, and a preparation containing, among other things, Rauwolfia. Thirty-three patients responded favorably to amobarbital, twenty-five to meprobamate, twenty-five to the Rauwolfia preparation, nineteen to chlorpromazine, and eighteen to benactyzine. But twenty-two patients responded just as favorably to the placebo.

Physical pain, as well as mental anguish, is amenable to placebo therapy. Its susceptibility has been established by numerous double-blind investigations, including, as it happens, the first. In their introductory study of 1937, Harry Gold and his associates compared the effectiveness of two conventional analgesics (theobromine and aminophylline) with that of a placebo in the treatment of cardiac pain. They found "no appreciable difference." In 1950, a similar study, undertaken by a team that again included Gold, produced exactly the same result. Khellinine, a drug derived from bishop's-weed, had earlier been informally described in the pages of the *American Heart Journal* as a superior means of relieving the pain of angina pectoris. Gold and his collaborators subjected khellinine to a formal double-blind evaluation, and found, as they reported to the *American Journal of Medicine*, that its powers were no greater than those of the placebo. Of thirty-nine patients participating in the test, slightly more than a third obtained complete relief from both. A drug no more effective than a placebo is, like a placebo, no drug at all. If khellinine had truly possessed the analgesic vigor envisioned by its original proponents, the result of Gold's evaluation would have been, of course, quite different. The khellinine would have relieved the pain of not merely a third but all (or practically all) the patients who received it. In 1953, a control appraisal of the usefulness of the anticoagulant heparin in blocking cardiac pain, also reported to the *American Journal of Medicine*, again affirmed the power of the placebo. A third of one group of patients were relieved of pain by intravenous injections of heparin. But so were a third of a group who received injections of saline solution. (Heparin has since been returned to its proper function as a specific anticoagulant.) And so—according to a report published in the *Annals of the New York Academy of Science* in 1949—were five of nineteen cardiac patients who were maintained for several weeks on lactose tablets alone.

The pain of coronary-artery disease is not the only pain over which the placebo has a certain sovereignty. It can also blunt the agonizing pain that often follows major surgery. "In [thirteen] studies of severe, steady postoperative wound pain," Henry K. Beecher, professor of anesthesiology at Harvard University Medical School, notes in a recent report to the *Journal of the American Medical Association*, "we have found that rather constantly thirty per cent or more of these individuals get satisfactory pain relief from a placebo." ("Satisfactory relief" is defined by Beecher as "fifty per cent or more relief of pain at two checked intervals—forty-five and ninety minutes after administration of the agent.") A total of four hundred and fifty-three men and women, all patients at Massachusetts General Hospital, participated in these tests. The number of patients who obtained relief ranged from a low of fifteen per cent in one study to a high of fifty-three per cent in another. Moreover, Beecher adds, the studies produced "strong evidence that placebos are far more effective in relieving early postoperative wound pain when [the pain] is severe than when it is less so." The impact of the placebo on clinical headache, according to a classic study conducted by E. M. Jellinek, professor of biometrics at the Yale School of Medicine, in 1946, is even more emphatic. In this study, a hundred and ninety-nine general-hospital patients were regularly given a lactose placebo upon complaint of headache. Approximately sixty per cent of the patients reported prompt relief. Stewart Wolf, of the University of Oklahoma School of Medicine, and Harold G. Wolff, professor of medicine at the Cornell University Medical College—in a monograph entitled "Headaches"—cite an arresting instance of how promptly a placebo may act. "A forty-three-year-old businesswoman, who had dedicated much of her life to a domineering and often disapproving mother whom she said she 'adored,' began to realize as she talked [in a psychiatric consultation] that she really resented her mother's tyranny," they recount. "Pulse recordings made from the right superficial temporal artery were of relatively low amplitude at first . . . but as she [continued to speak of her mother], the recorded tracing of a cranial artery pulsation increased in amplitude. A pounding began on the right side of her head. Within a few minutes, she had a full-blown [migraine] headache. At the height of her headache, [she was given] a hypodermic injection of dilute salt water. . . . She was told that it was a powerful drug which could constrict her arteries and remove the pain." It did. "Almost immediately," the report goes on, "the headache began to subside and within a few minutes was gone entirely. At the same time the recorded artery pulsation [demonstrably] reduced in amplitude." Another pain syndrome that readily responds to placebo therapy is that of rheumatoid arthritis. "The number of rheumatic patients found to benefit from placebos is about the same as the number favorably influenced by salicylates [aspirin and related salicylic-acid compounds] or even cortisone," E. F. Traut and E. W. Passarelli, investigators at the arthritis clinic of the Cook County Hospital, in Chicago, recently reported to the *Annals of the Rheumatic Diseases*. "Eighty-eight patients were studied in detail. Lactose placebo tablets [taken after each meal] benefited one half of all patients—twelve per cent of them for longer than six months. Placebo tablets benefited most of the patients with the severer grades of arthritis. Placebo injections benefited sixty-four per cent of thirty-nine patients resistant to placebo tablets." In addition to relief of pain and "stiffness," the benefits included improvement in sleeping, eating, bowel action, and general well-being. A reduction in swelling was also noted among most of the responsive patients. This, the authors pointed out, was—like the artery constriction observed by Wolf and Wolff—a "purely objective improvement."

Other investigators have reported equally pure objective reactions to placebos in other ailments. One of these is motion sickness. In an experiment described in the *Bulletin* of the Johns Hopkins Hospital in 1949, two Johns Hopkins clinicians—L. N. Gay and P. E. Carliner—induced motion sickness in a panel of thirty-three volunteers. When the patients were properly prostrated, each was given a lactose placebo. Within thirty minutes, more than half of them (approximately fifty-eight per cent) were visibly recovered. They had ceased to vomit, they were no longer cold and clammy, and the ghastly pallor characteristic of such seizures had been replaced by normal color. Gastric hyperacidity, according to a study reported by Stewart Wolf and a group of associates to *Gastroenterology* in 1952, is another condition that manifestly yields to placebo therapy. The study was done on a patient with a gastric fistula (an opening into the stomach through the abdominal wall), and consisted of thirteen trials. On eight occasions, the observers noted, the administration of a placebo produced a measurable decrease in the gastric acid level. Two independent studies—one by B. R. Hillis, assistant in the Department of Materia Medica and Therapeutics at the University of Glasgow, and the other by J. S. Gravenstein, resident physician at the Massachusetts General Hospital, and a group of associates —have demonstrated the power of the placebo to suppress cough. Hillis, whose study was published in the *Lancet* in 1952, induced coughing fits in six volunteers. Four of them were quickly relieved by a subcutaneous injection of saline solution. The Gravenstein study—reported to the *Journal of Applied Physiology* in 1954— involved forty-eight patients with clinical cough. A lactose placebo was effective in eighteen members (or about forty per cent) of the group. The placebo can also conspicuously cure the common cold. Or so Harold S. Diehl, dean of medical sciences at the University of Minnesota, reported to the *Journal of the American Medical Association* in 1933. Thirty-five of a hundred student victims of acute attacks whom he treated with lactose tablets were promptly freed of their sniffles, fever, and malaise.

Nor are these several soothing services the only measure of the placebo's wide-ranging power. They merely manifest one aspect of it. It has, no less emphatically, another, and harsher, side. Toxic placebo effects as real as those produced by any genuine drug have been recorded by many investigators in the field. As a rule, like most other drug-induced dishevelments, these effects are relatively mild. In one of the numerous studies undertaken by Beecher and his associates at Harvard, thirty-six of seventy-two participating patients were made drowsy by a lactose tablet. Seven actually fell asleep. Of ninety-two patients in another Beecher study, twenty-three developed headache following the administration of a placebo. Fourteen others complained of mental confusion. Nine were nauseated. Nausea, together with faintness and diarrhea, was also reported, after treatment, by seven of the hundred Minnesota students in Diehl's common-cold experiment. Serious reactions are not, however, unknown. Three of thirty-one patients in a test conducted by Stewart Wolf became violently ill. "One of the three," he recounts, "had sudden overwhelming weakness, palpitation, and nausea within fifteen minutes of taking her tablets. In a second patient, a diffuse, itchy, erythematous maculopapular rash developed after ten days of taking [placebo] pills. A skin consultant considered the eruption to be a typical dermatitis medicamentosa [or drug-induced reaction]. After use of the pills was stopped, the eruption quickly cleared. In a third patient, within ten minutes of taking her pills, epigastric pain developed, followed by a watery diarrhea, urticaria [hives], and angioneurotic edema of the lips." In an evaluation of streptomycin as an adjunct to chest surgery, made by William B. Tucker, director of the tuberculosis service of the Veterans Administration Central Office, in Washington, two-thirds of a group of patients who received only placebos developed every sign (including blood-cell changes and hearing loss) of streptomycin toxicity. And Arthur Shapiro, whose strictures against the indiscriminate use of placebos have already been mentioned, has reported a case in which a lactose placebo brought about a shattering impairment of liver function.

Although the placebo is rightly reckoned an agent of infinite range, the powers it manifests are less than absolute. In contrast to the results obtained by a genuine drug, its potential reach exceeds its predictable grasp. The effectiveness of the placebo is almost chaotically variable. It is determined by the interplay of several multifaceted forces. Environment has an important bearing on the result. A placebo administered in a hospital, where the patient lies surrounded by symbols of authority and care, is more likely to have an effect than one taken by someone alone at home.

Another factor is the amount of stress engendered by the complaint. Placebos are "most effective when the stress (anxiety or pain, for example) is greatest," Beecher has postulated. There is no ready explanation of this phenomenon. One possibility is that the ability to respond to suggestion increases with the urgency of the desire for relief—for, as Beecher, among others, has also observed, the power of the placebo tends to slacken with use and diminishing need. On the other hand, it may simply be that exquisite stress, in the form of fear or foreboding, is itself a product of suggestion, and hence is exquisitely amenable to counter-suggestion. A third, and crucial, factor involved in the placebo effect is the nature of the patient. "There are personality characteristics and habits of mind which predispose a person to respond to a placebo," Louis Lasagna, professor of clinical pharmacology and medicine at the Johns Hopkins University School of Medicine, has noted. "The psychological predisposition to respond is probably present in varying degrees in all of us. But some persons are very likely to respond positively in a wide variety of situations. Others will almost never respond, whatever the situation." In Lasagna's opinion, which is shared by most investigators in the field, the traits that distinguish the former group have a strong neurotic cast. The people most receptive to the magnetic pull of faith tend to be "emotionally expressive and to speak freely, most frequently of themselves and their problems." They exhibit "somatic symptoms (nervous stomach, diarrhea, headache) during periods of stress," and are habitual consumers of cathartics and aspirin. They are "anxious, self-centered, and emotionally labile." Few of them are college graduates, and most are regular churchgoers. Such factors as sex and age appear to be irrelevant. So does intelligence. The trait that chiefly distinguishes those who seldom respond to the placebo is emotional stability. That and sophistication.

Just how the placebo achieves its effects has not yet been determined. Some twenty years of intensive research have established little more than the vigor, the variety, and the limitations of the phenomenon. The nature of the neural alchemy that enables the credulous mind to transmute illusion into reality remains very largely obscure. Its significance, however, seems clear enough. It indicates that medicine, despite a century of scientific progress, is still an art as well as a science. It also suggests the composition of the many therapeutic triumphs of other, less rational approaches to the treatment of disease.

[*1960*]

CHAPTER 10

The Most Delicate Thing in the World

WE HAD JUST SAT DOWN—Harold Cousminer and I—in his gritty little first-floor office at the New York City Health Department, in lower Manhattan, when the telephone on his desk gave a shattering peal. Cousminer raised his eyebrows. "Well, here we go," he said. "But that's the way it generally is on Saturday night. Don't ask me why." He plucked the receiver from its cradle, and cleared his throat.

"Poison Control," he said. There was a pause. "Oh?" He reached for a pencil, glanced at his watch, and scribbled something on a pad of paper. "Well, I think you ought to have a gastric lavage done." He listened patiently, and nodded. "I understand, Doctor. And I agree. It's fortunate he vomited. Very fortunate. But to be on the safe side . . . You're dealing with the carbolic family, you know. That's the toxic agent there." He listened again. "O.K. Hold on a minute. I'll see what I can find." Cousminer swung around to a table at his elbow. It held a metal filing cabinet, two black leather satchels of the sort carried by doctors, a large cardboard box labeled "Calcium Gluconate for Black Widow Spiders," and a row of medical texts. He felt along the row of books, pulled out one called *The Symptoms and Treatment of Acute Poisoning*, and spread it open on the desk. After a moment, he picked up the receiver. "Hello? Well, here's the procedure— take down what you want of it. Gastric lavage as soon as possible. The choice is vegetable oil or a ten-per-cent solution of alcohol. Followed by lavage with water. Followed with demulcents such as egg albumen, egg yolk, milk, or gruel. No specific antidote. Further treatment is symptomatic and supportive. Good results have been reported from the intravenous injection of five-per-cent glucose in saline." Cousminer closed the book. "I guess that about does it," he said. "Not at all, Doctor. Glad to be of help."

"What was that?" I asked.

Cousminer shrugged. "Nothing very unusual." He leaned back in his chair. "An interne up at Roosevelt Hospital with a problem on his hands. He's got a five-year-old boy in there whose mother fed him a teaspoonful of CN disinfectant an hour or so ago. I told him what he was up against. CN is largely phenol—carbolic acid. And how to handle it, as you heard. That's what I'm here for— to answer questions like that. Primarily, anyway. A night emergency inspector also has other duties. I take complaints from the public on coal gas, carbon monoxide, and contaminated food, and when necessary I go out and investigate the situation. It all comes under the general heading of poison. But that kind of trouble accounts for only a fraction of our calls. Most of the trouble I hear about comes from toxic drugs and household chemicals. Everybody's house is full of both—especially the latter. Detergents, for example. There must be a hundred of them on the market. And deodorants, insecticides, stain removers, laundry bleaches, paints, mouthwashes, shoe polish. All plainly labeled with a big brand name and full instructions on how to use. But you very seldom see anything about the ingredients—toxic or otherwise."

"Isn't there any legislation covering that?" I asked. "Something like the Pure Food and Drug Act?"

"Apparently not," Cousminer said. "I understand the American Medical Association has appointed a committee to work for a law, but those things take time. There's always a certain amount of resistance. Meanwhile, to put the matter gently, things are sometimes rather awkward for a doctor when he gets an emergency call. It can turn what might be only a minor misfortune into a real calamity. It often did until a few years ago. The idea of a clearinghouse where doctors and hospitals could get information about ingredients originated in Chicago. They established the first Poison Control Center there in 1953, and almost every large city in the United States and Canada has one now. Our center opened in the spring of 1955. The results, I'm told, have been very satisfactory. Not that there's been any decline in drug and household-chemical poisoning. The average for the country is still over a hundred and fifty thousand cases a year. But there has been a drop in deaths—from upward of fifteen hundred a year to around a thousand. The reason is that the doctors don't have to work blind any more. They don't have to guess at the nature of the toxic substance in the box or bottle with the fancy label. All they have to do is step to the telephone. They know that we will probably have the answer. If the product in question is well established, the chances are it's fully discussed in one of the standard toxicological texts, and we've got them all—the best, the latest. We also have a laboratory upstairs that keeps abreast. When something new appears on the market, our chemists break it down, and the analysis goes into that filing cabinet over there. They keep an eye on the old products, too—the manufacturers change their formulas from time to time. So, one way or another, we can generally rise to the occasion. Not that we've never been stumped. We are— every now and then. But that's to be expected. You can't have a file on everything that might possibly find its way into somebody's stomach. I'm talking about accidental poisoning, of course. People don't often try to kill themselves by eating a can of Kiwi. We only hear two stories here. One is ignorance—not realizing the danger of leaving drugs or chemicals around where children can get at them. The other is carelessness. Like the case of that boy up at Roosevelt. His mother is one of the many who seem to live in a trance. She didn't notice that she was giving him CN. She thought it was his cough medicine."

"That isn't unusual?" I inquired.

"Oh, they're all unusual," Cousminer said. "It's a matter of more or less. CN seems to turn up a little more often than most. It ranks pretty close to Clorox, Zonite, and the pine deodorants.

In the drug field, the chief offenders are the barbiturates and, of course, aspirin. But none of them happens every day. Or even every month. The only thing you can expect on this job is the unexpected. That's one thing I like about it. It keeps you on your toes. If it weren't for the unpredictable, the job would be hard to take—for me, anyway. The time would hang too heavy. We have a peculiar setup here, you know. It hasn't much in common with the average night-shift routine. There are five of us night inspectors, and we take our tours of duty in rotation. We work a night, lay off for four, and then come on again. But the tours we work are really tours. We start at 5 P.M., when the rest of the department goes home, and we stay with it until nine o'clock the next morning, when the day men in the various categories we combine —Environmental Sanitation, Food and Drugs, and the rest—take over. If that sounds strenuous, believe me, it is. Sixteen hours is a long time, especially at night, and in a godforsaken part of town like this. It's endless. It's also lonely—lonely as hell—although that doesn't bother me as much as it seems to bother some of the others. I've got a few resources. In fact, the hours are mainly why I took the job. This isn't my career—I've made other plans. Which means I have to have my days and most of my evenings free. I'm thirty-two years old, I'm married, and I've got two children, but the war gave me a late start in life, and I'm still going to school." He smiled. "Graduate school at N.Y.U. I've got a master's degree in science from there, and in another two years I'll have my Ph.D. My field is geology—paleontology, to be exact. I also teach a little —I have a couple of classes at N.Y.U. and one at Cooper Union —but not quite enough to keep me afloat. I need a job, and this one perfectly fits the need. It makes the whole thing possible."

"I supposed you were a doctor," I said. "I thought you'd have to be."

"The department thinks otherwise," Cousminer said. "So does Jerome Trichter. He's the assistant commissioner who set the night-inspector service up and keeps it going. As a matter of fact, we don't need doctors on this night job. We're not here to prescribe to the general public. Our information is strictly for doctors and hospitals—"

The telephone cut Cousminer short. He sat up with a jerk, took a deep breath, and reached for the receiver. "Poison Control," he said, and paused. "I see—yes. About what time was that?" For a long moment, he was silent. He sat absorbed, gazing blindly at the wall, occasionally nodding. Then, abruptly, he said, "Oh, definitely. Very bad. Especially in a child that young. I'd say you ought to do a gastric lavage at once. But let me take a look." Opening the book he had consulted before, he found what he wanted, and frowned. He turned again to the telephone, and said, "Sorry—I was wrong. Standard procedure is Universal Antidote to start. Five or six heaping teaspoons suspended in a glass of water. *Then* lavage, with three hundred cc.s of potassium permanganate. Or an emetic—the choice is mustard or salt—to be repeated until vomiting occurs. Also, three heaping teaspoons of magnesium sulfate may be left in the stomach as a saline purgative. Acidosis is usual. It may be relieved by injecting sodium r-lactate solution intravenously until the carbon-dioxide combining power is restored, or until urine is alkaline to phenolsulfonephthalein or to litmus paper. Intravenous normal saline may be sufficient to combat mild acidosis. But I hardly think that applies in this—" He nodded. "That's right. . . . Of course—any time. . . . Absolutely. Good-by."

Cousminer pushed the telephone away. His eyes had a distant look. It was a moment before he relaxed again in his chair.

"That sounded serious," I said.

"It is," Cousminer said. "Very much so. A case of methyl-salicylate poisoning in an eight-month-old girl. Oil of wintergreen, they call it on the market. It's used as a rub for muscular aches and pains. Her parents just brought her into St. John's Hospital, in Brooklyn, which was sensible, but a little late. It happened about an hour and a half ago." He glanced at his note pad. "Around eight, the hospital said. How it happened isn't clear—except that the mother accidentally fed her a tablespoonful of the stuff. A tablespoon averages about fifteen cc.s. And six cc.s is the minimum fatal dose for children."

"You recommended something called Universal Antidote," I said. "What is that?"

"The book recommended it," Cousminer said. "I just passed it on. Although I must say I'm pretty well acquainted with it. Universal Antidote isn't actually universal, but it takes in a lot of territory. It's generally useful as a counteractive to most drugs and household chemicals. Depending on the poison, it either neutralizes the toxic agent or alters it in some way that stops or slows up its absorption until it can be eliminated. That's why it's usually followed by lavage or an emetic. The remarkable thing about it seems to be its simplicity. All it is is two parts of activated charcoal and one part each of magnesium oxide and tannic acid." The telephone rang again. Cousminer came briskly erect. "I've often wondered who thought it up," he added, and, turning, caught the receiver to his ear.

"Poison Control," he said. "Yes?" A look of incredulity crossed his face. "I'm sorry, but where did you say—" He broke off and listened. His expression cleared. "I see. Yes, of course." There was a longer pause. "Well, frankly, no. It isn't one of the big brands. But unless the label says different, it's probably acetone. Hold on, and I'll make a check." Cousminer opened *The Symptoms and Treatment of Acute Poisoning*, but after a glance at the index he pushed it aside and stood up. He moved along the table to the filing cabinet and slid out a narrow drawer. I caught a glimpse of a file of dog-eared cards, and then his shoulders blocked my view. He gave a grunt of triumph or surprise. The drawer slammed shut, and he returned to his desk and the telephone. "Hello? Well, that's the problem—acetone. Do you want the treatment? . . . That's right. An emetic—sodium chloride is preferred—or lavage. In either case, followed by stimulants to combat collapse. The choice is strong coffee, caffeine with sodium benzoate, or aromatic spirits of ammonia. If necessary, transfusion of whole blood. O.K.?" He shook his head. "Not at all. That's what we're here for."

Cousminer hung up. "Very odd," he said, and sat back, smiling. "Not the case, particularly. A six-year-old boy got hold of his mother's nail-polish remover. Fortunately, the bottle was practically empty, so he didn't get too much. Why he did it, I can't imagine. Six is a little old for that kind of foolishness. But what got me was the hospital. They took him to Lying-In. I'm surprised the staff up there had even heard of us." He smiled again, and then gave a sudden laugh. "That reminds me of a call I had one night last fall. No connection with Lying-In, of course, but also on the odd side. It was a woman—a nurse, from the sound of her voice. You can usually tell by that air of command. Was this the New York City Department of Health? I told her it was. The Poison Control Center? Yes. Were we open twenty-four hours a day, seven days a week? Yes. And the telephone number—was Worth 4-3800 correct? Yes. Then she thanked me very kindly and started to hang up. I stopped her. What was this all about? Oh, just a routine check, she said, to make sure their information was correct and up to date. Well, might I ask who was calling? Why, certainly. She thought she had told me. This was the Something-or-Other Sanitarium, in Something City, California. Apparently, they keep a list of the leading Poison Control Centers all over the country."

A heavy door slammed in the distance, and the sound of footsteps echoed down the corridor. Cousminer looked at his watch. "Coffee break," he said, and jumped to his feet. "Be back in a minute." He vanished through the door. I gazed after him into the shadowy hall, and waited. The lonely clamor of silence settled over the room. I could hear the moan of the wind in the court beyond the window. The table stretched and creaked, the wall behind me tapped, a paper stirred in the wastebasket under the desk. Overhead, the light gave a pulsating tick and seemed for a moment to dim. The room began to have a subterranean feel.

Cousminer reappeared with a lumpy paper bag. He put it on the desk, extracted two cardboard containers of coffee, and handed one to me. "Kindness of the night watchman," he said, dropping into his chair. "He remembers me when he goes out to lunch, and later on, when my time comes, I do the same for him. He answers the phone whenever I'm called out, and takes messages. Or gets someone to cover for me if a problem turns up. He's the one who let you in tonight. So he knew I had company and brought two coffees."

"Very nice," I said.

"It helps," Cousminer said, and took a long swallow. He set the container on the desk. "I don't suppose you've got a cigarette?" I had, and held out the pack. Then I took one myself. "I quit smoking a couple of months ago," he said. "It gave me something to wrestle with. But now I've had my fun. I think I'll go back again."

The telephone rang. Cousminer dropped his cigarette into an ash tray and extended a hand. "Poison Control," he said. "Yes, this is the Health Department." He recovered his cigarette. "They prepared food without a permit—was that it? . . . Oh. . . . Oh, I see. Well, I'll tell you what. Call back on Monday morning and ask for the Bureau of Food and Drugs. That's the best place to file this sort of complaint." He hung up with a tolerant snort.

"What was that about?" I asked.

"Pizza pie," Cousminer said. "A member of the lunatic fringe wants us to close down a lunchroom somewhere out in Queens because they keep their pizzas in the refrigerator and heat them up on order. He's got some notion about frozen food. Thinks it's contrary to nature, I gathered. We get a good many calls like that. Outraged cranks. Drunks with a grudge. And just plain nuts. People who wake up and smell carbon monoxide—which, of course, is completely odorless, as well as colorless and tasteless. People who complain that the janitor has siphoned all the air out of their room. People who think their neighbors are trying to asphyxiate them with poisonous incense. They'd almost be funny if they weren't so sad."

Cousminer stubbed out his cigarette and sat back with his coffee. "I remember one call I got about a year ago," he said. "I'll never forget it. A woman over in Brooklyn. Said her apartment was full of fumes. She'd been smelling them all evening—this was around 2 A.M.—and they were getting stronger and stronger. It was all she could do to breathe. I asked her to describe the odor, but it seemed she couldn't. Nobody could, she said. It was indescribable—oh, too revolting for words. Well, I wasn't much impressed by that. It had a fairly fishy sound. On the other hand, she was obviously sober. No more excited than you'd reasonably expect. Gave me her name and address in a very businesslike way. So I said O.K., I'd be right out. You can't take chances on anything involving gases or fumes. You have to go and see. Which I did. It was a run-down building in a run-down neighborhood— a Chinese laundry on the first floor, a roaring saloon across the street, and a used-car lot on the corner. A perfect environment for trouble. And when I got upstairs and she opened the door, I was sure of it. She was just as sensible-looking as she sounded. I put her down for a retired schoolteacher—around sixty-five, and as neat as a pin. So was her apartment. I went through it room by room. No odors, not a sign of gas—nothing. I don't mean I just thought so. I knew it for a fact. We don't guess or estimate on a gas investigation. We use instruments. Our equipment includes an explosimeter, to see whether the gas content of the air is near the exploding point; a manometer, for measuring gas pressure; and a CO meter, which will detect even the faintest concentration of carbon monoxide. Along with various tools. They're all in that satchel over there on the table—the fat one. The other bag is Food and Drugs paraphernalia. Bottles and cartons for samples. Embargo forms. Et cetera. Well, it took me about an hour. I even went down in the cellar and poked around the furnace. She had me that convinced. But finally I was satisfied, and I told her so. She gave me a look that curled my hair. Did I mean to say I still couldn't smell the fumes? That's when I first saw the light. I didn't say no. Instead, I asked where they seemed to be coming from. No answer. Just another look. Then she took me by the arm and marched me over to the front window and pointed across the street—at the saloon. Now could I smell it? I obliged her by sniffing, but that wasn't enough. I had to say something. I asked her what it was she smelled. 'The odor of rotting souls,' she said."

Cousminer drank off the last of his coffee. He crushed the empty container and pitched it into the wastebasket. "Maybe she did," he said.

"I wouldn't know," I said.

"No," he said. "Neither would I. I've got a speculative turn of mind. At least, I like to use my head. But not in that direction. I suppose that's why I'm a paleontologist, and a night inspector. The problems that interest me—and the kind I usually get—are a little more down to earth. I don't care how tricky they are. All I ask is that when you finally put two and two together, the answer turns out to be four. Not x. I've had some tricky ones, too. I remember one not long ago that gave me a certain amount of mental exercise. As a matter of fact, I can think of two. The first was another Brooklyn case, and it also involved a saloon. That's where the story began. The scene had changed, however, by the time I came into the picture. My introduction was a telephone call from King's County Hospital—a doctor in the emergency room, with the usual request for help. Only it wasn't exactly usual. It was a case of vegetable poisoning. The victim was a Puerto Rican, a man about thirty, and the history he gave the doctor was this: He had dropped into a bar on his way home from work. After a couple of drinks, he got to talking with the bartender, and somehow the conversation got around to a big decorative plant in the window. It had been there for years, the bartender said, but he had never known what it was. The Puerto Rican said it looked like sugar cane. Another drink and he was certain. To prove his point, he broke off a piece of the stalk and started chewing it the way they did when he was a boy back home. The next thing he knew, his mouth was on fire. Then his throat. He had never felt such pain. Then his face began to swell, and he realized what had happened —he'd been poisoned. So he headed for the nearest hospital. By the time the doctor saw him, his face was so swollen he was hardly able to talk. Examination showed a violent inflammation throughout the mucous membrane of the mouth, tongue, and throat, and he was very obviously in agony. He was also, it seemed quite clear to the doctor, in very serious trouble. But what kind of trouble? What was the plant? What was its toxic principle? And what, if any, was the antidote or treatment?

"I told the doctor I'd see what I could do, and call him back. Not, however, with much enthusiasm. It looked hopeless. To be frank, I didn't even know how to begin. There wasn't much point in searching the files or trying one of the texts we have on poisonous plants. You can't look something up unless you know its name. The only possibility I could think of at the moment was Harry Raybin. Raybin is technical director of the center and one of the men we can call on for help in an emergency. Another, of course, is Mr. Trichter, but his field is primarily environmental sanitation. So I put in a call for Raybin, and got him at his home. That's all, though. He was as stumped as I was. Which left me with a choice between Trichter and a needle-in-the-haystack hunt through Muenscher's *Poisonous Plants*. But before I could make

up my mind, one of those nice things happened. I had an idea—
a hunch. I called the Bronx Botanical Garden. It was after hours
and the office was closed, but eventually somebody answered. A
watchman, and very obliging. When I hung up, I had the names
and telephone numbers of all their top botanists. As it turned out,
one was enough. Or perhaps I simply picked the right man first.
Anyway, I told him the story and he told me the answer. It was
as simple as that, and almost as quick. It sounded, he said, like
Dieffenbachia seguine. Sometimes known as dumb cane, and indigenous to tropical America. In fact, it couldn't be anything else.
Moreover, he added, I could rest assured that there was nothing
to worry about. *Dieffenbachia* was not a poisonous plant. It took
me a minute to absorb that piece of information. Then I reminded
him that, after all, the man was in the hospital. In a great deal of
pain. Swollen up like a pumpkin. Only just able to speak. No
doubt, he said, but that was not the result of chemical damage. It
was purely mechanical, and essentially harmless. One of the characteristics of *Dieffenbachia* was its secretion of very sharp crystals
of calcium oxalate. And one of the consequences of chewing the
plant was temporary loss of voice. That's why it was called dumb
cane."

Cousminer smiled a fleeting smile. I had left my cigarettes on the
desk, and he helped himself to one. "The other case I mentioned
was less exotic," he said. "And quite a bit grimmer. It started, for
me, with a police report. That was one evening last January. I'd
just come on duty when they phoned it in. A couple of hours
before, the superintendent of a tenement over on East Broadway
had found one of his tenants—a bachelor around thirty-five or
forty—dead in bed. I've forgotten how he made the discovery, but
that part isn't important. He did, and called the police, and they
came up, and one look was all they needed. No question about the
cause of death. The man was sprawled on his back in a very untidy
tangle of bedclothes, and his face was cherry-red. A classic picture
of carbon monoxide. The medical examiner placed the time of
death at about 7 A.M., and said there was good reason to believe
that the man was an alcoholic, or at least a heavy drinker. Well,
those were the facts, except for one thing. It wasn't suicide. There

were no gas outlets open. That made it an accident, and a case for us. So I got out my bag of tools and went over to East Broadway. It turned out to be a three-story building of cold-water railroad flats, built about 1910, and in fair repair. The dead man's apartment was top floor rear, but my first stop was the super's—on the floor below—for the keys and anything else that might be useful. He told me the man had lived there for years, originally with his parents. They were both dead now. His father had died two years before, and his mother just the previous month. Since her death, the son hadn't spent much time at home. Had all his meals out, and only rolled in to sleep. The apartment confirmed that much. It was the usual three-room layout, with the kitchen in the middle, and a lot of gas equipment—refrigerator, kitchen range, and two or three space heaters. But, as the police had found, they were all turned off or out of use. The refrigerator was even disconnected. However, none of the things were in very good shape. For all I knew, they were leaking at every joint. I unloaded and went to work. I spent an hour or more on the fittings alone. Then I covered every inch of the place with the CO meter. But no soap. I didn't find anything that might even hint at trouble. The apartment was safe, and, that being the case, my job was done.

"This was around seven-thirty. I remember looking at my watch when I finished packing my bag. Then, all of a sudden, I smelled smoke—coal smoke. It came from the kitchen, and by the time I got there, it was already good and thick—too thick for comfort. The source was plain enough. It was seeping out of an unused stovepipe vent that was capped with an old pie tin on the wall above the gas range. Buy why? How come the smoke wasn't going on up the flue? I opened a window to clear the air, and decided I'd better find out. There was a ladder at the end of the hall that led through a hatch to the roof. I climbed up and out, and went over to the chimney. It was letting off smoke, but not much—just a little wisp. I flashed my light down the flue, and you never saw such a rat's nest. Sticks, old rags—all kinds of trash. I don't know who did it—kids, probably—but it was a very thorough job and, from the look of the junk, one that had been going on for quite some time. Well, that explained the smoke in the dead man's kitchen, and maybe a whole lot more. Coal smoke is an excellent source of carbon monoxide. At any rate, I had to locate the fire, if only to put it out. The super's apartment seemed the place to start. One reason, of course, was its location, directly below the dead man's rooms. But I really think the super's help was all I had in mind at first. Until he opened the door. Then I caught a whiff of burning coal. I followed my nose to the kitchen, and there it was—a potbellied stove, going to beat the band. The rest, after I'd put out the fire, took about three minutes. I learned that the super only used the stove to take the chill off his flat. His usual time was now, in the early evening. But sometimes he used it for an hour or two in the early morning. That morning, he recalled, had been one of those times. I didn't need any more. When I added that to what I already knew about the dead man's habits, the picture was in focus. The tenant came home and fell into bed. Let's say around midnight or so. A few hours later, the place began to fill with smoke, but he was too drunk to wake up, and slept right through to eternity." Cousminer shrugged. "That's my theory, anyway."

"It sounds very reasonable to me," I said.

"It fits the facts," Cousminer said. "I've also got another theory. Or maybe suspicion would be a better word. On the way back here, I got to thinking about the dead man's parents. I wondered if there might be some connection between their deaths and his. Particularly his mother. It was simply curiosity, but I wanted to know. Several days later, I dropped in at the Bureau of Records and Statistics here in the Health Department and had a look at their death certificates. They made rather interesting reading. I don't mean I found any proof—none whatever. But the cause of death in both was something that could have been brought about by a dose of carbon monoxide."

The telephone rang. Cousminer discarded his cigarette and took up the receiver. "Poison Control," he said. "That's right." He listened, and frowned. "I'm afraid I don't follow you. . . . Yes, I got that—it's spelled D-e-l up to where the label's torn. But what's it supposed to be used for? There must be some hint on the bottle. I mean—" He nodded attentively. "I see. Clear as mud. However —hold on while I check our file." He rose and went over to the cabinet and pulled out a drawer. After a moment, he slammed it shut, and walked thoughtfully back to the phone. "Sorry," he said. "We've got nothing of that description in the files. Must be something very new. But, judging from what you say, it's almost certainly a solvent. Which would probably make it benzine or one of the chlorinated hydrocarbons. . . . Oh? It does, eh? Well, if it smells like benzine . . ." He reached for *The Symptoms and Treatment of Acute Poisoning* and heaved it open. "O.K. The thing to do is empty the stomach by lavage. Saline solution. And that's it. Not much else you can do in the way of emergency treatment. . . . Yes, I hope so, too. Good night."

Cousminer sat for a moment gazing at his notes. Then he shook himself and slumped back in his chair. "Well, that's one way to build up the file," he said. "I can think of better ones, though."

"What happened?" I asked.

"A two-year-old out in Manhasset got hold of what sounds like some sort of benzine preparation," he said. "I gather it's used for cleaning radio parts—'to restore volume control and contact' is the way the label puts it. That's about all I know, except that she just arrived at the North Shore Hospital, and her chances are pretty slim. Nonexistent, I should imagine. According to the doctor, she swallowed about two ounces of the stuff."

"Oh," I said.

Cousminer gave me a curious look. "Yes," he said. "Very sad." He hesitated. "That's the standard reaction, isn't it? But somehow I've never felt that way. I don't mean that I'm hardhearted. Or hardboiled—like a Bellevue interne. And I'm certainly not indifferent. It's just that my viewpoint is a little out of the ordinary. I told you I was in the war. I was a gunner on a B-24, and I flew thirty-five missions. That experience was part of it. The rest is what I've seen on this job, and what I've learned as a paleontologist. Most people take life for granted. My feeling is that it's not that dependable. In fact, it's the most delicate thing in the world. It's a miracle. And one false step and it's over."

[*1957*]

CHAPTER 11

A Certain Contribution

————————◆————————

AMONG THE NUMEROUS scientific problems under investigation in the laboratories of the Midwest Research Institute, at Kansas City, Missouri, in the fall of 1959 were two involving snakes. One was a study for an industrial firm of the effect on snakes of certain chemical compounds. The other had been commissioned by the New York Zoological Society, and its purpose was to develop a satisfactory method of controlling the parasitic snake mite *Ophionyssus natricis*. Both these projects were under the general direction of William B. House, principal chemist at the Institute, but the bulk of the laboratory work, which included the care and handling of some thirty snakes, was carried out by a young herpetologist named Gary K. Clarke. Most of the snakes in his charge were harmless—bull snakes, coachwhips, corn (or red rat) snakes, speckled king snakes, prairie king snakes, Eastern yellow-bellied racers. Nine, however, were venomous. This group consisted of three prairie rattlesnakes, two Southern Pacific rattlesnakes, a timber rattlesnake, a Western diamondback rattlesnake, a red diamond rattlesnake, and a copperhead. All, as required by the studies in progress, were excellent specimens of their kind, but the red diamond was in every way outstanding. It was the oldest (about ten years of age), the longest (fifty-two inches), the heaviest (nearly six pounds), and, since the species is restricted in range to the southernmost tip of California and the more desolate reaches of the upper Baja California peninsula, by far the rarest. It was also, for a rattlesnake, an uncommonly docile creature. Or so Clarke was inclined to think until the afternoon of November 4th.

"I haven't really changed my mind," Clarke says now. "Not altogether, anyway. What happened was the product of a certain set of circumstances. I don't mean it was inevitable—one thing led to another, but only up to a point. The deciding factor was chance. However, there was a pattern. To begin with—to begin some-where—I was alone in the laboratory that day. I have an assistant who helps with the routine, but he was at home with a cold. Ordinarily, that wouldn't have mattered much. Snakes need very little care. You only have to feed them once a week. In fact, they can go without food for a month and not be seriously harmed. They're also naturally clean and neat. But November 4th was not an ordinary day. It was a Wednesday—the first Wednesday of the month. And the first Wednesday of every month was when we weighed our snakes. That posed a problem. I like to have help on that particular job. I can do it myself, and I have—any number of times. I've been handling snakes since I was eleven or twelve. The first real pet I ever had was a seven-foot boa constrictor. Still, the weighing is a lot less trouble with someone helping out. I'm talking, of course, about venomous snakes. The others are noth-ing. On the other hand, I hated to put it off. I couldn't put it off too long. My regular monthly project reports were due in a couple of days, and I had to have the data on weight before I could finish them up. I finally decided, What the heck, I've done it often enough, I might as well go ahead.

"I started in right after lunch. The herpetological laboratory is in the basement of a wing of the Institute building. The entrance is through my office. A door at the rear of the office leads into a big workroom. Beyond that are two serpentariums. One of them houses non-poisonous snakes. The other is reserved for venomous species. Our snakes are separately confined in rectangular wooden cages mounted on tables set around the wall. The cages are mostly my own design. They vary in size according to need, but each has a screened ventilation porthole at the back, a hinged lid with a hasp fastener on top, and a fixed Plexiglas observation panel along the front. Those designed for venomous snakes are equipped with double padlocks, and the Plexiglas panels are three-quarters of an inch thick. That's only partly to keep the snakes from busting out. Snakes aren't lions or tigers. The main reason for those precautions is to protect the snakes from nosy people, and to prevent accidents. I don't want some janitor poking his mop handle through the glass. My plan that afternoon was to weigh the snakes in the venomous-snake room first. I was there and ready to go at one-thirty. I remember the time because I looked at my watch to estimate how long the job would take. Weighing a snake can be tricky, but the procedure is fairly simple. You lift him out of his cage. You've got a sack handy—an ordinary cotton flour sack is what we generally use—and you drop him in, tail first. You twist the sack closed, tie a knot in it, and hang it on a balance scale. His weight is the total minus that of the empty sack. Then you return him to his cage. My assistant and I had it down to a system. He opened up the cage and held the sack to receive the snake. I did the rest. We usually ran the whole job off in around an hour and a half. I couldn't hope to breeze along like that alone, but I'd still be through by four o'clock or thereabouts, and we don't close up until five. I had plenty of time.

"So I didn't hurry. I didn't want to hurry. The first snake to be weighed was the red diamond rattler. Big Red, I call him. And he's a handful to handle alone. A good many snakes—even rattlesnakes—you can pick them up with one hand. That leaves your other hand free to manipulate the sack. But not Big Red. I knew from experience I'd need both hands for him. I don't mean simply to lift him. Six pounds of snake isn't all that heavy. I mean to lift him properly, to hold him nice and steady. Otherwise, he might thrash around and maybe break his neck. That meant I had to rig the sack in advance. I have a method that works pretty well. I take a straight chair and drape the sack over the back in such a way that the neck hangs open just right. Which I did—very carefully. I got it arranged exactly to my satisfaction. Then I unlocked and opened the cage. Big Red was lying there in a resting coil with his head pillowed on his back. He looked at peace with the world. But that didn't mean I could just reach in and pick him up. You don't try that with any rattlesnake. I had to secure his head, and for that you use a snake hook. A snake hook is a long-handled tool with a crook at the end. It looks something like one of those grass whips. I took the hook in my left hand, and gently—very gently, so as not to rile him—I pushed his head off his body and onto the floor of the cage. Red hardly twitched. When I had his head in position, I pinned it there with the hook. I then went in with my right hand and grabbed him by the back of the neck. There's only one safe place—directly behind the wedge of his head. Anywhere else, he could twist around and reach me with his fangs. As a rule, in the pit-viper family—the venomous genera that include rattlesnakes, copperheads, and cottonmouths—the larger the snake, the longer his fangs. The biggest North American pit viper is the Eastern diamondback rattlesnake. According to Laurence Klauber, of the San Diego Zoo, the leading authority on rattlers, its fangs may measure more than an inch in over-all length. Big Red wasn't quite in that class. However, I will say this. His fangs were long enough to inspire my deepest respect. I made sure I had the right place. Then I got rid of the hook and brought my left hand back and caught him at mid-body and lifted him out of the cage. He squirmed a little, but nothing much—nothing at all unusual. I pointed his head well out of reach and carried him over to the chair.

"There's a trick to getting a snake into a sack. It's far harder than getting him out. We have a tool for that. When you're ready to free a snake, you simply return him—sack and all—to the cage. You take a long pair of forceps and work the neck of the sack open. Then you move the forceps down toward the bottom of the sack, and pull. It usually peels right off. You then lift it out and drop the cage lid, and you're done. Sacking a snake is a bare-handed job. As I said, a snake goes into the sack tail first. It isn't hard to ease him in. The problem is how to release his head and get your hand away and close the sack—in time. You can't imagine how fast a snake can move. If you just let go, he'll be up before you even blink. But here's something else about snakes. A snake resents being held by the neck. He's helpless, and he hates it. And that's the basis of the trick you use to get him safely sacked. You jerk his head up a bit. You sort of stretch his neck. His instinct is to pull back with all his strength. The instant you feel him respond, let go. His pull does the rest. He loses his balance and tumbles to the bottom of the sack. Now's your chance. You snatch out your hand and give the sack a twist. Then you tie a quick knot in it and swing it away from your body. You want to be sure you keep it there, too. He's very apt to be riled.

"Well, that's the sacking procedure. It usually goes off like clockwork. The snake is out of the cage and into the sack and ready for weighing in very little more than a minute. Even Big Red. He's harder to handle than most of the others, but only because of his size. His disposition is the sweetest of any snake I know. I have no idea what got into him that afternoon. He wasn't upset—not at first. He just didn't seem to want to coöperate. I hoisted him over the sack and began to slide him in. For a moment, everything went fine. Then, all of a sudden, he curled up his tail and swung it out of the sack. That was a bit odd, but hardly alarming. Snakes have their whims. I got him straightened out, and tried again. Same thing. He went halfway in, then doubled back and out. It was as though he were being playful. So I started all over again. With exactly the same result. I don't know how many tries I made. At least a dozen. I finally decided the reason must be the sack. I released my grip at mid-body and reached down with my left hand and widened its mouth. That meant I was holding him just by the neck. When he felt himself slump, he gave a violent wrench. I almost thought I'd lost him. But I let the sack go and grabbed him again in time. The trouble was, the damage was done. Big Red wasn't used to that kind of treatment, and he was beginning to lose his temper. And before he lost it, I wanted him safely sacked. I lifted him up and started him in once more. But this time he wouldn't go in at all. Instead, he gave it a slap with his tail, and the sack slipped off the back of the chair and fell in a heap on the floor. And now he was really mad. He opened his mouth to striking width. That's wide. When a snake wants to strike, his jaws flatten back as wide as a pair of shears. I'd never had such a ringside look at his fangs—the two big functional fangs knifing out from the upper jaw and the two smaller reserves. All four were unsheathed and fully erect.

"I've given a lot of thought to that particular moment. I know now what I should have done. I should have faced the fact that everything was going wrong. I should have hustled him right back to his cage to cool off, and moved on to one of the others. And the idea did occur to me. But then I thought, No, I'm not going to give up yet. I'll try it one more time. I knew it wouldn't be easy —not with the sack where it was now. Nevertheless, I thought I could manage. There was no question of using my hands. I needed them both to control Big Red. Pointing his head as far out of reach as I could, I knelt down on the floor and leaned across his back. I caught the edge of the sack in my teeth. I pulled it and yanked it and finally fumbled it flat. The next step was to open the mouth of the sack. I scrunched around and found it with my teeth and lifted up a corner. So far, so good. I brought Red into position and worked his tail through the mouth of the sack. Then I very carefully drew the sack up over his back. I had to be careful. He was getting madder by the minute. And stronger. I was puffing and blowing, but not old Red. His struggles didn't seem to faze him. I kept on working at the sack, and he was finally well enough in to let me get my left hand free. I changed the sack from my teeth to my hand—and gave his head that little jerk. Down he went. Out came my hand. I twisted the neck of the sack and knotted it tight with a quick half hitch and sat back on my haunches. I lifted the sack to the proper upright position. Then, holding it there on the floor about a foot in front of me, I got to my feet. I must have been off balance for an instant. Big Red thrashed out, and the sack swung up and at me. I felt a stab of pain in my left leg. His fangs were sunk in the underside of my knee.

"I didn't panic. I don't mean I wasn't frightened. I mean I wasn't anything. I was simply and completely dumfounded. It had happened so quickly, so unexpectedly. My mind just seemed to go numb. But I functioned. Some part of me did—some instinct or reflex or something. Because the next thing I knew, I had broken his grip and wrenched the sack away. It was seeing the venom that started my mind working again. There was a big yellow stain on the sack where Red's fangs had pierced it, and another on my trouser leg. There was also some on the floor—a teaspoonful, it looked like. I knew Red's venom glands had been full. He'd never been milked—never had his venom artificially extracted. And he had never been fed live food, so it hadn't been necessary for him to discharge his venom to eat. We feed our snakes freshly killed mice and rats from one of the biology labs. But even so. The amount of venom spewed around was fantastic. It didn't seem possible that I could have received very much of a dose. In fact, I almost considered going on with the weighing. Almost, but not quite. My leg was on fire—it was like somebody was carving it up with a red-hot razor blade. I decided I needed help. That was my first real thought. My second thought is a little hard to explain. It makes me sound so cool. But I had it, and it went like this. I thought, Well, if I had to be bitten, I'm glad I got it from Red. There's practically no clinical literature on bites by red diamonds —particularly, Klauber says, in which all the early symptoms are recorded. The species is too rare. So at least I've got a chance to make a certain contribution. It isn't pure disaster.

"My immediate responsibility, of course, was Big Red. I had to get him back in his cage. On the way, I looked at my watch. It was exactly one-forty-five. We'd been struggling for fifteen minutes. That pretty well tells the story. No snake will take that amount of handling without getting good and riled. It wouldn't be natural. And while I'm at it, I want to say this. I don't think Red was specifically mad at me. He was just mad, and I had the bad luck to get within his reach. He was still mad. He was still dangerous, too. But I didn't let that bother me. I got him caged in nothing flat. I untied the sack and peeled it off. I couldn't leave him in it. He had to be comfortable, and free to get at his water. Then I locked him up. We always keep a snake-bite kit in that serpentarium. I stuck it in my pocket and headed for the nearest telephone—in the corridor just outside my office. My knee was beginning to hurt like heck. I mean really hurt. My whole left leg felt on fire. I didn't dare hurry, though. I knew enough to realize that I mustn't stir up my circulation. In a way, I didn't want to hurry. To get help, I had to call my supervisor, Dr. House, and I hated to. It was embarrassing. A herpetologist really shouldn't be bitten, you know. There's even a term for a bite of that kind. When a professional handler of snakes is bitten, it's called an illegitimate bite. It isn't a true accident. The man is expected to know better. Well, Dr. House answered the phone himself. I'll never forget our conversation. It was so awful. He said hello in such a cheerful voice.

"I said, 'Dr. House, this is Gary Clarke. I've just been bitten by a rattlesnake.'

"I can't really say what he said next. It wasn't a word. It was like a moan, only worse. Then he said, 'Oh, no.'

"I told him I was afraid so.

" 'All right,' he said. 'O.K. I'll be right down.'

"Whichever way he came—down the stairs or by the elevator —it would take him a couple of minutes. His office is on the third floor. I decided I'd better start helping myself. Favoring my left leg all I could, trying to keep it rigid, I hobbled back to my office and sat down at the desk and got out the snake-bite kit. The time was then one-forty-eight. There was blood all over my trouser leg. I rolled it up and had a look at the wound. It was bleeding freely —which, of course, was all to the good. The fang marks were roughly parallel to my foot. Strictly speaking, I hadn't been bitten, since Red had struck my leg in such a way that he couldn't bring his jaws together for a full bite. I'd only been stabbed. Still, it looked like a heck of a stab. It felt like one, too. It was burning hotter and hotter. I took a rubber-tubing tourniquet from the kit and whipped it around my leg just above the knee. That would stop the venom from travelling on to the rest of my body. The next step was to make an incision at the site of the wound for faster drainage. I cleaned the wound with an antiseptic solution from the kit. I was all set to go to work with the blade when I heard a commotion down the hall, and Dr. House came galloping in. Fred Baiocchi, the first-aid representative for our section, was right behind him. Then came Curtis Sandage, a senior chemist, and a whole raft of others. They all looked pretty wild. It seemed to me that I was the calmest man in the room. But maybe not, because I remember Fred Baiocchi saying, 'Relax. Sit back and try to relax.' Maybe I just thought I was calm.

"Fred took the blade and made the incision. It was a good big one—about an inch and a half long—but I hardly felt it. It was just another pain among many. Then he handed me a suction cup, and I went to work with that to increase the flow from the fang stabs. Everybody was talking to beat the band. I gathered that Dr. House had called one of the doctors the Institute retains, and an ambulance. The ambulance was coming from Menorah Hospital, only a few blocks away, where the doctor was on the staff. I looked at my watch: one-fifty-five. While we were waiting, Dr. Sandage broke open an antivenin kit. He asked me if I was sensitive to horse serum—to antivenin. Some people are, and in that case there's the possibility of a toxic reaction more serious than the bite. I told him that I'd had a routine sensitivity skin test some months before, with negative results. However, to be on the safe side, he gave me another test. It's a very quick test. The results would be ready to read by the time I got to the hospital. A couple of minutes later, the ambulance men walked in. They lifted me out of the chair and laid me on the stretcher, and just then the Institute public-address system gave a squawk. The operator announced that I was wanted on the telephone. I remember turning to Fred Baiocchi. 'Would you mind taking it?' I said. 'Tell them I'm busy right now. Tell them I'll be back in a couple of hours.' I actually thought I would be."

Clarke was carried into the emergency room of Menorah Hospital at seven minutes past two. The physician summoned by Dr. House was waiting there to receive him. It was, as it happened, the first time that he had been called upon to treat a case of snake bite, but his procedure was unexceptionable. He briefly loosened the tourniquet, to restore sufficient circulation to prevent necrosis of tissue. He next noted the result of the serum-sensitivity test. It was negative. Thus reassured, he injected five cc.s of antivenin near the puncture site and another five cc.s in the left buttock. He then made a second incision, just above the knee. After an interval of ten minutes, he administered two more injections of antivenin— at the site of the wound and in the upper left thigh. This was followed by a prophylactic injection of tetanus antitoxin and (as a general supportive measure) an injection of ACTH, and then by a routine diagnostic examination. The findings revealed no immediate cause for alarm. Clarke's blood pressure was 138/80, or approximately normal for a man of his age. His temperature was 99.2 degrees. His pulse rate was 88. The physician dressed the several wounds, removed the tourniquet, and administered a soothing injection of morphine. That completed the emergency treatment. At two-forty-five, or exactly one hour after he was bitten, Clarke was formally admitted to the hospital and rolled into a surgical ward and put to bed.

"I will say this," Clarke says. "I was very glad to be there. By the time they'd finished with me in the emergency room, I'd lost all desire to get back to the lab. It wasn't just the pain. I felt so weak. I remember at one point asking the nurse for a pencil and paper and trying to make some notes. It was too much for me. I didn't have the strength to hold the pencil. The only notes I made that afternoon I dictated to my wife. Dr. House or the hospital or somebody had notified her, and she came running in a little after three. But even talking was an effort. And the hospital made it worse. You know how it is—they keep after you every minute. Somebody was always jabbing me with a thermometer. Or bringing me something to eat or drink that I didn't want. I wasn't hungry. Or taking my blood pressure. They did that every hour. They had to, of course. In snake bite, there's always the danger of shock, and they had to be on guard. Fortunately, that didn't happen. My blood pressure reached its lowest level early the following morning. It went down to one-ten over seventy-four. That's low, as I understand it, but still above the danger point. They also kept giving me injections—penicillin, antivenin, morphine. I suppose the morphine helped, but if it did, I didn't notice. It didn't give me what I'd call relief. Around five o'clock that first afternoon, I tried to describe the pain to Margaret Ann, and I still have the notes she took. I said, 'My leg feels like it was run through a meat grinder and then had acid poured over it.' But that was just the beginning. It got worse. My leg began to swell, and every stretch exposed another nerve. The doctor looked in on me at six-forty-five. When he pulled back the covers and changed the dressing, it was all I could do not to yell. The feel of his breath on my knee was something I can't describe.

"So was the next twelve hours. What I remember of it, anyway.

At about eight-thirty in the evening, my leg began to jerk. I tried to hold it stiff. I gave it all the strength I had. But I couldn't. I'd feel the muscles begin to contract, and—wham! Another jerk. That went on for an hour or more. Then somebody came in and gave me another shot of morphine. I must have dozed after that. At least, I don't remember much of anything until sometime after midnight. One of the nurses was taking my blood pressure. Suddenly, I felt an awful wave of nausea, and vomited. Oh, I was sick! I vomited and vomited. I was completely out of control. And every heave was like a blowtorch on my leg. The nurse ran out and came back with an interne. He gave me an injection of Dramamine. The retching finally stopped, but by then I was past caring. I really didn't care if I made it or not. The scientist in me was gone and the patient had taken over. I began to pray. I don't know exactly what for. It wasn't either to live or to die. I think I just prayed to take my mind off my misery. It was a distraction. It was a way of making time move. I lay there praying and looking at my watch. You don't know what time is until you've spent a night like that. But I made it move. My goal was seven o'clock. I don't know why. Maybe I was a little delirious. When I got there, it was like a glorious victory. I told myself, 'I've been in almost unendurable pain for six or seven hours. And endured it. So I can stand it from now on out. It can't possibly get any worse.'

"I don't know whether it did or not. Pain is pretty hard to measure beyond a certain point. I do know it didn't let up. All day Thursday was just like Wednesday night. I was still too sick to eat. My breakfast that morning was raspberry Jell-O and tea. I only drank the tea. It was the same at lunch. I swallowed a little broth. I was still too weak to write. It was still torture to move, but I couldn't keep from moving. My leg kept jerking, and every now and then my whole body would give an agonizing jump. I still didn't have any interest in life. Before Margaret Ann left on Wednesday evening, I had asked her to bring me some things from home. I thought I wanted some books, to read up on my case, and my camera and a box of flash bulbs. My idea was that it might be instructive to take some pictures of my leg. She arrived about noon with everything, including all my favorite books—'Poisonous Amphibians and Reptiles,' by Floyd Boys and Hobart M.

Smith, and 'The Natural History of North American Amphibians and Reptiles,' by James A. Oliver, and Klauber's two-volume 'Rattlesnakes: Their Habits, Life Histories, and Influence on Mankind.' I let them sit on the table. The scientist in me was dead. Well, missing, anyway. He did come back in time. Margaret Ann sat with me until they brought my dinner in at five o'clock, but I hardly said a word. I didn't even have the strength to grumble. Or eat. My dinner was a little broth and a couple of bites of Jell-O. The one thing I really remember about that day was the doctor's evening visit. I only remember that because it was so horrible. The first thing was that I got a look at my leg. It didn't look much like a leg any more—it looked like a log. It was swollen from just below the hip all the way down to my foot. And I mean swollen. It was so puffed up that my calf was actually bigger than my thigh. It was also a dozen different colors. The second thing was this. The doctor decided to make some more incisions—a series of six longitudinal cuts at intervals around my thigh. But first, on account of the pain, he shot my leg full of procaine anesthetic. I'll never forget the feel of those stabs. He knew what he was doing, though. I could never have lived through the incisions without an anesthetic. Every time he touched my thigh with the scalpel, it burst open like an overdone sausage.

"I spent another nightmare night that night. Even a full grain of morphine—I'd never had more than a quarter grain before—seemed to have no effect on the pain. It was Wednesday night all over again, except that I didn't vomit. That was the only real difference I can remember. But the next morning—Friday, November 6th—I began to feel a little better. I wasn't out of my misery. Far from it. My leg still hurt like heck. It throbbed and ached with every breath I took. But an ache isn't quite the same as pain. You can stand it. And my appetite came back. The reason for that, I think, was largely cortisone. They gave me an intravenous infusion at about ten o'clock that morning, and by noon I was actually hungry. When dinnertime came, I was starved. I cleaned my tray—a bowl of Jell-O, a cup of broth, a pot of tea—and I could have easily gone on and put away a steak. The most important change, though, was my attitude. My will to live returned. I began to care.

"You might call that the turning point. Not in the sense of passing a crisis. I don't mean that. There wasn't any crisis. It seems to be generally agreed that my recovery was never seriously in doubt. I didn't get a big enough charge of venom, and the treatment I received could hardly have been more prompt or efficient. I simply mean that by then the worst was over. I still had a long way to go. It was another week before I could leave the hospital, and much of that time I felt awful. But I was never in such pain again, or so low in mind and spirit. On Saturday, I started writing up my notes myself, and every day I noted some improvement. My blood pressure climbed gradually back to normal. My white-blood-cell count dropped from a high of nearly twelve thousand to a normal of sixty-five hundred. My leg began to look like a leg once more—by Sunday, I could even bend it a little. The following day, it was nearly normal in size. Around eight-thirty that night, they gave me a pair of crutches, and I was able to hobble into the bathroom. I almost enjoyed the rest of my stay. I read and rested and ate like a horse. I would have enjoyed it if they had given me a little peace. But now that I was feeling better, I had visitors all the time. Everybody in the hospital flocked around—internes, nurses, orderlies, even other patients. They all wanted to see what a snake bite looked like. They also wanted to know what I was going to do to Red. They thought I was counting the days until I could get my revenge. And when they learned that I wasn't even mad, they looked disgusted. They shook their heads and walked away. They thought I was some kind of monster."

Clarke was discharged from the hospital on Friday, November 13th. He spent the next four days at home, recovering his strength, learning to walk without support, and bringing his clinical notes up to date. The final entry in his record reads: "Area immediately around bite is still tender. Able to walk fairly well now. If my calculations are correct, I was punctured with the hypodermic needle more than sixty times after I had been bitten!" On the morning of Wednesday, November 18th, Clarke returned to work. After reporting to Dr. House, he hurried down to the laboratory, briefly conferred with his assistant, and then limped into the venomous serpentarium. "I wanted to see Big Red," he says. "I wanted to make sure that he was clean and comfortable. But there was also something else. I wanted to see what I felt. I wanted to make sure of myself. I looked at Red for quite a while. And it was all right. I didn't feel anything about him—only a deep and abiding respect."

[*1961*]

CHAPTER 12

S. Miami

<hr/>

AROUND FIVE O'CLOCK on Friday morning, June 4, 1954, an Upton, Massachusetts, garage mechanic whom I'll call Alfred Edison—a married man and the father of a three-year-old daughter—was wrenched from sleep by a grinding pain in the stomach. It doubled him up and turned him over and almost took his breath away. He began to groan, and his groans awakened his wife. He heard her asking what had happened, but before he could answer, a wave of nausea and diarrhea overwhelmed him. When he emerged from the bathroom some ten minutes later, the light was on in the nursery. His wife was holding the baby in her arms. The child was flushed and whimpering, and she had vomited in her bed. She was also, it soon developed, diarrheic. Frightened into a fleeting convalescence, Edison helped his wife calm and comfort the child, and presently she fell asleep. The Edisons then headed back to bed. At the door of their room, Mrs. Edison stopped. Her face went green. She turned and ran for the bathroom. Edison got as far as the nearest chair. He tumbled into it, gagging and retching, with another seizure of cramps. The baby awoke again and began to cry. There was no more sleep for anyone in the Edison house that night. Even the baby only dozed. Finally, toward seven o'clock, they decided to call the doctor. Edison dragged himself downstairs and telephoned a general practitioner named Bernard F. McKernan.

"Not that he had much choice," Dr. McKernan says. "I mean, if they wanted a doctor. Upton is a fair-sized village. It has a population of around three thousand. But I'm the only physician in town. Don't ask me why. It isn't my doing. I could use some help—in fact, I'd welcome it. I'd be more than happy to share the strain. I certainly would have been back there in June of 1954. However, I'm the doctor, and he called me. I was up and dressed —you have to get up early to handle a practice like mine—and was just sitting down to breakfast. It wasn't hard to get the picture. The symptoms told the story. I couldn't see much cause for alarm, but I already had one house call to make in that neighborhood, so I told him I'd drop around. I got there a little after eight. I found no reason to change my first impression. It looked like a routine gastroenteritis. What I call summer diarrhea. Moreover, by then the worst appeared to be over. No more cramps and no more vomiting. Nobody had any fever. The only remaining symptom was diarrhea. I gave them each a dose of kaolin for that, and prescribed the usual bland diet and rest. Then, as a matter of course, I asked them what they had been eating in the past twenty-four hours or so. They couldn't think of anything unusual. They couldn't seem to think of anything at all. Just what they always ate, they said. I let it go at that. I told them to give me a ring the following day if the diarrhea continued, and went on to the next call on my list. They didn't call me on Saturday, so I put them out of my mind.

"Until Sunday. Sunday is nominally my day of rest. I realize that people can't always arrange their illnesses to suit my convenience, but I don't have office hours on Sunday, and I'm very much obliged when nobody calls me at home. Needless to say, that seldom happens. And it didn't happen that Sunday. My holiday ended at about three o'clock in the afternoon with a call from a man named, I'll say, Smith. He sounded pretty frantic. Could I come over right away? Both of his children—an eight-year-old boy and a girl of four—were violently ill. So was his wife. So were two members of her family who were spending the weekend with them—her father and one of her brothers. I asked him what seemed to be the trouble. Cramps, he said, terrible stomach cramps. Nausea and vomiting. Diarrhea. That made me perk up my ears. Summer diarrhea is a common complaint, but it isn't all that common. Two family outbreaks in less than three days in a village this size was something to think about. I told him I was on my way. I saw Mrs. Smith and the children first. Smith hadn't exaggerated. They were sick—really sick. Far sicker than the Edisons had ever been. Along with everything else, they were flat on their backs, too weak to lift a hand, and running quite a fever. Both children had a temperature of a hundred and three, and Mrs. Smith's was almost that high. I then had a look at her brother. The old man, it turned out, wasn't there. He didn't believe in doctors. When he heard I was coming, he left and went home—to Hopkinton, as I recall. No matter. His is another story. He died a week or two later, but not of gastroenteritis, although that might have been a contributing factor. The cause of death was a tibial-artery thrombosis. Well, to get back to the Smiths—I did what I could to make them comfortable. I also revised my original diagnosis. This was obviously no mere summer diarrhea. It was a full-fledged case of food poisoning—bacterial food poisoning, most likely.

"In the first place, it couldn't be chemical poisoning. That usually comes on within minutes of ingestion, and the time lapse is never much more than a couple of hours. These people, however, took sick before breakfast. They didn't eat any breakfast. Their last meal was dinner on Saturday night. And the dinner menu eliminated the possibility that they had been poisoned by some inherently poisonous plant or animal substance. Toxic mushrooms, for example. Dinner was steak and fried potatoes, bread and butter, carrots and peas, and coleslaw, with milk for the children and watermelon for dessert. It had to be some form of bacterial poisoning. To judge from the clinical picture, the organism responsible could be either a staphylococcus or one of the salmonella group. My guess, in view of the onset time, was the latter. The staphylococcus toxin makes itself felt within two to seven hours. Salmonella takes from twelve to thirty-six hours. The next step was to try to determine just what food had served as the vehicle of infection. At a glance, there were three possibilities—the milk, the coleslaw, and the steak. But only at a glance. The children didn't eat any coleslaw, and they alone drank milk. That left the steak. Meat is an excellent medium for the growth of salmonella. Raw or rare meat, that is. Thorough cooking will safely destroy the organism. The Smith steak was fried to a crisp. Well, maybe the trouble went back to an earlier meal. I took up Saturday lunch and Saturday breakfast and dinner on Friday night. Lunch was out of the question. The boy had lunched at a neighbor's house, and the brother had also eaten somewhere else. Breakfast was completely innocuous. It consisted of fruit juice, doughnuts, and coffee. The children drank milk. Friday-night dinner was even less promising than the dinner on Saturday night —fried fish and boiled potatoes, bread and butter, and stringbeans, with the usual milk for the children. Dessert, as on the following night, was watermelon.

"I've seldom felt so stumped. Or, a moment later, so stupid. I was just about ready to call it quits when the obvious suddenly dawned. The children were sick. Mrs. Smith was sick. Her brother was sick. And so, apparently, was her father. But Smith himself was well. How come? There was only one reasonable explanation. He hadn't eaten something that all the others ate. I was right. I asked him and he told me. It was watermelon. He never ate watermelon. He simply didn't like it. I don't know what I expected, but I'm sure it wasn't that. I'd never heard of watermelon as a vehicle for food poisoning. Nobody ever had. Nevertheless, it had to be considered. I asked Smith a few more questions and got a few more answers. They had bought the watermelon—it was half a melon, actually—at the supermarket in Milford, about five miles southeast of here, on Friday. There was some of it left. It was out in the refrigerator, if I wanted to take a look. I told him to keep it there. I'd probably want to have it analyzed.

"I got back home a little after four. I put the car away and went in the house and dropped my bag, and the doorbell rang. It was a woman I knew—Mrs. Brown, I'll call her. She and her husband and their four young children lived just down the street. Well, she hated to bother me on Sunday, but it couldn't be helped. It was mostly on account of the children. They had been sick and vomiting since nine or ten o'clock that morning. And now they were violently diarrheic. So was she, but it was the children that really concerned her. What did I think was the matter? I let that go for a moment. I had some questions of my own that I wanted answered first. She hadn't mentioned her husband. Did that mean that he wasn't sick? No, she said. Or, rather, yes—he was fine. I began to get a rather creepy feeling. Had they by any chance eaten any watermelon recently? She gave me a very odd look. Why, yes; they'd had watermelon for dinner only last night. I wondered if it might have come from the supermarket at Milford. It did—yes. That's where they always traded. And they had all eaten some of it? No. She and the children had, but not her husband. He didn't like watermelon. Neither did she, particularly. They had really bought it mainly for the children. I picked up my bag and opened the door and followed her out of the house.

"The first thing Monday morning, I put in a call to the Milford supermarket. I identified myself to the manager, and told him I had an outbreak of food poisoning on my hands that was tentatively traced to watermelon bought at his store within the past two or three days. Until the matter was settled, I'd be much obliged if he would withhold all watermelon still in stock from sale. All things considered, he took it very well. He didn't try to argue. He stuttered and stammered a little, but that was largely from shock. Or maybe just plain disbelief. If so, I could hardly blame him. I didn't entirely believe it myself. The idea of watermelon as a source of infection in food poisoning still seemed a trifle far-fetched. There was reason to suspect it, but the evidence was purely circumstantial, and it was based on just two sets of circumstances. It could be a mere coincidence. I don't mean I really thought so, but it was possible to wonder. It was possible on Monday morning. By Monday afternoon, however, it was wholly out of the question. Two things accounted for the change. One was that I saw the Edison family again. I was called back there around noon. The kaolin hadn't seemed to help. They were all still miserably diarrheic. In view of what I now suspected, that wasn't too surprising. An attack of salmonellosis can hang on for four or five days. In fact, I've known of cases where the symptoms kept recurring for weeks, and even months. I did what I could—what I'd done for the others. I prescribed another adsorbent, and a regime of penicillin and sulfasuxidine. I then brought up the subject of food again. With a little prompting, their memory revived. Enough to recall that on Thursday night they'd had watermelon for dessert. It was all gone now—they had only bought a slice. But, yes, it had come from the supermarket at Milford. Then came another outbreak—a young couple I'll call Miller. The Millers had been sick since Sunday with cramps, vomiting, and diarrhea. Mrs. Miller had a temperature of a hundred and two. On Saturday night, they had entertained another couple at dinner. Dessert was a slice of watermelon, from the Milford supermarket. There was some of it left in the refrigerator. Their guests, as it happened, hadn't eaten any. I took down the name of their friends, and when I got back to the office I gave them a ring. The wife answered the phone. Her husband was at work—and quite well. So was she.

"Well, that was the end of the argument. The watermelon was clearly in the picture. It was also clear that I had gone as far as I could alone. The rest was up to the State Department of Public Health. Food poisoning is a reportable disease in Massachusetts. I filled out a notification form and sent it off to the health officer for this district, in Worcester."

The district health officer to whom Dr. McKernan addressed his report was a physician named Gilbert E. Gayler. It reached Dr. Gayler on Tuesday. The following morning, he drove down to Upton for a preliminary survey of the outbreak. He first conferred with Dr. McKernan. There were now, he learned, not four but five stricken families. The fifth was an elderly couple named (I'll say) Green. They had shared a slice of watermelon from the Milford supermarket on Friday night, they had become ill on Saturday, and on Tuesday, after nearly four days of misery, they had summoned Dr. McKernan. The Greens brought the number of cases to a total—the final total, as it turned out—of seventeen. Dr. Gayler spent the rest of the morning on a round of clinical calls. Accompanied by Dr. McKernan, he visited the Greens, the Smiths, and the Millers, and left with each of the several patients an enteric-specimen kit. The patients were instructed to mail the kits as soon as possible to the Diagnostic Laboratory of the Massachusetts Department of Public Health, in Boston. In addition, Dr. Gayler obtained from the Millers the remains of their Saturday night watermelon. His next stop, after a hurried lunch with Dr. McKernan, was the supermarket at Milford. He interviewed the manager, the assistant manager, and three clerks assigned to the fruit-and-vegetable department. All five were in their normal state of health. None were, or recently had been, afflicted with any sort of skin, respiratory, or gastro-intestinal trouble. An examination of the fruit-and-vegetable department indicated that it was, if anything, better kept and cleaner than that of the average market. As requested by Dr. McKernan, the store's stock of watermelons— both whole and sliced—had been withdrawn from sale, but all the cut melons were still meticulously wrapped in cellophane, as they had been all along. Dr. Gayler took one of the slices with him to be analyzed along with the Miller sample. He then returned to his car, and headed for Boston and the Diagnostic Laboratory.

Dr. Robert A. MacCready, the director in charge, was not at the laboratory that afternoon when Dr. Gayler turned up with his samples of melon. He was attending a conference at the State House. It was not until his return the next day that he learned of the visit and its purpose. He heard the news from his senior bacteriologist, Mrs. Marion B. Holmes, and he heard it with incredulity.

"I had no opinion of Dr. McKernan," Dr. MacCready says. "I didn't know him. I did know Dr. Gayler, though. I knew him well enough to know that he was a sound and sensible man. That's about all that kept me from scoffing at Dr. McKernan's hunch. There are innumerable vehicles of salmonella infection. The literature is full of outbreaks spread by almost any food you can name —meat, poultry, fish, eggs, milk, cheese, salads, pastries. Almost any food, that is, except fresh fruit. The incidence of salmonella in fresh fruit is so rare as to be almost negligible. Especially watermelon! That thick hide! The notion was almost whimsical. Mrs. Holmes thought so, too. Or, rather, she did at first. But now, after thinking it over, she wasn't entirely sure. She didn't attempt to explain just how a watermelon might come to harbor a colony of salmonellae. She simply pointed out that watermelon is rich in sugar and moisture. It could thus serve the organism very nicely as a medium for growth and proliferation. Which, of course, was perfectly true. I had to agree that watermelon was within the range of possibility. In my opinion, however, it still seemed quite unlikely. The inside of a whole watermelon is presumably sterile, and the cut melons had been carefully wrapped by clerks who were all in good health. I'd believe the implication when I saw some proof—when and if the laboratory could demonstrate the presence of salmonella in those melons. The procedure involved in such a test is a standard one. Specimens of the suspected material are planted in certain culture mediums that especially favor the growth of salmonella. Then nature takes its course. The results, if any, can usually be obtained in two or three days. This was Thursday. We should have an answer by Saturday or Sunday. Meanwhile, there was nothing to do but wait.

"The only trouble was I didn't feel like just waiting. It wasn't impatience. I got over that long ago. It was simple curiosity. I was intrigued. Watermelon or no watermelon, it was a most unusual case, and I wanted to know a good deal more about it than Mrs. Holmes had learned from Dr. Gayler. That meant a trip to the scene. I made the necessary arrangements that afternoon, and drove down on Friday morning. For company, among other reasons, I took along a colleague—Joseph P. Reardon. He was, and is, the epidemiologist in the Department's Division of Communicable Diseases. As it turned out, Dr. Reardon more than paid his way. Our first stop was Dr. McKernan's office. Dr. Gayler joined us there. They gave us a full report. Dr. Gayler's contribution was a poll of the other doctors in the Milford area. I don't remember just how many he called, and it doesn't matter. The responses were all the same. None of the doctors had seen a case of acute gastroenteritis in the past ten days or two weeks. So the outbreak was confined to Upton. Before moving on to Milford, we had a look at some of the patients. That was mere routine. We didn't expect any revelations and we didn't find any. We did pick up another sample for the laboratory—the melon that Dr. McKernan had instructed the Smiths to save. Dr. Gayler had been favorably impressed by the look of the supermarket. So were Dr. Reardon and I. We inspected it practically foot by foot. There was no evidence of rats or mice. Animal droppings—particularly those of rodents—are a frequent salmonella reservoir. The store was as clean as good management could make it. Then we settled down in the fruit-and-vegetable department. We talked with the clerks and arranged for sample stools. The watermelons were still under embargo—some of them whole and some sliced and covered with cellophane. We were shown the knife that was used to slice them, and I took a sample swab of the blade for laboratory analysis. Dr. Reardon suggested a swab of the shelf where the knife was kept. I thought that was pretty futile—there was nothing there but dust. The possibility of salmonella's even existing there—let alone multiplying—was exceedingly remote. But I humored him. There was no harm in one more sample. We had little enough to show for the day.

"We left Dr. Gayler at Milford, and Dr. Reardon and I drove back to Boston. After dropping him off, I stopped by the office. The only news from Mrs. Holmes was the arrival of the first lot of stool samples. I handed over our harvest of swabs and melon and went home. I wasn't exactly depressed. I just didn't feel quite comfortable. It was obvious that Dr. McKernan had done an excellent job. So good, in fact, that I hardly knew what to think. I still had certain misgivings about the watermelon theory. It still went against my grain. And yet, if the melon wasn't responsible, what was? The answer to that was: Nothing. There wasn't anything else. It had to be the melon.

"Our laboratory is on a skeleton basis over the weekend. We don't have the funds to function at full strength seven days a week. As a rule, however, there's always somebody there—the bacteriologists take turns—and this weekend it was Mrs. Holmes. She kept me in touch with developments. As expected, there were several, and, as hoped, they told the story—the only possible story. Dr. McKernan was right. By Sunday night, the laboratory had confirmed him on every point. It confirmed his clinical diagnosis of salmonellosis. All of the patient stools were teeming with salmonellae. So were the Smith and Miller watermelon samples. That confirmed the melon as the vehicle of infection. It also pretty definitely linked the outbreak to the Milford supermarket. Then, thanks to Dr. Reardon, the shelf swab completed the chain. It produced a magnificent culture. I still find that hard to believe.

The odds against it were literally astronomical. It was an extraordinary stroke of luck. And a very fortunate one, as well. Because the swab I'd taken of the knife itself was negative. What happened, I suppose, was that the knife had been washed after Dr. McKernan embargoed the melons. The knife was our only disappointment. We got one other negative culture—from the melon slice that Dr. Gayler had picked up at the store—but that was hardly a blow. Just the reverse, as a matter of fact. It provided an acceptable answer to one of the two big questions that the positive cultures raised. It explained why the outbreak was confined to just those seventeen customers of the Milford supermarket. Dr. Gayler's melon was clean because the bulk of the melons were clean. If all, or most, or even many of the melons had been contaminated, the outbreak pattern would have been quite different. There would have been cases scattered all over the Milford area. But none of the doctors polled by Dr. Gayler had seen a sign of gastroenteritis. The conclusion was practically unavoidable. There must have been only two or three contaminated melons, and by some freak of circumstance they ended up in Upton.

"The other question was, of course, the essence of the problem. It was also the essence of my discontent—the root of all my misgivings. How did the contaminated melons get that way? How *could* something with so thick a hide have ever got contaminated? To answer that—to even attempt an answer—we needed to know a little more about the organism involved. We knew it was salmonella, but we didn't know the serotype—the species. When we did, we might have a lead. However, serotyping calls for antigenic analyses that most laboratories—including ours at that time—are not equipped to perform. We relied for such work on the New York Salmonella Center, at Beth Israel Hospital, in Manhattan. Accordingly, on Monday morning we prepared a sample culture and sent it off to the Center for specific identification. If all went well, we would have a report in a couple of days or so.

"The salmonella is a curious group of pathogens. It differs in many important respects from the other bacteria commonly associated with food poisoning—such as the staphylococci and *Clostridium botulinum*, the botulism organism. For one thing, salmonella is inherently infectious to man. The ingestion of food containing a quantity of living salmonellae commonly results in illness. Morever, because salmonella is perfectly adapted for growth and reproduction within the human body, the quantity need not be an enormous one. With the others, the mechanism is quite different. Botulism and staphylococcus food poisoning are intoxications rather than infections. Their cause is not the living organism but a toxin excreted in the food by the organism in the course of its proliferation there. In other words, the food itself is poisonous. That largely explains why staphylococcus food poisoning comes on so much faster than salmonellosis. Botulism takes longer—sometimes three or four days—but it isn't a gastroenteritis. It's primarily a disease of the central nervous system. And an extremely serious one. Fortunately, it is easily controlled. *C. botulinum* lives in the soil and can grow and elaborate its toxin only in a total absence of oxygen. Most outbreaks of botulism in this country are traced to home-canned vegetables inexpertly washed and processed and eaten without further cooking. Although heat has little or no effect on the botulism organism itself, proper cooking will safely destroy the toxin. The staphylococci enterotoxin, on the other hand, is highly heat-resistant. In addition, the staphylococcus organism is ubiquitous in nature. It's even been isolated from the air of rooms. And it is perhaps the commonest cause of boils and other skin and wound infections. Nevertheless, the control of staphylococcus food poisoning is not —at least potentially—too difficult. Refrigeration will prevent the development of the toxin, and good common-sense hygiene on the part of food handlers will do the rest. Salmonellosis would seem to be as easily controlled. Cooking, refrigeration, and cleanliness are all helpful precautions. The first will destroy the organism, and the others will retard its growth. But the problem is more complicated than that. Infected human beings are not alone responsible for the spread of salmonellosis. Salmonella can live in the intestinal tract of almost any animal, including those that are closest to man—dogs, rats, mice, cows, chickens. And, to make matters worse, it appears to be a perfect parasite. It can live and propagate in most such animals without any visible signs of harm to the animal.

"Nor is that all. New species of salmonella turn up every year.

Since 1885, when the first member of the group was described—
by an American pathologist named Daniel E. Salmon—literally
hundreds of species have been identified. The total now known is
well in excess of four hundred. So far, I'm glad to say, most of
them don't exhibit any unusual pathogenic powers. They produce
a disagreeable but not usually fatal illness. But that doesn't mean
they never will. A more virulent species might emerge tomorrow.
The multitude of species is not in itself particularly disturbing. It
actually has a certain epidemiological value. Many apparently
unrelated outbreaks of salmonellosis have been linked through
identification of the species involved. It also sometimes happens
that the identity of the species will indicate the ultimate source of
the trouble. It has been the custom for many years to name a
newly discovered species for the place where it first was found.
The names of some no longer have any geographical significance.
In the intervening years, the species they denote have been found
in many different places. *Salmonella montevideo* is one of that
increasingly widespread group. So, among others, are *S. oranienburg, S. newport, S. derby, S. bareilly*, and *S. panama*. A good
many more, however, are still essentially regional species. Such as,
to mention just a few, *S. dar-es-salaam, S. moscow, S. bronx, S.
israel, S. marylebone, S. ndola, S. oslo*, and *S. fresno*. Another is
S. miami. And that was the one we got. That was the Upton
organism.

"I had a telegram from Dr. Ivan Saphra, the chief bacteriologist
at the New York Salmonella Center, around four o'clock on Tuesday. The late Dr. Saphra, I should say—he died in 1957. A great
pity. He was a fine man, and an outstanding one in his field, as
his work in this case plainly testifies. Our culture didn't reach him
until sometime Tuesday morning, but he had it typed that afternoon. It often takes longer than that to identify a relatively common species. To even think of *S. miami* in this part of the country
was remarkable. The implications of his report were even more so.
S. miami, as its name suggests, is a Florida organism. It has been
recovered in several human outbreaks in that area, and from many
different animals. We could hardly have hoped for a more provocative lead. Or one that so comfortably simplified the problem. It
was only necessary to find a link between Florida and Massachu-

setts. What might have transported *S. miami* from way down there to here? An animal host? Not likely. Our examination of the supermarket had produced no evidence of rodent infestation. A human carrier? The answer to that was on my desk in a laboratory report on the specimen stools from the fruit-and-vegetable clerks. They were negative for salmonella. What else? Well, unless I was very much mistaken, Florida was a major source of produce for the Northeastern market in the spring and early summer. I put in a call to the supermarket at Milford and had a word with the manager. He was most coöperative. Their melons were Florida melons.

"That seemed to tell the story—the only reasonable story. We could scratch the store off the list. The trouble didn't originate there. It came up with the melons from Florida. To be sure, that was largely an inference, but it had the ring of truth. No other explanation was warranted by the facts. It wasn't, of course, the whole story. It didn't tell us how the contaminated melons got contaminated. That basic question still loomed. But it helped. We had sufficient data now to at least make a stab at an answer. We began with a train of assumptions. Suppose a melon had come in contact with infected animal droppings down there in some Florida field. Or, for that matter, after it was harvested and stacked in the local jobber's warehouse. Suppose some of that material adhered to the skin of the melon. Suppose it was still there when the melon arrived at the store. And suppose it was still there when the clerk took his knife and sliced up the melon for sale. What then? It was easy enough to find out. All we needed was a watermelon.

"I picked one up on the way to the office on Thursday. We lugged it into the laboratory, and Mrs. Holmes prepared a dilute suspension of *S. miami* from one of the positive cultures. She swabbed some of the material on the skin of the melon. Then, using a clean knife, she cut a slice out of the melon at that point. That pretty well reproduced our hypothetical situation. The next step was to demonstrate the result. We made two sets of cultures from the meat where it had come in contact with the knife. The first was made immediately after the melon was cut, and the second a few hours later—when the organism would have had time to establish itself better. We then tried a different approach. We deliberately contaminated the knife with our *S. miami* suspension and cut off another slice of melon and made a culture from that. The idea, of course, was to see if a knife could spread the infection from one melon to another. At that point, we called it a day. For good measure, however, we left the original slice of melon overnight on the laboratory table. Fifteen hours or so at room temperature would give the remaining *S. miami* a really good chance to grow. The following day, we made a culture from that exposed slice.

"We got the first results on Saturday. They weren't exactly discouraging. I went down to the laboratory and read them myself. On the other hand, they fell a bit short of convincing. The first set, made right after the first slice was cut, was practically nothing —just a hint of *S. miami.* There was a little more life in the two other Thursday cultures. They each produced a colony or two. That left the overnight culture. I won't pretend that we waited for Sunday with bated breath. The results of the other cultures were an indication that we might expect something fairly conclusive. So I was fully prepared for the best. But I wasn't prepared for what we actually got. It wasn't just a good solid cluster of colonies. It was any number of colonies—innumerable colonies. It was an *S. miami* metropolis."

[*1961*]

CHAPTER 13

Leaves of Three

THROUGHOUT MOST of temperate North America, *Rhus toxico-dendron* Linnaeus, or poison ivy (or poison oak or poison creeper or climbing sumac or three-leaved ivy), flourishes. It is found from Canada to the West Indies and from Mexico to Maine, and in almost every kind of environment. It grows in boggy glens and upland pastures, in hedgerow thickets and open woods, in cornfields and on ocean dunes, in back yards and city parks, and on railroad rights-of-way. Few plants are less demanding. Its basic needs are a little sun, a little soil, and a little rain—ten inches a year is enough. It is also, with its pale and subtly scented blossoms, its mistletoelike berries, and its gleaming trifoliate leaves—rich copper in early spring, emerald green in summer, mottled pink and yellow in fall—a plant of singular beauty. Indeed, except for its toxic touch it is a thoroughly admirable plant.

The poisonous nature of poison ivy is generally conceded. Only one dissenting opinion is prominently on record, and it is also the earliest known allusion to the plant. It was set down in 1624 by Captain John Smith in his "The Generall Historie of Virginia, New England, and the Summer Isles." "The poysoned weed is

181

much in shape like our English Ivy," he noted, "but being but touched, causeth rednesse, itching, and lastly blisters, the which howsoever after a while passe away of themselves without further harme; yet because for the time they are somewhat painfull, it hath got it selfe an ill name, although questionlesse of no ill nature." Captain Smith's opinion was clearly altogether his own. Not even the aboriginally stoical Indians of his time took so nonchalant a view of poison ivy. The Onondagas called it *ko-hoon-tas*, meaning "stick that makes you sore," and their Cherokee cousins were conciliatory as well as respectful; they always addressed it as "my friend." Captain Smith's assumption that poison ivy is a member of the ivy genus, Hedera, though equally mistaken, is less difficult to understand. It so much looks—and climbs—like ivy that most seventeenth-century authorities made the same assumption. The French botanical explorer Jacques-Philippe Cornut, whose pioneering "Canadensium Plantarum" appeared in 1635, was one of that number. He called it *Hedera trifolia canadensis*. It was not until the middle of the eighteenth century, when the plant came to the more sophisticated attention of Linnaeus, that it found its proper taxonomic niche, as *Rhus toxicodendron*, in the uniformly toxic Anacardiaceae family. Its companions there include the poison sumac, the cashew, the doctor gum, the mango, and the Japanese lacquer tree.

The most distinctive aspect of poison ivy is its leaves. Linnaeus, in his classic study, described them as "three'd, leaflets petioled, egg'd, naked, most intire." It is possible that his familiarity with poison ivy was limited to the inspection of a few dried specimens, but more probable, since poison ivy was cultivated as an eerie curiosity by many European horticulturists in the late seventeenth and early eighteenth centuries, that he had an opportunity to observe the living plant. In any case, it seems certain that he based his description on a rather scanty sampling. For the leaves of poison ivy, as those closer to its native habitat have always been aware, are anything but uniform. "I know few plants the form of whose leaves is so various," Thomas Horsfield, a Pennsylvania physician and the first American to make a comprehensive study of poison ivy, noted in a monograph in 1798. They range in length from one to four or five inches. They are as often elliptical as egg-shaped, and as often hairy as hairless. Moreover, their margins are only sometimes entire, or smooth. This trait varies widely, even on the same plant. Poison-ivy leaves may be lightly saw-edged (like an elm's) or deeply toothed (like a sycamore's) or, occasionally, softly lobed (like certain oaks'). In addition, the plant itself takes different forms. It usually occurs as a low, ground-cover creeper, but it climbs as handily as woodbine or bittersweet, and in richly favorable circumstances it evolves into a bushy waist-high shrub. It may even—to judge from a fourteen-foot specimen found in California—become a tree. The only reliably regular feature of poison ivy is the arrangement of its leaves. They grow in groups of three on a common stem in the form of a fleur-de-lis. It is this telltale characteristic that inspired the warning couplets that are the only celebration of poison ivy in verse:

> Leaves of three,
> Quickly flee.
> Berries white,
> Poisonous sight.

The poison of poison ivy is a phenolic (or carbolic) substance formally known to science as $C_{21}H_{32}O_2$. Its purpose has yet to be established. Some authorities have suggested that it is produced to protect the plant against destruction by herbivorous animals, and some consider it a waste product, but the theory most widely held depicts it as a substance generated at some particular stage of the metabolic process. Since 1896, when its constituents were first identified by Franz Pfaff, an inquiring American physician, it has had a succession of names—toxicodendrol, lobinol, and urushiol. The last of these, and the name now generally preferred, derives from the Japanese "*urushi*," meaning "lacquer," and commemorates an extensive illumination of the identically toxic properties of the Japanese lacquer tree by a group of Japanese research chemists in the early nineteen-twenties. Urushiol, appearing as a sticky, resinous, saplike fluid, is ubiquitously present in poison ivy. It has been found in the leaves, flowers, fruit, twigs, stems, and roots. Its toxicity is as constant as its presence. It is unaffected by age, situation, or season, and it is always high—virulently high. Experiments (by Pfaff and others) have shown that as little as one one-thousandth of a milligram of urushiolic sap will produce a typical dermatitis. Nevertheless, the virulence of poison ivy is more apparent at certain times and places than at others. It is most apparent in the spring, when the plants are young and frail and easily bruised, and the poisonous sap is most readily released. As the season advances, the vulnerable leaves and stems mature and toughen. Those on plants growing in the full light of the sun become particularly tough and resistant to injury. Autumn leaves, wherever grown, are even tougher, and in winter the virulence of poison ivy is confined to the twigs and roots. The virulence of the urushiol itself, however, continues undiminished.

The isolation of urushiol did more than clarify the poisonous nature of poison ivy. It also broadly clarified the nature of poison-ivy poisoning. The most intimate of these secondary elucidations had to do with how poison-ivy poisoning is contracted. Until urushiol was riddled, both science and common sense were sat-isfied that the plant emitted a miasma as pernicious as its touch. Thomas Horsfield discussed this characteristic in his monograph of 1798. "The manner in which the eruption is excited, like its degree of violence, is subject to many variations," he noted. "It is [often] produced by the exhalation of effluvium of the plants. To what distance the exhalation is capable of extending its influence, I have not been able accurately to determine. My observations lead me to believe that in very excitable habits it extends at least to fifteen or twenty feet." A generation later, in 1829, R. Dakin, a New Jersey physician, described much the same phenomenon in a contribution to the *American Journal of the Medical Sciences* entitled "Remarks on a Cutaneous Affection Produced by Certain Poisonous Vegetables." Dakin, who thought he was breaking new ground ("I do not recollect ever having seen a treatise upon the subject"), reported, "It [the cutaneous affection] is contracted by touching certain plants and shrubs, and not improbably, some-times by inhaling, or swallowing with the saliva, the odour arising from them." Even the great Harvard botanist Asa Gray accepted this vaporific notion. "I . . . am very sensitive to the fresh plant," he remarked in a letter to a colleague in 1872. "Then the poison is volatile, as shown by its affecting persons who do not touch it actually." And as late as 1894, in a book called "According to Season," Mrs. William Starr Dana, a popular horticultural writer, warned, "If we are wise we tarry here [near poison ivy] no longer than by the carrion-vine, for the small white flowers, which are now fully open, are said to give forth peculiarly poisonous emanations under the influence of the June sun." The belief that the poison of poison ivy can express itself as a gas has not yet vanished from the earth, but it is no longer sustained by science. Pfaff's historic experiments (and those of many others) have plainly shown that, far from being so helplessly volatile as to vaporize in the heat of the sun, urushiol is among the most stable of substances.

The stability of urushiol both limits and enlarges its range. It enables one to scrutinize or smell or even (if care is taken not to bruise the leaves) handle a poison-ivy plant with impunity, but it has a less attractive side. Burning will destroy the plants in a poison-ivy patch but not their poisonous sap. The poison adheres in almost microscopic droplets to the bits of soot and ash that rise with the smoke, and thus is broadcast through the air. A cloud of poison-ivy smoke can be at least as baleful as a crushed and bleeding plant. ("I was on a railway train which for some reason stopped near where workmen were clearing off a swamp and burning the bogs and brush, which would in this latitude pretty certainly contain a considerable amount of . . . *Rhus*," J. H. Hunt, a Brooklyn physician, reported to the *Brooklyn Medical Journal* in 1897. "The smoke came in through the open car windows, and in about twenty-four hours I began to feel as if I had been sunburned, and swelling and vesication rapidly appeared, so that by the third day I was completely blind from the tumefaction closing my eyelids.") Urushiol is equally impervious to other destructive forces. It is insoluble in water and resistant to drying, and time has little effect on its potency. Poison-ivy leaves have been stored at room temperature for as long as five years without any loss in toxicity, and clothing—sweaters, topcoats, trousers, shoes—accidentally contaminated with poison-ivy sap has retained the power to produce a full-blown dermatitis for well over a year. So have golf balls, garden tools, kites, and the hair of dogs and cats.

Poison-ivy twigs immersed in water have retained their original urushiol vigor for sixteen months. In an experiment described by Walter C. Muenscher and J. M. Kingsbury, of the botany department at Cornell, a quantity of poison ivy was cut and spread out on the roof of a garage. It lay there exposed to the wind and weather for eighteen months. At the end of that time, its sap was found to be as virulent as ever. Another experiment known to Muenscher and Kingsbury would seem to be definitive. It involved a white canvas glove that had been worn during the collection of some poison-ivy plants for laboratory use and then put away in a closet. After an interval of ten months, the glove was brought out and washed for ten minutes in hot water with a strong laundry soap. It was then pressed with a hot iron, dried, and given to a volunteer to handle. The following day, the volunteer developed a classic case of poison-ivy poisoning.

The interval between exposure to poison ivy and the appearance of symptoms varies with the nature of the exposure. In general, the greater the exposure, the more quickly the rash erupts. It usually comes on in about twenty-four hours, but it may show up in ten or twelve hours, or not for two or three days. On the basis of this apparent incubation period, some early American proponents of the germ theory of disease—among them Thomas J. Burrill, a pioneer plant bacteriologist—were inspired to attribute the poisonous action of poison ivy to a microörganism. Burrill has the double distinction of being the first to propose this sinister hypothesis (in a contribution to the *American Naturalist* in 1883) and (in a manly letter to *Garden & Forest* in 1895) the first to withdraw it: "It must be acknowledged that I do not know as much about the matter as I once supposed I did." The reason for the procrastinated onset of poison-ivy poisoning is that the rash is not a superficial irritation. It originates in the epithelial tissue, and to reach that sensitive area the urushiolic sap must penetrate the protective keratin layer that chiefly forms the surface of the skin. There are also other factors that may affect its progress. They include body hair, scars and calluses, and heat. Hair and hardened skin inhibit the absorption of urushiol, but heat appears to promote it. The role of heat in poison-ivy poisoning is another phenomenon whose recognition stems from the isolation of urushiol.

Until then, the effects of the toxin were attributed empirically to sweat. "A state of increased perspiration at the time of exposure to the poison," Thomas Horsfield noted in his monograph, "has a most powerful influence in rendering persons more susceptible of the eruption." Sweat, according to this long-unquestioned view, dissolved the poison and thus hastened its absorption. The truth is very different. Urushiol is no more soluble in sweat than it is in water, but it does dissolve in fats and oils, including those secreted in the skin, and a body temperature high enough to bring on sweating will release these natural solvents. That partly explains the matter. Another and more significant explanation is that heat tends to increase the range of the poison by removing the protection of gloves and shirtsleeves and socks. Nevertheless, for all the protective value of clothes, the extent of poison-ivy poisoning bears little relation to the amount of body surface exposed. "It should be remembered," Bedford Shelmire, professor of dermatology at the Baylor University College of Medicine, told the annual meeting of the American Association for the Study of Allergy in New York City in 1940, "that poison-ivy dermatitis over the face, body, and genitals is usually caused from contact with the patient's own contaminated hands and rarely from direct contact with the plant. The thickness of the epidermis of the palms and palmar surface of the fingers usually inhibits a reaction at these sites. The manual transference of [urushiol] to other areas of the body where the epidermis is thin results in the typical vesicular ivy reaction."

Not everyone who touches poison ivy has the same reaction. People differ greatly in their susceptibility to urushiolic poisoning. Fully confirmed responses range from a tolerance that borders on immunity to a sensitivity so exquisite that the slightest contact is excruciating. These varying reactions were once confidently explained in terms of sex, age, and constitution. Thomas Horsfield was persuaded that "children are more readily poisoned than adults" and that "females are more easily affected than males." He was further inclined to believe that the poison took hold "more readily . . . immediately after than before a full meal." Dakin, in his 1829 report, observed that "susceptibility recedes as age advances," and added, "I do not recollect of ever having seen a pale-looking person poisoned." Later in the nineteenth century, investigators proposed that feeble health was a predisposing factor, that sensitivity increased with weight, and that blonds were more susceptible than brunets. Poison-ivy dermatitis is now defined as an allergy. It is, however, an allergy of a somewhat unusual sort. It differs from the classic allergic diseases (asthma, hay fever, eczema, hives) in two important respects. One is prevalence. At least half the adult population of the United States has a susceptibility to poison-ivy poisoning, while the total of American allergics to the four classic diseases is hardly eleven million. The second difference is that people allergic to urushiol are seldom afflicted with any other allergy. Conventional allergics, on the other hand, are generally prone to more than one allergic disease, and may be subject to many. Yet poison-ivy poisoning is a true allergic disease. It has the definitive characteristics. Like every other allergy, it may involve an inherited predisposition (hence the rugged tolerance that some people manifest), its symptoms appear only after two or more exposures, and frequently repeated exposures tend to sharpen its bite. Few people have any recollection of their first exposure to poison ivy. The reason for this is only partly that it usually occurs in childhood. It is largely because it causes no pain and leaves no visible mark. The first exposure (or, in cases of muted susceptibility, the second or third or tenth) does nothing more than sensitize the skin and render it vulnerable to urushiolic attack. It is the next assault that introduces one to poison-ivy poisoning. Just what produces the symptoms has not yet been established. The most persuasive evidence suggests a specific distortion of the normally protective antigen-antibody reaction. If such is the case, it may help explain the role of heredity in the matter. It may also help account for the equally curious fact that hypersensitivity to poison ivy tends to diminish over the years if further exposure is avoided.

Avoiding poison ivy is one sure way of avoiding poison-ivy poisoning. In fact, for those not endowed with a natural immunity of armor-plate strength and permanence, it is the only way. The belief that immunity can be acquired by chewing or eating poison-ivy leaves is a persistent and pernicious delusion. As recently as

1957, the author of Bulletin 680 ("Poison Ivy") of the University of Missouri College of Agriculture considered it advisable to warn: "An ungrounded and risky bit of folklore . . . is the belief that immunity can be gained by chewing poison-ivy leaves in the spring. This is an extremely dangerous practice." A more rational version of this backwoods expedient involves a course of graduated injections of poison-ivy extract, but (thus far, at least) its results are merely innocuous. Nor are any of the protective salves and ointments perennially on the market any more effective. Their apparent success is only apparent. "Extravagant claims for the value of numerous preparations . . . have been made from time to time, and some of these have their foundation in medical experimentation which seemed at first to show them useful," the Cornell botanists Muenscher and Kingsbury noted in a study. "In such experiments, patients who have had serious cases of ivy poisoning are usually chosen. Such persons usually avoid poison-ivy plants much more carefully than the average person, and any medication that they employ therefore usually appears to be beneficial. No preparation yet discovered . . . completely prevents the occurrence of poison-ivy symptoms in sensitive individuals."

There is also no satisfactory way of dispelling poison-ivy poisoning in sensitive individuals once exposure has occurred. "It may be said that because of the absorbent nature of the skin, all measures to get rid of the poison must be taken immediately," William M. Harlow, professor of wood technology at the New York State College of Forestry, observed in a recent monograph. "None of these measures [including the conventional thorough scrubbing with strong laundry soap], however, appears to be very practical, since those persons who can recognize the poisonous plants avoid them and are not poisoned (except perhaps indirectly), while those who do not [are unaware] that they have contracted the poison until it is much too late to use these remedies." A series of experiments conducted by J. B. Howell, a Dallas clinician, has demonstrated just how little late "too late" may be in poison-ivy prophylaxis. "A fresh poison-ivy leaf was rubbed between the thumb and forefinger of a non-sensitive individual," Howell reported in a communication to the *Archives of Dermatology and Syphilology* in 1943. "[He] then stroked in two places, respectively, the arms of nine sensitive volunteers. After an interval of one minute, one contaminated streak [on each volunteer] was vigorously washed with strong laundry soap, while the other was left as a control. Those mildly sensitive developed no dermatitis on the washed area, those moderately sensitive developed a somewhat reduced reaction, while in the extremely sensitive, there was little if any difference between the reaction developed on the washed and unwashed sites. When a time interval of five minutes elapsed between contact with the contaminated finger and washing, all nine volunteers developed an eruption on both washed and unwashed areas. In four of the patients, washing reduced the severity of the reaction, while in the remaining five, washing made no difference."

There is no specific treatment for poison-ivy poisoning. Once its grip is fixed, the most that medicine can do is help the victim endure it. Certain creams and lotions have certain soothing powers, but the only effective palliative drug is cortisone or one of its numerous derivatives. Cortisone is not, however, a fully sovereign remedy. Its many awkward side reactions, its disruptive impact on pregnancy, and its sinister capacity for intensifying or even reactivating a variety of disorders (tuberculosis, peptic ulcer, hypertension, diabetes, some heart conditions, most psychiatric ailments, and practically all infections) encourage physicians to prescribe it, if at all, with caution. The only safe and sure remedy for poison-ivy poisoning is time. After a while, as Captain John Smith so precociously observed, its symptoms "passe away of themselves." But, as a great many other observers can as accurately testify, their passage is often long and always highly uncomfortable.

One of the most experienced of these observers is a Long Island matron named Eunice Juckett. Mrs. Juckett and her husband, Charles, are both teachers at the East Hamptom high school, and several years ago, when Veterans' Day, November 11th, fell on a Monday, they took advantage of the holiday weekend to drive upstate to the village of Westport, on Lake Champlain, for a visit with Mr. Juckett's parents. Westport is a good ten hours from East Hamptom. The Jucketts left home early Friday afternoon and arrived at Westport around midnight. Saturday was dark and cold, and except for a morning walk through the village, they spent the day indoors. The weather cleared on Sunday, and that afternoon they took a drive in the country. A couple of miles from the village, Mrs. Juckett asked her husband to stop. They were passing a stony field, and the stones looked just right for a rock garden she had in mind to build. (Long Island stones are unsuitably round and smooth—as round and smooth as potatoes.) Mr. Juckett pulled over, and they got out and dug up several suitably angular stones and loaded them into the back of the car. Then they continued their drive. On Monday morning, directly after breakfast, they said their goodbyes and headed for home. They were almost there when Mrs. Juckett became aware of an itch on the underside of her right wrist. She pushed back her coat sleeve and inspected it.

"My heart sank," Mrs. Juckett recalls. "I knew I was in for trouble. I've had poison ivy too many times not to recognize the symptoms. I'm one of those terribly susceptible people. Charlie is the other extreme. Poison ivy doesn't seem to bother him at all. At least, he's never had it. But I was also rather baffled. So was Charlie when I told him. I mean, who ever heard of getting poison ivy in November? Besides, my experience had been that poison ivy showed up within about twenty-four hours of exposure, and I hadn't been out of the house on Sunday except to take a drive. And then I remembered digging up those stones. I hadn't seen any poison ivy there, and you may be sure I looked. I always look. It's an instinct we develop. But now I remembered something. The stones were tangled up in a lot of old roots of some sort, and I'd had to tear them loose. That must have been it—those roots. They must have been poison-ivy roots. Charlie agreed. There just wasn't any other explanation.

"We got home a little after eight. We had supper and unpacked and got ready for bed. By then, of course, the rash had begun to spread. It had spread on up my arm and down between my fingers and across to my other hand. I did what I always do—I got out the calamine lotion. I went to bed itching, but it wasn't too bad. It didn't really keep me awake. I woke up the next morning scratching my ankle. My hands were burning and beginning to swell. Charlie thought I ought to stay home. I wanted to, but I couldn't. I hated to report sick for something like poison ivy. So I went. I hope I never have to endure another day like that. I could feel the poison ivy creeping up my arms and legs. Then, just before noon, my face broke out. I'll never know how I got through the rest of my classes. By the time school was over, I was in absolute agony. I was on fire. I went home and crawled into bed, and Charlie called the doctor.

"I don't remember the next two weeks. I mean that literally. My mind is a total blank about anything that happened. They had me under sedation to keep me from losing my mind. I was poison ivy from head to foot. It covered nine-tenths of my body. My eyes were swollen shut and I could only just open my mouth—they had to feed me through a straw. I couldn't do anything for myself. My mother came over, and the doctor got three nurses to help her. I just lay there wrapped in dressings, and talked. They say I talked incessantly. It was mostly delirium talk—fever talk. I had a temperature at one point of almost a hundred and four. All I do remember is a succession of horrible dreams about spiders and snakes and long, trailing roots and vines. I was flat on my back for almost the whole of November. I didn't get up until just before Thanksgiving. The swelling was gone by then, and also the worst of the rash, and I really felt pretty good. It was another week, though, before I looked presentable."

[*1964*]

CHAPTER 14

In the Bughouse

———◆·◆·◆———

ONE OF THE CONTINUING perplexities of medicine is the nature of epidemics. The epidemic diseases themselves are no longer much of a mystery. Their causes (microbial, fungal, metazoal), their modes of transmission (by respiration, by ingestion, by insect or animal bite), and the means of controlling their spread (immunization, sanitation, isolation) have all been pretty well established. What still remains to be fathomed is the dynamics of the interplay of pathogenic virulence and human susceptibility that determines their comings and goings. It is not yet known just why certain diseases will suddenly appear, rapidly proliferate, and gradually peter out, and then—two years or three years or five years later—as suddenly reappear. It is also unclear just why, as sometimes happens, a disease will simply vanish.

There are several such disappearances reliably on record. Those of leprosy (which ravaged Europe as a plague of pandemic proportions in the thirteenth and fourteenth centuries, and then, in the early sixteenth century, spontaneously withdrew to its native Asia and Africa) and a frequently fatal complex of high fever, prostration, and ubiquitous aches and pains called the sweating sickness (which made five epidemic appearances in England between 1485 and 1551, and has never been heard of there, or anywhere, again) are among the most notorious. Others include scarlet fever (which, after several centuries of epidemic vigor and violence, transformed itself in the nineteen-forties into a generally innocuous disease of almost total immobility), von Economo's encephalitis (which was first described in Rumania in 1915, blazed its way around the world for a decade, and vanished in 1926), and the incomparably savage species of influenza whose only documented visitation was the worldwide epidemic of 1918-19. A more recent member of this fugitive company is a cosmopolitan curiosity variously known as Akureyri disease, benign myalgic encephalomyelitis, epidemic vegetative neuritis, Iceland disease, acute infective encephalomyelitis, atypical poliomyelitis, and epidemic neuromyasthenia. The last of these is the name most epidemiologists prefer.

Epidemic neuromyasthenia, as its name proclaims, is an epidemic disease whose more conspicuous clinical manifestations include a derangement of the nervous system (neuro) and muscular (my) weakness (asthenia). It was first recognized as an entity in Iceland in 1948. In the fall of that year, an epidemic of what appeared to be poliomyelitis broke out in Akureyri, Iceland's second-largest city, and when it finally ended, some four months later, a total of four hundred and sixty-five cases had been reported. An inquiry undertaken early in the outbreak by a team of public-health investigators under Björn Sigurdsson, director of the Institute for Experimental Pathology at the University of Iceland, at once eliminated poliomyelitis as the probable cause of the trouble. In fact, Sigurdsson and his associates noted in a report published in the *American Journal of Hygiene* in 1950, "The clinical and epidemiological characteristics of the Akureyri disease . . . do not fit in well with any of the epidemic diseases with which we are familiar." They then described its several peculiarities: "This disease was characterized by pains in the nape and back, accompanied by fever that was usually low. Paresthesias and hyperesthesias [extremes of skin sensitivity] were common, and approximately 28 per cent of the patients showed muscular paresis [an incomplete paralysis] that usually was light, but in a few cases very severe, and could hardly be distinguished from regular polio-myelitis. The disease, in some cases, ran a rather chronic course in that the fever sometimes lasted for several weeks, and relapses of fever, paresis, and sensibility disturbances were noticed in several instances some weeks after the initial attack. Even the slightest physical exertion or exposure to cold during the earlier stages of illness tended to aggravate the symptoms and bring on new manifestations of the disease. . . . Disturbances such as nervousness, sleeplessness, and loss of memory were rather common complaints after this disease in otherwise normal persons many months after the acute attack." In addition, the investigators pointed out, the Akureyri disease, unlike poliomyelitis, which has a predilection for the very young (most adolescents and adults having acquired a certain immunity), took the great majority of its victims from the teens and twenties, and—as a further distinction from poliomyelitis—none of the cases were fatal. A final reason for supposing the existence of a new disease was provided by the laboratory. Blood and other material taken from patients at various stages of illness were tested for evidence of poliomyelitis and a number of other possibilities—Coxsackie-virus infection, influenza (three strains), equine encephalomyelitis (two strains), St. Louis encephalitis, Japanese B encephalitis, rabies, chorio-meningitis, and Q fever. All the tests were negative.

Sigurdsson's supposition that the disease he and his associates encountered in Akureyri was a new one has been amply confirmed by time. In the fifteen years since their ambiguous find was introduced to medicine in the pages of the *American Journal of Hygiene*, some twenty outbreaks of a disease closely answering its description have been reported in seven widely scattered countries—Australia, Denmark, England, Germany, Greece, the Union of South Africa, and the United States. Time has also shown, however, that the appearance of epidemic neuromyasthenia in Akureyri in 1948 was probably not its first appearance. It was merely the first appearance at which it was confidently recognized as something new and different. Most investigators are now persuaded that its distinctive features can be plainly discerned in at least three earlier epidemic episodes.

The first of these occurred in 1934 in Los Angeles, and affected a hundred and ninety-eight people. All the victims were employees of the Los Angeles County General Hospital, most of them were nurses, and all of them recovered. An investigation of the outbreak was conducted by an assistant surgeon of the United States Public Health Service named A. G. Gilliam, and he recorded his findings in a report somewhat equivocally entitled "Epidemiological Study of an Epidemic, Diagnosed as Poliomyelitis, Occurring Among the Personnel of the Los Angeles County General Hospital During the Summer of 1934." The tone of Gilliam's title reflected that of his report. "Coincidentally with an epidemic of poliomyelitis in the City and County of Los Angeles, Calif., in the summer of 1934, there occurred among the employees of the Los Angeles County General Hospital an epidemic of illness diagnosed at the time as poliomyelitis," he observed in an introductory note. "If this diagnosis may be accepted in any large proportion of the cases, the epidemic is unique in the history of poliomyelitis because of the altogether unusual symptomatology and the extraordinarily high attack rate in an adult population. If the disease was not poliomyelitis, the epidemic is equally extraordinary in presenting a clinical and epidemiological picture which, so far as is known, is without parallel." Gilliam's report included thirty-two detailed clinical portraits, and the reasons for his uncertainty are apparent in any and all of them. Case No. 131 ("W. F., 27, attendant") reads:

On June 18 [the patient] developed a peculiar, diffuse headache which was not particularly severe, and was nauseated and felt generally "rotten" and extremely restless. There was also moderately severe pain along the ulnar distribution of both arms and in both thumbs. The following day her neck and back were definitely stiff. While working, she found that her arms were generally weak and she could hardly lift a baby or carry a tray, so she was admitted to the hospital. Physical examination confirmed the stiff neck and back and also discovered tenderness in the right deltoid, biceps, and right thigh. The temperature was 99.4° (the highest during this hospitalization). . . . The patient vomited after admission. On June 20, orthopedic examination revealed "numerous muscle groups weak or tender"; she was placed on a Bradford frame with all extremities immobilized. . . . She stated she was delirious during the day. . . . About June 24, severe muscle twitching, cramps, and pain developed, and lasted 10 days. She also had peculiar position sensations: "the feet felt like they were clear across the room" and she "couldn't wriggle the toes"; "when the eyes were closed, I felt like I was falling." Orthopedic note states on June 29, "muscles of the left arm normal; lower extremities tender; muscles right arm still tender." . . . Routine physiotherapy muscle tests being completely normal on July 12 and July 19, the patient was discharged on the latter date. Following her discharge, she had repeated episodes of terrific headache, fever, chills, vomiting, general aches and pains, and stiff neck, and she spent most of the time in bed at home. On September 18 she was readmitted, because, in addition to the general symptoms, she developed painful, burning urination. Her temperature had been recorded on the outside as 101° but the highest while hospitalized was 100°. No muscle weakness was detected on careful muscle check, but hospitalization was continued until October 30 because of intermittent headache, pain, general malaise, and nervousness. Following discharge, she had frequent insomnia, headache, and nervousness, and easy fatigue and calf pain after exertion. These symptoms gradually disappeared and she was considered able to return to duty on December 30.

Gilliam was nevertheless inspired to end his report on a somewhat more positive note. "Despite the peculiar clinical character of many of these cases," he wrote, "there appear to be good grounds for assuming that the majority of them resulted from infection with the virus of poliomyelitis."

The other earlier outbreaks that hindsight has identified as epidemic neuromyasthenia occurred near Fond du Lac, Wisconsin, in 1936, and in Harefield, England, in 1939. The scene of the Fond du Lac outbreak was a Roman Catholic convent, and thirty-five girls between the ages of fourteen and twenty-one were involved, all of them novices or postulants. The cause of the trouble was thought at first to be some form of encephalitis, and the United States Public Health Service was so informed. The symptoms, as reported to the Surgeon General by a Public Health Service investigator named Charles A. Armstrong, were rich and varied—chills and fever, headache, sore throat, pain in the back and chest, sweating of the hands and feet, tingling in the hands and feet, leg pain, difficulty in moving the legs, ringing in the ears, dizziness, confusion, apathy—but the picture they presented was diagnostically opaque. Armstrong could find no convincing evidence of encephalitis or of any other disease he knew, and he frankly acknowledged defeat: "The condition . . . is not explainable on the basis of any infection or intoxication with which I am familiar." The Harefield outbreak occurred in a hospital—the Harefield Sanatorium—and it felled a total of seven. All were women, all were young, all were nurses. Their complaints included fatigue, sore throat, muscular aches and pains, paresis, muscle cramps, nausea, urinary retention, depression, and nervous tension. As usual, they all recovered. In a report to the *Lancet*, entitled "Persistent Myalgia Following Sore Throat," two members of the sanatorium staff attributed the outbreak to "an unidentified virus."

The exhumation of these early outbreaks does more than simply swell the list of the probable appearances of epidemic neuromyasthenia. It serves to further document two singular aspects of the disease. One, of course, is its striking predilection for young women. The other is its almost equally striking predilection for closed, or cloistered, communities. Of twenty-four accepted outbreaks of epidemic neuromyasthenia, ten have occurred in hospitals and among hospital personnel, one (at Fond Du Lac) in a convent and one (in Germany) in an Army barracks, and in many of the others there were doctors and nurses among the victims. Thirty-four of the four hundred and sixty-five victims in Akureyri were students at a boarding school.

Ten epidemics of epidemic neuromyasthenia have been reliably recorded in the United States since its discovery at Akureyri. They have ranged in size from an outbreak of seven cases (in Pittsfield and Williamstown, Massachusetts, in 1956) to an explosion (in Tallahassee, Florida, in 1954) that totalled four hundred and fifty. The first of the ten (nineteen cases, fifteen of them young women) occurred in Alexandria Bay, in northern New York; in the late summer of 1950, or only a few weeks after the publication of the Akureyri study. Its resemblance to the disease described by Sigurdsson and his associates was almost immediately apparent, and this prompted two physicians of the area—D. Naldrett White and Robert B. Burtch—to write an account of the visitation. Their paper, entitled "Iceland Disease: A New Infection Simulating Acute Anterior Poliomyelitis," appeared in *Neurology* in 1954, and was the first corroborative celebration of Sigurdsson's discovery. The most recent American outbreak of any considerable size occurred at Punta Gorda, Florida, in 1956. It is also the only one of any considerable size that the United States Public Health Service has had an opportunity to investigate thoroughly.

The Punta Gorda epidemic came to the attention of the United States Public Health Service by way of a request for help from an epidemiologist on the staff of the Florida State Board of Health named James Bond. His request, as is customary in such cases, was addressed to the chief of the Epidemic Intelligence Service at the Communicable Disease Center of the U.S.P.H.S., in Atlanta. In 1956, that was Donald A. Henderson. Dr. Henderson (now an executive of the Epidemiology Branch at the C.D.C.) found it on his desk on the morning of Wednesday, May 9th.

"Dr. Bond's letter didn't tell us very much," Dr. Henderson says. "It was just a note. He was reporting sixty-four cases of what he called Iceland disease. The term 'epidemic neuromyasthenia' hadn't yet come into general use. The outbreak had begun in the early part of March, and he had been on the scene for about a week. He would be grateful for any advice or assistance we might be able to give him. That was about the gist of it. But it was quite enough to arouse my interest. I'd never seen a case of epidemic neuromyasthenia, but I knew about it. I'd read the literature. And I knew that Bond knew what he was talking about. He'd been in on the big outbreak of epidemic neuromyasthenia down in Tallahassee a couple of years before. So I put in a call to Bond at his office in Jacksonville. We had a little talk, and he told me what he could. All but one of the cases were women—white women— and their ages ranged from thirty to sixty. The other case was a seventy-year-old man—also white. Punta Gorda was a predominantly white community. It had a population of around three thousand, only about five hundred of them Negroes. The town was situated on the southwest coast, on Charlotte Harbor, and was the seat of Charlotte County. It was a shrimp-fishing port, with some farms and cattle ranches inland, and it drew a few vacationers in the winter. It had a twenty-three-bed hospital and three practicing physicians, and it was on their appeal that Bond had come into the case. The clinical picture was almost exactly what he had seen in the Tallahassee outbreak. The principal presenting symptoms were recurrent sharp pains in the muscles of the back and neck, severe headache, disturbances of coördination, and some transient motor and sensory dysfunctions. Plus a strong emotional overlay —tension, anxiety, depression. The physical findings were essentially unimportant, and the results of certain routine laboratory tests had all been within the normal range. At the moment, the situation was stable—no new cases in almost a week. Well, that suggested that maybe the outbreak was waning. If so, there was no particular hurry about our getting down there, since the best time to carry out an investigation is during the acute epidemic phase. When that phase has passed, time is not of critical importance. I was disappointed, of course, but I was also rather relieved. An immediate investigation would have imposed a bit of a strain. We were very shorthanded right then, and our annual Epidemic Intelligence Service conference was coming up in a couple of weeks. So I proposed a visit in June. Bond thought that would do very well. Meanwhile, he said, he would keep me in touch with developments.

"Which he did. And very promptly. I got a call from Bond the following week—the following Wednesday, in fact. The wane had turned out to be only a lull. Five new cases had just been reported. He thought we might want to make a change in our plans. The best I could manage was a compromise. We were still shorthanded, but no longer desperately so. I had an investigator more or less available—a young E.I.S. physician named David C. Poskanzer. I said I would get him off as quickly as possible. I got him off on Sunday, and he was down in Punta Gorda most of the week. That was the week before the E.I.S. conference. Poskanzer returned to Atlanta on Friday, and his report was a feature of the meeting. One thing that particularly struck him about the disease was its enormous and confusing array of symptoms. They were protean—absolutely protean. He stressed that over and over again. I thought I knew what he meant. That is, the point had been emphasized in all the literature I'd read. But I was mistaken. The symptomatology of epidemic neuromyasthenia is extremely hard to picture. You really have to see it for yourself.

"Well, I got to see it a few days later. Once the conference was out of the way, I was free to recruit a team for a real investigation —a comprehensive clinical and epidemiological study. I didn't need an army. I knew from Bond and Poskanzer that we could count on a lot of local help. The team I picked consisted of Poskanzer and me and two others. They were E. Charles Kunkle, a professor of neurology at Duke University School of Medicine who also serves as a Public Health Service consultant, and Seymour S. Kalter, the chief of the diagnostic-methodology unit of the virus-and-rickettsia section of our Laboratory Branch. Kalter, Poskanzer, Kunkle, and I got to Punta Gorda on Sunday, May 27th, and checked into a motel that Poskanzer knew about. Then we had a meeting with Bond and the local physicians, and on Monday morning we got to work. We stayed at Punta Gorda four days—through Thursday. That was our first visit. One of the characteristics of epidemic neuromyasthenia is a prolonged and relapsing course. We learned that early on. A patient seems to shake it off, and then it comes back again. So we made two followup visits to see it through to the end. We returned for two days in October, and again, for another two days, in November of the following year.

"I think, on the whole, the study was worth the time and effort. It was well worth it. All the same, it was a bit maddening. We learned everything, and nothing. The point is, though, we had everything *to* learn. We were up against a new disease, and essentially still a completely mysterious one. The literature—the earlier studies—hadn't done much more than establish it as an entity. That gave our investigation a very special character. Diagnosis is the key in most investigations. Once that is accomplished, the rest is usually only a matter of time. The cause is implicit in the nature of the disease, and the cause suggests the source of the trouble. It tells us what to look for and where. In this case, we had a diagnosis —a kind of diagnosis—but it told us hardly anything. It was only a name—a label. We had to begin at the absolute bottom. First of all, we had to examine the diagnosis. We had to determine whether a specific disease entity was actually present in epidemic form. That involved the phenomen that Poskanzer had stressed at the conference—the enormous and confusing array of symptoms. The significant symptoms had to be determined and the clinical picture clearly defined. Then we had to determine the scope of the outbreak. The next step was to determine the cause and the source of the trouble.

"Nobody seriously questioned the presence of an epidemic in Punta Gorda. The local medical records showed that, beginning around the end of February, a gradually increasing number of mostly women patients had been observed and hospitalized with a complex of more or less prostrating symptoms that seemed to fit the entity we now call epidemic neuromyasthenia. There was a total of sixty-nine such patients on record at the time of our arrival. About thirty of them were still sick, and from that group we selected twenty-one cases—seventeen women and four men— for definitive clinical analysis. At the same time, with the help of neighborhood volunteers, we organized a house-to-house survey in order to get a clearer notion of the actual incidence and distribution of the illness. Medical records are only an indication of the scope of an epidemic. There are always a number of victims who can't or won't see a doctor. This was particularly true in Punta Gorda. Our interviewers visited nearly four hundred homes and talked to more than a thousand people, and they turned up sixty-two additional cases. They were very definitely cases, too. The interviewers accepted as cases only those that met a fairly rigid set of criteria. These criteria were our own, developed from our preliminary clinical findings, and they established three diagnostic points. A definite change in physical or emotional status, or both, indicating an onset of illness—that was the first criterion. The second was an illness of at least seven days. The third was the presence of at least six out of nine relevant symptoms of recent occurrence or exacerbation. They were fatigue, neck pain, headache, aching-limb pain, loss of appetite, nausea, impairment of memory, depression, and paresthesia. I was in on several of the interviews, and I can testify that we managed to get the facts— one way or another. I remember one case in point. It was a preacher—white, middle-aged, and married. His wife had been eliminated—no significant symptoms—but we weren't quite sure about him. He had been sick, and his symptoms were generally provocative. Except on the emotional side. He insisted that there was nothing wrong with his mind or his memory. As we rose to go, the interviewer asked him if she could have a glass of water. Of course, he said, and left the room. But almost at once he was back. The interviewer had asked him for something—what was it? She told him. Oh, yes. He started out of the room again, and then stopped and called upstairs to his wife. Where did they keep the ice cubes? She told him, and he went on out to the kitchen. But a moment later he called her again. This time he wanted to know just how many cubes should go in the glass. We added him to the case list.

"I called our criteria fairly rigid. That's all they were, I'm afraid. They were as rigid as we could possibly make them, and I think they were reasonably effective, but they fell a bit short of scientific excellence. Epidemic neuromyasthenia is a most ungrateful disease in that respect. Its manifestations are subjective rather than objective. It produces all kinds of symptoms but—to the best of our present knowledge—very few signs. That was the first and possibly the most important thing we learned from our twenty-one detailed clinical studies. There was practically nothing that we could see or touch or measure. I mean, there were no lesions to examine, no big livers or tender spleens to feel, no jaundice, no classically paralyzed limbs, no cloudy chest X-rays, no laboratory data to analyze. We used to sit in my room at the motel after dinner and puzzle it over and over. None of us had ever seen anything like it. We just couldn't put it together. It was bizarre. Even the signs that did turn up were fantastic. Most of the patients complained of paresthesia—areas of decreased or increased skin sensitivity. They could generally guide us to the specific patch, and when the patch was on the back—out of the patient's sight—we always marked it in color. The next day, we would question the patient again, and invariably he guided us to a different—an unmarked—area. But the curious thing was that none of the areas encompassed by these paresthesias corresponded to any recognized area innervated by a nerve or nerves. One woman patient complained of nodules on her arms. We looked where she told us to look, but there was nothing there that we could see or feel—no sign of any kind of lump. That's funny, she said, they *were* there. She said she knew because the site was still tender. We humored her. We asked her to let us know if and when another nodule appeared, and we went on to the next examination. She called us the very next day. She had another nodule. We trotted around to her room, and—holy Christmas! She was right. She did have a nodule. In fact, there were two of them—little pea-sized swellings on the underside of her left wrist. There was no discoloration, but they were sensitive to the touch. Or so she said. Well, this was getting interesting. It seemed possible that we were on to something that the laboratory could test and maybe identify. We persuaded her to let us take a sliver of one of the nodules for a biopsy examination, and one of the hospital staff came in and did the job. But, oh dear!—he didn't go deep enough, and nothing showed up. That was a crushing defeat. It was maddening. Because that was the end of her nodules. They never came back. I tell you, we began to feel that we were living in the bughouse.

"The bughouse possibility actually occurred to us. We simply couldn't put together a pathophysiological explanation. We got no help from the laboratory, and the results of our physical examinations were just as useless. That left us with nothing to go on but the histories—what the patients themselves could tell us. And the more of their complaints we heard, the more we began to wonder about a functional explanation. So many of the symptoms were psychoneurotic symptoms. I'll give you an example—a more or less typical case. She was a young unmarried woman, a beautician by trade, and one of our twenty-one closely studied cases. The course of her illness was especially characteristic. It came on quite insidiously toward the end of April. There was a gradual onset of fatigue, accompanied by intermittent headache and neck pain. At about the same time, she became aware of a peculiar sensation in her right leg. It felt numb and weak, and every now and then she seemed to stumble. She began to feel clumsy at her work, and her hands began to shake. It got harder and harder for her to write. Then her memory began to fail. She would forget the names of her regular customers, and she couldn't remember what to charge for the various regular services. That went on for about a month.

Then, suddenly, her headache and neck pain increased in severity, and she developed a crippling backache. Her headache was practically prostrating. So she went to see a doctor. She described the symptoms I've mentioned, and added that she felt as if she were shaking all over inside. Four days later, she developed diarrhea, nausea and vomiting, and vertigo, and was hospitalized. She remained in the hospital a month. During that time, she complained of a feeling of choking, difficulty in swallowing, and hyperventilation—the feeling of being unable to take a deep breath. She complained of pain around her eyes and intermittent double vision. There were times when it seemed to her that her heart doubled or tripled its beat. She constantly complained of fatigue and depression, and she often cried without provocation. She also complained of swellings in her arms and legs, her abdomen, and her face, but there was no objective evidence of this. Nor was there any apparent explanation of her trouble in swallowing or in taking a deep breath, and there was no electrocardiographic confirmation of her accelerated heartbeat. The only positive physical finding was tenderness in two small areas in her back. She was given aspirin for her headache and other pains, but it didn't seem to do much good. Around the end of June, she began to improve, and she was discharged to convalesce at home. We got the next installment of the story when we saw her again in October. For about a week after her discharge, she seemed to be almost well. And then she had a relapse. All her symptoms recurred, and she was laid up in bed at home for three weeks. In August, she again felt better, and returned to work. Her headaches and neck pains continued intermittently, and the slightest exertion exhausted her. She needed at least ten hours of sleep every night, and she took a nap every afternoon. Her most disabling complaint, however, was depression. She was still depressed when we saw her that October, and her mind was conspicuously slowed. She was unable to perform various simple tests—repeating a set of five numbers in reverse, or subtracting serially from one hundred. There was also still some tenderness in her back, and we noted a slight insensitivity to pain in her lower right leg. Her difficulties in mentation were a bit equivocal. This was true, of course, in most of the other cases, too. We had no basis for comparison. It was quite possible that her memory was normally bad. And maybe she was just naturally a bit thick in the head. But the third visit cleared that up. When we saw her in November of the following year, she was fully herself again. And she was a conspicuously bright young woman.

"You can see why the possibility of a psychoneurotic explanation came so readily to mind. Every symptom that poor woman had was conceivably psychogenic, and the same was true of the symptoms of all the other cases. Depression. Terrifying dreams. Crying without provocation. Nausea and headache and diarrhea. Back and neck pains. Imaginary fever. Problems of memory and mentation. Vertigo. Hyperventilation. Menstrual irregularities. Difficulty in swallowing. Fatigue. Fast heart. Imaginary swellings. Paresthesia. And paresis. But paresis of a very curious sort—an unwillingness, rather than an inability, to move an arm or a leg. Almost a fear of movement. It was like a hysterical paralysis. But there are no waves or epidemics of hysterical paralysis. They simply don't happen. And that was the trouble with a psychoneurotic explanation of the epidemic. There were plenty of psychoneurotic symptoms, but they weren't enough in themselves to support a mass-reaction hypothesis. There was, in fact, every objection to such an explanation. For one thing, so far as we could discover, nothing had happened in Punta Gorda that could have excited a mass reaction. For another, the separate illnesses appeared at scattered intervals. That was clearly spelled out in the histories of both the reported cases and those we turned up in the house-to-house survey. The illnesses were scattered all the way from February to June. Moreover—and this is most significant—there was hardly a ripple of apprehension among the general population of the town. Nobody even suggested that the schools be closed. Or the movies or the beaches or anything. Nobody seemed in the least alarmed by what was going on. It was just the reverse of a panic situation.

"So we dropped the bughouse theory. But if it wasn't a question of mass-reaction hysteria, what *was* the anatomy of the epidemic? We went to work on the possible sources of trouble. Could it be something transmitted by insects? Most of the recorded outbreaks of epidemic neuromyasthenia had occurred in the insect season.

But the answer here was no. There had been few mosquitoes or any other possible insect vectors in Punta Gorda until the second half of April, and the epidemic was well under way by then. We checked the usual urban sources of mass illness—the drinking water, the milk, the general food supply, the beaches. The answer again was negative. There wasn't a hint of contamination anywhere. We considered the possibility of a toxic product of some sort. We searched the case histories for some provocative coincidence—the common use of a certain cosmetic or household chemical. But nothing came of that, either. There weren't any likely links. There was no single factor of any kind uniquely common to the group affected. The only kind of coincidence we found was one for which the literature had rather explicitly prepared us. That was a disproportionately high rate of illness among hospital and medical personnel. The attack rate for the general adult population was around six percent—which, by the way, is quite high. But it was *forty-two* percent for the hospital and medical people. Sixteen of a total of thirty-eight doctors, nurses, technicians, and hospital receptionists, cooks, maids, and janitors were on our roll of cases.

"We were left with one possibility. It was also, of course, the likeliest explanation. The pattern of the epidemic, the apparent absence of any common exposure factors, and the high incidence of illness among medical and hospital personnel were consistent only with an infectious disease transmitted from person to person. Just how the microörganism responsible might travel from one person to another was not at all clear. It is still wide open to conjecture. We were able, however, to postulate the general nature of the microörganism. It was probably a virus. It almost certainly wasn't one of the rickettsia. We did laboratory studies for all known rickettsial agents, and they were negative. Besides, the symptoms were wrong—most rickettsial diseases are characterized by high fever and a rash. Moreover, most of them are insect-borne. And it probably wasn't a bacterium. The laboratory studies were uniformly negative. It's true that they were negative for viruses as well as for bacteria, but the techniques for detecting bacteria are far better than those for detecting viruses. There is, of course, the possibility that the infection in epidemic neuromyasthenia may occur quite early on and that by the time the patient sees a doctor he has stopped excreting the organism. That's not unheard of, you know. It happens in several virus diseases. And rheumatic fever follows a precipitating streptococcal infection by as much as a month. So does acute glomerulonephritis. Nevertheless, if bacteria were involved, the chances are that we would have got something growing in the laboratory. Some hint of something would have sooner or later shown up. But not with a virus. The viruses are different. It's hard enough to find them in the best of circumstances. There are virus diseases in which no detectable change occurs in the white-blood-cell count, and they're extremely hard to cultivate. They're extremely numerous, too. Umpteen new ones are discovered every year.

"There was a certain satisfaction in forming that hypothesis. It's nice to come to even the most tentative conclusion. One gets a sense of accomplishment. But it wasn't much of a comfort. I mean, it didn't really explain a thing. The case was still a mystery. As a matter of fact, it was more than that. It was eerie. There's something a bit unnerving about a new communicable disease— a disease whose cause and means of transmission are essentially unknown. I'll never forget the end of that first visit to Punta Gorda. We were able to relax later on, but we didn't know about that yet. It was the only time I've ever felt uneasy after an investigation about going straight home to my wife. For all I knew, I might have been exposed to epidemic neuromyasthenia, and I was worried about passing it on to her. I actually considered stopping over somewhere for several days and waiting to see what happened. The reason I didn't was that the incubation period was also a total mystery. I didn't know how long it would be advisable to wait.

"And yet, by the end of the investigation—by the end of our third and final visit—we did have a real sense of satisfaction. We could truthfully say that we had accomplished something. Our work here at the C.D.C. is with communicable disease. We want to know all we can about it. And now we had had the experience of studying an outbreak of a new and mysterious communicable disease in detail. Reading about a disease is hardly the same as actually working on it. There's obviously a world of difference. We still know painfully little about epidemic neuromyasthenia, but Punta Gorda gave us at least some sense of what it is and what it isn't. We'll know it the next time we see it. And we'll have some new approaches to employ. It is now perfectly clear that medical and hospital people are especially vulnerable to epidemic neuromyasthenia, so we'll concentrate on them. We'll get to them as early as possible, we'll keep them under the closest possible observation, and we'll recover every possible specimen for laboratory study. In other words, we're ready and waiting. But we have been for quite a few years, and I must say I'm beginning to wonder. I wonder if there will ever be a next time. The last reported outbreaks of epidemic neuromyasthenia occurred in 1958 in Athens, and in a convent up in New York State in 1961. Neither of them was recognized for what it was until it had almost run its course. We haven't heard even a decent rumor of it since then. It seems to have disappeared."

[*1965*]

AUTHOR'S NOTE: It has not disappeared. There have been several reported outbreaks of what appeared to investigators to be epidemic neuromyasthenia since 1961—in a factory in Franklin, Kentucky, in 1965; in Galveston County, Texas, in 1967; in a convent in Montgomery County, Pennsylvania, in 1967; in Virginia, in 1979; and in Fort Myers, Florida, 1980. The diagnosis of epidemic neuromyasthenia is difficult. This is because it is primarily one of exclusion. I have had letters from a number of people, mostly women, who believed they were suffering from epidemic neuromyasthenia. But the disease remains essentially as mysterious as ever.

CHAPTER 15

Shiver and Burn

———————◆—◆—◆———————

IT BEGAN WITH a touch of malaise. Mrs. Walter Wells (as I'll call her), the eighteen-year-old daughter of a recently retired Army sergeant, and the recent bride of a vacuum-cleaner salesman, woke up that morning—Saturday morning, May 22, 1965—at her home in Cataula, Georgia, a village some ten miles north of Columbus, feeling tired and achy and listless. Her husband was sympathetic and encouraging. He said it was nothing to worry about. She had probably been working too hard. That, she knew, was true enough. She *had* been working hard. She and her husband had only just moved to Cataula. Her father, a widower, had been stationed at Fort Benning, about five miles south of Columbus, and until April 15, when he retired from the service and moved to Florida, they had shared his quarters there. The move and the job of getting resettled had been exhausting work. Her husband was right; she was probably a little run-down, and she would take it easy for a while. She did, but her indisposition persisted. She felt no better the following day, or on Monday, or Tuesday, or Wednesday. On Thursday, she began to feel worse. She felt cold, and then flushed and hot. She took her temperature; it was 101 degrees. An hour later, it had risen to almost 102. Then it began to fall, and by evening it was back to normal. It was normal all the next day. Even the dragging malaise seemed to have lifted at last. For the first time in a week, she felt almost well. But the day after that—on Saturday, May 29—her temperature rose again. When her husband came in from a round of afternoon calls, it had climbed past 103. It was also well beyond any easy explanation. He went to the telephone and called the doctor.

The doctor whom Wells called was a general practitioner in Columbus whose name, I'll say, is John Henry Page. As it happened, however, Dr. Page was out of town that day, and the call was taken by an associate in the emergency room at St. Francis Hospital in Columbus. The nature of Mrs. Wells's illness, as her husband described it, was not at all clear to the doctor, but high fever is always decisive, and he told Wells to bring her right in. She arrived with a temperature of just under 103. The only other physical abnormality that a preliminary examination showed was some tenderness over the lower abdomen. That, together with the high fever, suggested the possibility of an infection in that area. So did her history. The doctor gathered from Mrs. Wells that some months before—in July 1964—she had been treated at the Martin Army Hospital, at Fort Benning, for a urinary-tract infection of some kind. This, it seemed quite possible, might be a recurrence of that.

Dr. Page took over the case on Sunday morning. He found Mrs. Wells sitting up comfortably and looking far from seriously ill. She said she felt pretty good, and her temperature was down to normal. The absence of fever was an acceptable surprise. A glance at the record showed him that she had been treated with tetracycline at the time of admission, and tetracycline has the power to promptly lower fever (by destroying its microbial cause). An examination of her lower abdomen was additionally corroborative: it was still tender—exquisitely tender. Dr. Page saw no reason to dispute his associate's definition of her trouble. The signs and symptoms were all generally consistent with a urinary-tract infection. On Monday, however, her familiar discomforts returned. She felt chilly and full of fugitive aches and pains, and her temperature began to climb. It climbed to 103. But it was back to normal on

Tuesday, and so was Mrs. Wells. Then, on Wednesday, her temperature rose again. It continued to fluctuate like that. It was up one day and down the next, and when it was down she felt fully recovered. She felt so well that she wanted to get up and go home. Dr. Page sat down in perplexity and reviewed the clinical and laboratory records of the case. There was nothing in either to explain its peculiar progress. The next time she asked to be discharged, he shrugged and made the necessary arrangements. It was not an unreasonable decision. A week of hospital care and treatment had achieved no apparent results. That was one reason. Another was that Mrs. Wells could not afford an indefinite hospital stay. She had no kind of hospitalization insurance. Before she departed, however, Dr. Page stopped by with a word or two of advice. He hoped she was on the road to recovery, but, in his opinion, she hadn't reached it yet. He wanted her to rest as much as possible, and he wanted her to keep a close watch on her temperature. If she had another attack of fever, he wanted to know at once.

Mrs. Wells was discharged from St. Francis Hospital on Wednesday, June 9. Three days later, on Saturday afternoon, she telephoned Dr. Page at his office. She reminded him that he had asked her to call if her fever came back. Well, it had. To tell the truth, she had felt a little feverish on Thursday, but— Anyway, this was different. She had just taken her temperature, and it was almost 103. Dr. Page heard her with more sympathy than surprise. He had half expected such a call. He gave a reassuring grunt, and told her not to worry. Nevertheless, he added, it seemed inadvisable for her to stay on at home. Didn't she agree? Very well. He wanted her back in the hospital that evening—in the Columbus Medical Center hospital this time. Mrs. Wells was admitted there at about six o'clock. Her temperature had dropped somewhat by then. The hospital reading was 100.8. The only other physical abnormality noted at the admission examination was continued abdominal tenderness. There was thus, as far as Dr. Page could see, no reason to revise his earlier diagnosis. Mrs. Wells still appeared to be the victim of a urinary-tract infection. He did, however, choose to revise his therapeutic attack. Instead of tetracycline, he prescribed a course of sulfisoxazole and chloramphenicol. They seemed, temporarily, effective. Mrs. Wells felt pretty well on Sunday, and her temperature was normal all day. But the following day, as so often before, the chills and fever and aches and pains returned. And the day after that, as equally often before, the symptoms all vanished. The results of the usual laboratory tests were also consistently uninstructive. Mrs. Wells's white-blood-cell count was 9500—a trifle high, but normal. Her hemoglobin levels were 10.2 and 9.5 grams percent—a trifle low, and indicative of some anemia. Her urine contained a few white blood cells, but not enough to be of any pathological significance. Toward the end of the week, another round of standard tests was made. With one exception, the immediate results were exactly as before. The exception was an insignificant decline in Mrs. Wells's white-blood-cell count.

That was on Friday, June 18. The next afternoon, Dr. Page received at his office a call from the Medical Center. His caller was the hospital pathologist. He was calling, he said, to make an addition to the laboratory report on Mrs. Wells. One of the laboratory technicians had been inspired to take a closer microscopic look at a sample of her blood. The pathologist cleared his throat.

"You know what that girl's got?" he said.

"I don't guess I do," Dr. Page said. "What?"

"She's got malaria."

"*Malaria?*"

"Malaria."

"No kidding," Dr. Page said. "Well, golly Pete."

"I'm sending a blood sample down to Fort Benning for a confirmatory study," the pathologist said, "but there's no doubt about it. It's malaria. I looked at the smear myself."

"You know something?" Dr. Page said. "I'll bet my granddaddy is squirming in his grave. My daddy, too, for that matter. They wouldn't know what to make of me. I mean, they both would have had her diagnosed by at least the second day. But I've never seen a case of malaria before."

Malaria (or ague, or marsh fever, or jungle fever, or Roman fever, or Cameroon fever, or Corsican fever, or intermittent fever, or paludism) is probably the greatest of the great pestilential fevers. It is certain that no other infectious disease has caused so much misery to so many millions of people for so many thousands of years. It is equally certain that none has had so great an impact on the course of human history. Malaria has changed the direction of history on innumerable occasions. It was largely responsible for the periodic decline of civilization in ancient Mesopotamia, and for the physical, intellectual, and moral debilitation that toppled Attic Greece and Imperial Rome. It was malaria that caused the death of Alexander the Great at thirty-three, at the apex of his conquest of Asia. Endemic malaria held back for many years the construction of the Panama Canal, and because it finally yielded to American rather than to French control, it made possible the precocious preeminence of the United States in Central American affairs. And it was chiefly because of malaria that Black Africa is still predominantly black. It made West and Central Africa the celebrated "white man's grave" of mid-Victorian lore.

The cause of malaria is a tiny protozoan microbe of the genus *Plasmodium*. Four species of this influential parasite find the human body a satisfactory habitat. They are *Plasmodium vivax*, *Plasmodium falciparum*, *Plasmodium malariae,* and *Plasmodium ovale.* The human body is not, however, their only dwelling place. They require for the full development of their parasitical potentialities a certain period of residence in the body of one or another of the sixty or seventy members of the ubiquitous *Anopheles* genus of mosquitoes. That is where they manifest the sexual side of their nature. It is also where most biographers of *P. vivax* and its fellow-plasmodia choose to open their inspection of the organism. The microbe reaches there in a droplet of blood drawn by a female anopheles (anopheline males are vegetarian) from some malarial man. The mating of male and female plasmodia occurs in the stomach of the mosquito, and at once. The ultimate progeny of this urgent, if haphazard, union are sporelike organisms called sporozoites. After two or three weeks, they gravitate by the thousand to stations in the salivary glands of the mosquito. From there, when next the mosquito feeds on human blood, they somehow insinuate themselves into the body of its victim. Once adrift in the bloodstream, these immigrant sporozoites move briskly with the circulation to a lodging in the functional cells of the liver. A leisurely period (six to twelve days) of growth and multiplication (by simple division) ensues. The fruits of this sojourn then burst from the ravaged cells and plunge into the bloodstream again. Some of these multitudes are recalled by chance or atavistic instinct to the liver, but most of them establish themselves in the red blood cells and settle down to another period of parasitic gourmandizing and asexual reproduction. This period, like the liver stage, ends with the disintegration of the victimized cells and the release of another generation of avid young plasmodia. It is the aim of each of these creatures to find and quickly penetrate another red blood cell and there repeat its reproductive cycle, but only a fraction succeed in doing so. About ninety percent of them are overwhelmed and destroyed by certain cells known as macrophages that the body summons into defensive action. Nevertheless, enough plasmodia survive this and subsequent macrophage attacks to ensure an almost infinite continuation of their red-cell reproductive cycle. Three or four cycles, however, are usually sufficient to complete the evolution of the organism. The third or fourth cycle produces, in addition to the usual red-cell parasites, a number of sexually differentiated plasmodia. It is the chance ingestion of these fully evolved plasmodia by a feeding anopheles that perpetuates malaria.

Although all plasmodia are equally bound to this stylized mode of life, the different species follow it in somewhat different ways. Their differences in man are most pronounced in the red-cell reproductive stage. One point of difference is the age of the cell they choose to parasitize. *P. vivax* confines its insinuations to young and newly fabricated cells. So, it is believed, does *P. ovale*. *P. malariae*, on the other hand, is partial to cells that have reached maturity. Red blood cells of any age are acceptable to *P. falciparum*. Another difference in the species is their reproductive rate. *P. vivax* produces an average of sixteen new organisms in each invaded cell, but the average for *P. ovale* and *P. malariae* is only eight, and *P. falciparum* produces variously from eight to twenty-four. A third difference is in the length of the reproductive cycle. It ranges from between thirty-six and forty-eight hours for *P. falciparum*, through forty-eight hours for *P. vivax* and *P. ovale*, to seventy-two hours for *P. malariae*. These differences, though unimposing, are not without significance. They have sufficient impact to shape four more or less distinctive varieties of malaria.

The immediate cause of the clinical symptoms of malaria appears to be an acute intoxication. It is precipitated by the explosive end of the red-cell reproductive cycle and the sudden flooding of the bloodstream with obnoxious foreign protein—swarms of new plasmodia and cellular flotsam. The paroxysm of chills and fever that classically marks an attack of malaria thus is probably a toxic reaction. This reaction continues until the body's macrophage defenses have checked the swarming plasmodia and a kind of filtering service situated in the spleen (an enlarged and tender spleen is one of the clinical indications of malaria) has gathered up the debris. The nature of the reaction is largely determined by the nature of the infecting organism. *P. falciparum* has the most ferocious nature of its kind, and it induces by far the severest form of malaria—a form that is frequently fatal. One reason for this is the ready acceptance by the organism of any red cell, its high fertility, and the speed of its reproductive cycle. Another, and more important, reason is that in *P. falciparum* infections the red blood cells are so seriously affected that they tend to adhere to the walls of the capillaries and build a strangling occlusion. *P. vivax* and *P. ovale*, whose generative eruptions occur every other day, and *P. malariae*, with a cycle that produces in its victims a paroxysm only every third day, lack this sinister agglutinative power (as well, perhaps, as other, still incompletely fathomed powers), and the malarias they produce are relatively (though only in comparison with falciparum malaria) less severe. They, too, can be fatal, they are almost always prostrating, and they tend (if untreated) to hang on for months, and sometimes even years.

The regular recurrence of chills and fever at intervals of a day or two or three is classically suggestive of malaria. With the possible exception of the afternoon rise in temperature that traditionally characterizes tuberculosis, a predictably intermittent fever occurs in no other disease. It sets malaria distinctly apart from fevers of other origin. The uniqueness of malaria in this respect made possible its early recognition as an entity. It seems to have been recognized as such at least as early as the fifth pre-Christian century. The Book of Leviticus which was written at about that time, contains a probable allusion to malaria in one of the several instances on record there of the Lord's exceptional truculence: "I will even appoint over you terror, consumption, and the burning ague." It is certain that malaria was specifically known to Hippocrates. In *Epidemics I*, his masterwork, he clearly distinguishes between continuous and intermittent fevers. He then defines the intermittent fevers as quotidian (daily), tertian (every third day), quartan (every fourth day), and semi-tertian. A semitertian fever is one that recurs about every thirty-six hours, like that of the falciparum malaria. "The least dangerous of all," he reports, "and the mildest and most protracted, is the quartan. . . . What is called the semi-tertian . . . is the most fatal." The first-century Roman encyclopedist Aulus Cornelius Celsus saw malaria even more plainly. "Of fevers," he wrote in *De Medicina*, a medical compendium, "one is quotidian, another tertian, a third quartan. . . . Quartan fevers have the simpler characteristics. Nearly always they begin with shivering, then heat breaks out, and, the fever having ended, there are two days free; thus on the fourth day it recurs. But of tertian fevers there are two classes. The one, beginning and desisting in the same way as quartan, has merely this distinction, that it affords one day free, and recurs on the third day. The other is far more pernicious. . . . Out of forty-eight hours, about thirty-six . . . are occupied by the paroxysm." An association between malarial fevers and swamps and marshes was also observed very early. One of the most precocious of these observers was a Roman scholar of the first pre-Christian century named Marcus Terentius Varro. In discussing the proper site for a farmhouse, Varro warns, "Note also if there be any swampy ground . . . because certain minute animals, invisible to the eye, breed there . . . and cause diseases that are difficult to be rid of. Said Fundanius: 'What shall I do to escape malaria, if I am left an estate of such a kind?' 'Why,' said Agrius . . . 'you must sell it for as [much] as you can get, or if you can't sell it, you must quit it.' " A century later, Lucius Junius Moderatus Columella, a Hispano-Roman writer on agricultural subjects, came independently to the same supposition. "Nor indeed must there be a marsh near the building," he declared, "for [a marsh] always throws up noxious and poisonous steams during the heats." And, he perspicaciously added, it "breeds animals with mischievous stings which fly upon us in exceeding thick swarms . . . whereby hidden diseases are often contracted."

The Roman implication of "certain minute animals" and "animals with mischievous stings" in the spread of malaria vanished from the European mind with the fall of the Roman Empire. It was lost, along with most of the rational arts and sciences of Greco-Roman culture, in the credulities of medieval Christianity until almost modern times. All that survived of the observations of Varro and Columella (and many others of their inquisitive kind and time) was a vague distrust of marshy places as a source of malarial steams. The name "malaria," as it happens, derives from this miasmal theory. It developed from the Italian *mala* (bad) and *aria* (air), and was introduced into English by Horace Walpole in a letter to a friend (". . . a horrid thing called mal'aria, that comes to Rome every summer and kills one") in 1740. The traditional French designation of the disease, *fièvre paludéenne* (or marsh fever), is equally miasmal. There was a time, however, in the deeps of the Middle Ages, when even the miasmal explanation of malaria slipped from common knowledge. Malaria then was taken to be a form of demonic possession. The sudden chill, the blaze of fever, the burst of sweating, and then the almost instantaneous recovery suggested to innocent imaginations the malicious coming and going of a fiend, and charms were composed to hasten his departure. One—to be chanted up the chimney—ran:

> Tremble and go!
> First day, shiver and burn,
> Tremble and quake!
> Second day, shiver and learn,
> Tremble and die!
> Third day, never return.

Almost two thousand years went by before the possibility of a connection between mosquitoes and malaria was once more glimpsed and recorded. Giovanni Maria Lancisi, an early-eighteenth-century Italian epidemiologist and physician to three popes (Innocent XI, Clement XI, and Innocent XII), is usually celebrated as Columella's most immediate successor. In 1717, in an examination of the miasma theory entitled "De Noxiis Paludum Effluvis," Lancisi confidently traced the source of malaria to marshes and other stagnant waters, and then proposed that the mosquitoes so abundant there might be the agents of its dissemination. He also described the nature of their role. Mosquitoes "do not cause death by the bite or the wound," he declared, "but infuse by the bite or wound a poisonous fluid into our vessels." Lancisi's recovery of the ancient Roman comprehension of malaria was widely read and warmly proclaimed, but it failed to excite emulation. "De Noxiis Paludum Effluvis" at once became the standard word on the subject, and it remained about the only one for well over a hundred years. Then, in 1854, a West Indian physician of French extraction named Louis Daniel Beauperthuy perceived a larger measure of the truth. "The absence of mosquitoes during cold weather explains the disappearance of malaria," he wrote at the end of a study in Venezuela. "Intermittent fever is a serious disease spread by and due to the prevalence of mosquitoes. . . . [It owes its] toxicity to an animal or vegetoanimal virus, the introduction of which into the human system occurs by inoculation. The poisonous agent, after an incubation period, sets up . . . a true decomposition of the blood." Beauperthuy (if he meant what he seems to say) was one of the brilliant guessers of prescientific medicine. He died, in 1871, on the eve of the establishment of the germ theory of disease causation, and the triumphant riddling of malaria in the closing years of the nineteenth century was—and could only have been—a product of modern medical science. It was also, as is usual in modern science, the work of many men in many parts of the world. They included Rudolf Leuckart, a pioneer German parasitologist (who showed, by way of a worm parasite of fish that also lived in a species of flea, that an insect could serve as intermediate host to an animal parasite); Patrick Manson, a Scottish physician working in China (who showed, through studies of a nematode infestation called filariasis, that a mosquito could extract a parasite from the blood of a man and then satisfactorily serve it as a host); the American pathologists Theobald Smith and F. L. Kilborne (who showed, in a series of experiments with cattle, that insects can transmit disease from one animal to another); Charles Louis Alphonse Laveran, a French

Army physician working in Algeria (who showed the presence of protozoa of the genus *Plasmodium* in the red blood cells of a malaria patient); Camillo Golgi, an Italian histologist (who showed that the malaria paroxysm coincides with the release of plasmodia from the parasitized red cells); and Ronald Ross, a Scottish surgeon in the Indian Medical Service. It was Ross's discovery of plasmodia in the stomachs and, a year or two later, plasmodia spores in the salivary glands of anopheles mosquitoes that had fed on malaria patients which completed the general elucidation of the disease. The first of these climactic discoveries was made on August 21, 1897, and on the evening of that day he cautiously announced the fact in a letter to his wife, in England: "I have seen something very promising indeed in my new mosquitoes." He then turned to his journal and, in the privacy of its pages, opened his heart in a poem:

> This day designing God
> Hath put into my hand
> A wondrous thing. At His command
> I have found thy secret deeds
> Oh million-murdering Death.
>
> I know this little thing
> A million men will save—
> Oh death where is thy sting?
> Thy victory oh grave?

Ross was, providentially, a better prophet than poet. His divinely directed discovery, by finally and firmly fixing attention on the anopheles mosquito as the vector in malaria, has unquestionably saved many millions of men. It is probable, however, that many millions more owe their salvation to modern adaptations of two weapons that have been at hand for centuries. One of these came into being as a natural corollary of the miasma theory. This, in its earliest effective form, was the draining of marshes. The other, of course, is quinine. Quinine is a complicated alkaloidal compound ($C_{20}H_{24}N_2O_2$) that was originally derived from the bark of the cinchona tree, a South American evergreen indigenous to Peru. The first malarial European to experience the power of an infusion of cinchona bark to block or terminate a paroxysm of chills and fever was a Jesuit missionary named Juan Lopez. That was in 1600. The healing draught was given to Lopez by a friendly Peruvian Indian, but how the Indian knew of its curative powers is uncertain. Malaria is not native to the Western Hemisphere. It entered the New World in the blood of the Spanish conquerors of Mexico and Peru in the sixteenth century, and it seems unlikely that the remnant Incas could have become sufficiently familiar with the new disease by the time Lopez was felled to know its specific vulnerability to cinchona bark. The probability is that his benefactor merely knew the bark to possess (as it does) a cooling touch in fever. Cinchona bark was introduced into Europe by Alonso Messias Venegas, another Jesuit missionary, in 1632. Its mastery of malaria was quickly confirmed and ardently endorsed by a succession of ailing Jesuits, including Cardinal Juan di Lugo, the illustrious confidant of Innocent X. Outside the society of Jesus, however, the bark was for a time rather differently received. Its Jesuitic genesis rendered it repellent to many seventeenth-century Protestants. Oliver Cromwell was an outstanding member of that fiercely sectarian company. He died, in 1658, of malaria, after refusing a proffered decoction of what he (and others of his kind) called Jesuits' bark. Cinchona bark, or Jesuits' bark, or (as it most generally came to be known) Peruvian bark, was also rejected on principle by much of seventeenth-century medicine. Orthodox medicine found its action not in harmony with the rationale of therapeutics then in vogue. This rationale was venerably rooted in the humoral theory of pathology, which held that disease resulted from an imbalance of the body's constituent fluids (originally blood, phlegm, yellow bile, and black bile), and it conceived the function of a drug to be the restoration of balance by seeking out and neutralizing harmful substances and then eliminating them from the body by means of violent purgation— by inducing vomiting, sweating, salivation, urination, hemorrhage. The conventional treatment of malaria included a powerful calomel purge. Humoral pathology dominated medicine until the establishment by Rudolf Virchow and others of cellular pathology around the middle of the nineteenth century, but the eventual acceptance of Peruvian bark—along with such other non-purgative specifics as colchicum (for gout) and digitalis—served to hasten its end. Peruvian bark was itself supplanted in the early nineteenth century. In 1820, the French pharmacologists Pierre Joseph Pelletier and Joseph Bienaimé Caventou discovered in quinine, an isolated essence of the bark, a more potent and more potable remedy for malaria, and within three years it was widely manufactured and almost everywhere available. The ingenuities of modern chemistry have since produced a synthetic quinine and a multitude of other remedies. Among the most esteemed of these are chloroquine, amodiaquine, and primaquine. Chloroquine and amodiaquine are substitutes for quinine. Like quinine, they are able, by destroying plasmodia of all species in the red-cell reproductive stage, to swiftly cure an acute attack of malaria, but they have no effect on the reservoir of plasmodia sequestered in the liver. The powers of primaquine are precisely supplemental to those of the quininelike drugs. Primaquine is lethal to the liver-dwelling plasmodia, and it can also kill or sterilize the sexually mature products of the red-cell stage—the organisms whose ingestion by an anopheles mosquito perpetuates the disease. Eight to ten days of quinine (or three days of one of its companion drugs) followed by fourteen days of primaquine will usually effect a radical, or total, cure.

Sanitary engineering, insecticides such as DDT, and the several antimalarial drugs have saved many millions of lives around the world, but they have also done more than that. They have made the lives of many more millions bearable. The menace of malaria is not so much its frequent lethality as its far more common capacity for taking the life out of living. No disease is more dulling, more depressing, more debilitating than chronic malaria. It was malaria in its chronic form that crushed the spirit of Attic Greece and wasted the strength of Rome, and practically every habitable part of the world (with the unexplained exception of New Zealand and most of the islands of Oceania) has at some time felt its enervating touch. "An intensely malarial locality cannot thrive," Ronald Ross wrote in a monograph in 1907. "The children are wretched, the adults frequently racked with fever, and the whole place shunned whenever possible by the neighbors. The landowner, the traveller, the innkeeper, the trader fly from it.

Gradually it becomes depopulated and untilled, the home only of the most wretched peasants." J. A. Sinton, another British malariologist with wide experience in India, has offered a more comprehensive definition. "There is no aspect of life in [a malarial] country which is not affected, either directly or indirectly, by this disease," he noted, in 1936. "It constitutes one of the most important causes of economic misfortune, engendering poverty, diminishing the quantity and the quality of the food supply, lowering the physical and intellectual standard of the nation, and hampering increased prosperity and economic progress in every way." An anonymous traveller on the Mississippi River in the eighteen-thirties (presented by Erwin H. Ackerknecht in *Malaria in the Upper Mississippi Valley: 1760–1900*) has durably described the look of chronic malaria. "As we drew near Burlington, in front of a little hut on the riverbank sat a girl and a lad—most pitiable-looking objects, uncared-for, hollow-eyed, sallow-faced," this memoirist wrote. "They had crawled out into the warm sun with chattering teeth to see the boat pass. To Mother's inquiries the captain said: 'If you've never seen that kind of sickness I reckon you must be Yankee. That's the ague. I'm feared you will see plenty of it if you stay long in these parts. They call it here the swamp devil, and it will take the roses out of the cheeks of these plump little ones of yours mighty quick. Cure it? No, Madam. No cure for it: have to wear it out.' " Children are particularly enfeebled by chronic malaria. "Chronic malaria in children retards normal growth," Paul F. Russell and his collaborators point out in *Practical Malariology*, the standard modern work in the field. "Such children are often listless, with sallow, puffy faces, thin, flaccid muscles, protuberant abdomen, and pale mucous membranes. Liver and spleen are enlarged, the latter sometimes enormously. Anorexia [loss of appetite], dyspepsia, and flatulence are common. Fever is recurrent. If untreated, the condition . . . may result in early death."

Malaria reached its broadest sweep around the middle of the nineteenth century. It was all but universal. It was endemic almost everywhere in Asia, Africa, and Latin America; in Mediterranean Europe (the fever of which Byron died at Missolonghi in 1824 was malaria) and in much of Russia, Germany, Holland, and England (malaria accounted for five or six of every hundred patients treated at St. Thomas's Hospital in London between 1850 and 1860); and in most of the United States. Its grip then somewhat loosened, and by the end of the nineteenth century the disease had largely disappeared from northern Europe, and in the United States it was still endemic only in the South. This salubrious, if circumscribed, decline has been variously explained, but most authorities attribute it to such fruits of industrialization as fewer swamps, better drains, less porous houses, more plentiful quinine, an intenser cultivation of land, and the displacement of riverboats by trains. In other, less dynamic parts of the world (including the American South), the spread of malaria was wholly unimpeded until shortly after the Second World War. As recently as 1940, some hundred and fifty thousand cases of malaria were reported in the United States, practically all of them in the South, and it is certain that there were many times that many cases not reported. Ten years later, in 1950, a more reliable method of reporting turned up a mere two thousand cases. There were fewer than two hundred in 1965. The therapeutic impact of growth and industrialization—and quinine and primaquine and DDT—has also been felt in other malarial countries. Since 1949, when the World Health Organization of the United Nations launched its continuing program of malaria eradication, the disease has been more or less uprooted in much of South America, in most of the Western Mediterranean world (including the once notoriously pestilential island of Sardinia), and even in parts of Pakistan and India. WHO has estimated that some three hundred fifty million cases of malaria—three and a half million of them fatal—occurred throughout the world (exclusive of China, North Vietnam, and North Korea) in 1955. In 1965, the total (for the same world) was around a hundred million cases, with about a million deaths.

Malaria thus appears to be going, and going pretty fast. Nevertheless, it is still very far from gone. "If we take as our standard of importance the greatest harm to the greatest number," Sir Macfarlane Burnet noted in "The Natural History of Infectious Disease," in 1953, "then there is no question that malaria is the most important of all infectious diseases." His appraisal remains unquestioned. "Malaria has a higher morbidity rate and is responsible for more deaths per year than any other transmissible disease," Martin D. Young, a leading American malariologist and a member of the expert panel on malaria of WHO, noted in a monograph in 1960. And in 1965, Marcolino G. Candau, director-general of WHO, declared, "From a world-wide point of view, communicable diseases must certainly be considered the No. 1 health problem, and among them malaria holds the most prominent place." Malaria still flourishes, as it always has, in all but Saharan Africa, in Central America, in the Middle East, in most of Southeast Asia, and on some of the islands of the southwest Pacific. The reasons for its prevalence there are chiefly ignorance and indifference. The causes of its lingering presence elsewhere in the world are more varied and more complicated and, it may turn out, more serious. They include—as many recent studies, among them the investigation that illuminated the case of Mrs. Walter Wells, have shown—the appearance of anopheles mosquitoes that are resistant to DDT and other insecticides, the appearance of plasmodia resistant to therapeutic (or tolerable) doses of all known anti-malarial drugs, the appearance of monkeys that can harbor malarial parasites to which man is also hospitable, and the fact that in many places from which endemic malaria has long since been banished the anopheles mosquito continues to live and breed.

The investigation into the case of Mrs. Walter Wells began on Tuesday, June 22. It was undertaken—at the invitation of the Georgia State Department of Health, and the medical authorities at Fort Benning—by two epidemiologists in the Epidemiology Branch of the Communicable Disease Center of the United States Public Health Service, in Atlanta. They were Robert L. Kaiser, chief of the Center's Parasitic Disease Unit, and James P. Luby, an Epidemic Intelligence Service officer assigned to Dr. Kaiser's office. The field work fell to Dr. Luby.

"That was only natural," Dr. Luby says. "This wasn't the first case of malaria down around Fort Benning that we had been asked to investigate. They'd had another civilian case—also a woman—down there the year before, in the summer of 1964. The investigation was headed by an EIS officer named Myron Shultz—he's up in New York now—but I was in on it. It wasn't a great success. We finally had to write it off as a cryptic case. In other words, we couldn't find the source of her infection. This time, I didn't ask for much—just somebody recently sick with an explicable case of malaria, and some anopheles mosquitoes in the right place at the right time to carry it to Mrs. Wells. But at least I knew the way to Columbus and some of the medical people there and out at the base. I got the assignment on Monday afternoon, and I drove down the following morning. Columbus is a good three hours from Atlanta. I checked in at one of those day-or-night motels that line the highway between Columbus and Fort Benning, and had an early lunch. Then I went on to the base and had a talk with the chief of preventive medicine there. That was Major Taras Nowosiwsky, one of the people I knew from the 1964 investigation. He showed me the laboratory data on the case. As expected, the base had confirmed the finding at the Columbus Medical Center. The only thing new was the type. Mrs. Wells's malaria was vivax malaria. Major Nowosiwsky then took me around to pay my respects to the commanding medical officer at the Martin Army Hospital, and I gave them a rough idea of what I planned to do. They promised me every possible assistance. The fact that Mrs. Wells was a former army dependent gave them a certain sense of responsibility. My next stop was the Muscogee County Health Department, in Columbus. Mary John Tiller, the deputy commissioner, was another of my old friends, and she made me feel right at home. I remember the greeting she gave me. 'Well,' she said, 'I was wondering when somebody from CDC was going to show up.' My purpose in seeing Dr. Tiller was to try to get some idea of the probable scope of the problem. She put my mind at rest on that. The local papers and the radio had given Mrs. Wells and her case all kinds of publicity, and she had been the subject of a medical grand rounds at the Medical Center—all of which, incidentally, gives you a pretty good idea of how times have changed in malaria—but nothing else had been brought to light. So the chances were good that Mrs. Wells was all I had to worry about. I decided it was time I had a talk with her.

"I found Mrs. Wells sitting up in bed and looking pretty good. They had started her on chloroquine as soon as the diagnosis was made, and she was now on primaquine. She was still a little weak, but her temperature had been normal since Sunday, and the worst was obviously over. She was very nice and helpful. We went over her history together. I couldn't really blame Dr. Page for missing the diagnosis. Nobody thinks of malaria around here anymore. But here in Georgia was where Mrs. Wells had contracted malaria. Her history settled that. She hadn't been in any of the malarial countries. The only time she had ever been abroad was a trip to Germany with her father in 1960. Since then, she hadn't even been out of the state. It was also certain that she had contracted malaria in the usual way—from the bite of an infected mosquito. It is possible, you know, to get malaria by way of a blood transfusion or through an injection of some kind. The literature is full of drug addicts with malaria. And you may remember all that excitement up in New York a few years ago when they found a blood donor with malaria. But Mrs. Wells had no recent injections or transfusions in her history. She had had some recent illnesses, though. The most recent was some menstrual trouble back in January, shortly after her marriage. In September, when she was still living at the base, she had an attack of strep throat. The most interesting illness was one that began on July 8. That was very interesting. Her symptoms included chills, fever, backache, weakness, and urinary frequency, and, the way she remembered it, the fever was intermittent. She consulted the outpatient department at the Martin Army Hospital on the second day, and, apparently on the basis of that urinary complaint, the examining physician made a tentative diagnosis of urinary-tract infection. She was treated with antibiotics, and in about ten days she was well. One of the things that made that illness interesting was, of course, the symptoms—chills and intermittent fever. They were compatible with a urinary-tract infection when taken by themselves, but not when the record showed a urinalysis negative for white blood cells. The other thing was the date of onset. July 8, 1964, struck a certain chord in my memory. It reminded me of that other case of malaria I'd been in on. I'll call her Mrs. Durham. Mrs. Durham's onset was July *10*, 1964.

"That gave me something to think about that evening after dinner. A good coincidence is always worth thinking about. Epidemiology is practically the science of coincidence. It was very hard to believe that those two cases of malaria were unrelated.

Mrs. Wells's history suggested very persuasively that this attack of malaria was not her first attack. The primary attack had occurred in July of 1964. This attack was a recurrence of that infection. The fact that she had recovered from the first attack without specific treatment didn't in the least embarrass that hypothesis. Untreated malaria recurs and recurs, but each attack is self-limited. After a certain length of time, the red-cell stage of the organism simply peters out. But onset wasn't the only coincidence. There was also the disease itself. Mrs. Wells had vivax malaria. So did Mrs. Durham. Another coincidence was proximity. Mrs. Durham was the wife of a second lieutenant, and they lived in Battle Park Homes, a duplex development at the base for junior officers. Mrs. Wells also lived at the base in 1964—in a development on Baker Street for noncommissioned officers. Battle Park Homes and Baker Street were only about a mile apart. Or so I gathered from Mrs. Wells. And most of the country in between was rough, heavily wooded, and full of damp, brushy hollows. It sounded just right for mosquitoes.

"I spent the next day in Cataula. Most of it, anyway. I would much rather have been poking around at Fort Benning, but it doesn't pay to cut corners. Before I went any further, I had to make completely certain that there hadn't been any other cases of malaria in the neighborhood. Cases that hadn't been diagnosed, that is, or asymptomatic cases. Dr. Tiller had arranged for the county sanitarian to show me around. A stranger, especially a stranger from up North—my home is Chicago—needs someone to vouch for him in those little Georgia towns. We met, and he took me around to meet the local physicians. There were two of them, a husband and wife in practice together, but they had nothing to contribute—no cases of malaria, no unexplained illnesses with fever, nothing in the least suspicious. That was as expected. They were mainly a courtesy call. If they had known any news, they wouldn't have saved it for me. Then we started in on our own. We started with Mrs. Wells's husband, then we saw his parents, then we called on the neighbors. Our procedure was this. We asked about any episode of fever in the recent past. If we got an affirmative answer, we asked about the cause. If the cause was unknown or uncertain, we took a sample of blood for definitive analysis. We visited forty-four homes within a mile-and-a-half radius of Mrs. Wells's home and we checked out a total of two hundred and fourteen people, but we didn't find a thing. There was one old man who had a suspicious history, and we got some blood and sent it back to the CDC laboratory in Atlanta. They did a malaria smear and a fluorescent antibody test, but the results were negative. Well, that, of course, was a great relief. Anything else would have been an awkward complication. This simplified the problem. It didn't tell us when Mrs. Wells got malaria. It was still possible that her present attack was her first. But it did tell us where. She got it at the base.

"I didn't believe that this was her first attack. But, as I say, it was possible. The incubation period in vivax malaria—the interval between the mosquito bite and the onset of symptoms—is usually about two weeks. Mrs. Wells moved off the base around the middle of April, and she didn't get sick until the twenty-second of May—almost six weeks later. That would seem to eliminate a 1965 infection, but it didn't. The reason was, she had gone back to the base. She went back several times. Her father had retired to Fort Myers or some such place in Florida, but Mrs. Wells still had her Baker Street friends. So 1965 was still at least conceivable. The only way to settle it was another fever survey. I might mention, by the way, that we hadn't forgotten the father. Dr. Kaiser had arranged for someone to look him up for an interview. I talked to Dr. Kaiser on Wednesday night and told him what I had learned and what I thought and what I planned to do next, and he completely shared my views. Then he told me about the father. His history and his blood were both negative for malaria.

"I drove down to the base the next morning and saw Major Nowosiwsky again. I told him I wanted to make a fever survey in the Baker Street area, and he OK'd the plan and arranged for one of his men to take me around. Then I asked about mosquitoes. I assumed they were there, they had to be there. But I wanted to know. Major Nowosiwsky took me in to see the base entomologist. He was a colonel—Colonel Petrakis—and he got out his records on the subject. The mosquitoes were there. Routine trapping in season for pest-control analysis regularly turned up several varieties of mosquito, and they included an anopheline—*Anopheles quadrimaculatus. A. quadrimaculatus* is one of about a dozen native American anopheles, and in this part of the country it's the most common. It had been trapped in several different traps, but the traps that interested me were those set up at the intersection of Fort Benning Road and Arrowhead Road and Custer Road, in Battle Park Homes. Fort Benning Road is one of the main thoroughfares in the reservation. Arrowhead Road is the only road to Battle Park Homes, and it's one of two roads to Baker Street. The other road to Baker Street is Custer Road. Colonel Petrakis's records also noted that larvae of *A. quadrimaculatus* had been found in a creek directly across from the Baker Street houses. I thanked the Colonel and picked up my guide and drove out to Baker Street feeling a whole lot better. You can't have malaria without a vector. The Baker Street survey was another Cataula. I had two opening questions this time. One was about unexplained fever. The other was about foreign travel—visits to endemic-malaria areas within the past three years. We visited sixty-one homes and talked to two hundred seventy-one people, and we found nineteen people who had been in endemic areas and two cases of recent and unexplained fever, but we didn't find any malaria. And that took care of 1965. Mrs. Wells's malaria was a 1964 infection. There was no other reasonable possibility. There was also no good reason now to doubt that her case and Mrs. Durham's were linked.

"The nature of the link wasn't hard to visualize. It couldn't have been one of the neighbors. My Baker Street survey and one just like it that was done the year before in Battle Park Homes eliminated that possibility. A common hypodermic needle or a common blood donor was also out of the picture. So, of course, was a visit to some endemic country. That seemed to identify the index case as a visitor to the general neighborhood of Battle Park Homes and Baker Street. It didn't much matter just where. Colonel Petrakis had demonstrated that there were potential vectors all over the area. I went back to Major Nowosiwsky, and he got out the records on all the men from overseas who had come down with malaria at the base in the past twelve months or so. There were quite a number of them, but only four were cases of vivax malaria. The others were mostly falciparum-malaria cases. Incidentally, that's the big malaria problem in Vietnam right now, and I gather it's quite a problem. They're seeing falciparum malaria out there that doesn't respond like the others. However . . . I was looking for vivax cases and found just four. Two captains and two sergeants. But worse than that, I knew them—all but one of them. I remembered both sergeants and one of the captains from the report on the Durham investigation, and the investigation had excluded them as possible sources of Mrs. Durham's infection. They were infectious—they had what we call parasitemia, they had the parasite in their blood—at the wrong time. I'll tell you what I mean. There are two incubation periods to be considered in malaria—one for the development of the parasite in the mosquito and another for the development of the parasite in the man. Both of these periods vary in length, but the mosquito period is the most variable. It varies with the temperature of the air. In vivax malaria in that part of Georgia, it ranges from a month or more in cool weather to a minimum of nine days in June and July. The minimum incubation period in man is eight days. The sum of those minimums is the minimum total incubation interval, or seventeen days. That's the shortest possible interval that could elapse between the infection of the mosquito and the onset of illness in Mrs. Durham and Mrs. Wells. So the man we were looking for should have had parasitemia in June, but no later than the twenty-fourth. Well, both the sergeants failed to satisfy that criterion, and for the same reason. Their onsets came too late. One was on June 28, and the other was on July 28. The captain was too early. His onset came on April 4. And the new case, the other captain, was even more hopeless. His onset date was March 21, 1965.

"I drove back to Atlanta that night. The next day was Saturday. I called Dr. Kaiser and told him the story. It looked as if we were up against another cryptic case. I know he was disappointed, but I felt worse than that. It made me uncomfortable, too, to think of that anonymous index case wandering around somewhere. He might very well be an asymptomatic carrier. I'd done my best, though. There was nothing I could think of left to do. I started in on my report on Monday morning. When I had my notes in order, I got out our general file on malaria. I wanted to take another look at the report on the Durham investigation. But I never got that far—not that morning. I came across something I'd never seen before. Or if I had, I didn't remember. It was a routine National Malaria Surveillance Report from the Third Army Medical Laboratory at Fort McPherson, Georgia. It was dated August 1964, and it reported cases of malaria diagnosed at Army installations in June of that year. I'd seen many such reports. The cases are identified by name, rank, and station, and there is always a short travel history. What made me stop and look at this report was a station—Fort Benning. I didn't even know I was looking until I saw it. It was cited in the travel history of a sergeant I'll call Sergeant Evans. Sergeant Evans was stationed at Fort Campbell, Kentucky, and his case had been diagnosed at the hospital there on June 27. He had arrived at Fort Campbell on June 24. Before that, he had been stationed at Fort Benning. He had been there from May 9 until June 23. Before that, he had been in South Korea.

"I picked up the phone and put in a call to Fort Campbell. It was practically automatic. And I was lucky. Sergeant Evans was still stationed there, and they finally found him and brought him to the phone. I told him who I was and what I wanted to know. His memory of his Fort Benning experience was vague. He lived there in barracks near the parachute-jump towers. That was a mile or two beyond the intersection of Fort Benning Road and Arrowhead Road and Custer Road. No, he didn't know Mrs. Durham or Mrs. Wells, and he had never been to Battle Park Homes or in the Baker Street development. Not that he remembered, anyway. His duties kept him mostly in the area near his barracks. But he had a car—a convertible—and he did get off the base a few times. And when he did, he naturally came and went by way of Fort Benning Road. How else? He supposed he had sometimes been stopped at the stoplight there at the Arrowhead Road and Custer Road intersection. Yes, he had been sick at Fort Benning. He'd had spells of chills and fever off and on during most of June. No, he hadn't reported for treatment—not until he got up to Fort Campbell. He kept hoping each remission was the end. One of his worst spells hit him one evening when he was off the base on a picnic. He remembered driving back to the barracks and shaking so hard he could barely drive. Yes, he usually drove with the top down. Or else why have a convertible? I laughed and agreed and thanked him for his help and coöperation, and hung up.

"I just sat there at my desk for a minute. I don't mind saying I felt pretty good. Then I got up and went in and told Dr. Kaiser what had happened."

[1966]

CHAPTER 16

The Case of Mrs. Carter

———————————•◆•———————————

THE CASE OF the woman whom I'll call Linda Mae Carter—Mrs. Joseph Carter—first came to the attention of Dr. Louis Cohen, an internist in Topeka, Kansas, on the morning of February 24, 1962. It was brought to his attention by a colleague on the staff of the Topeka State Hospital. Mrs. Carter, his colleague told him over the telephone, was thirty-three years old and the wife of a skilled machinist. The Carters had one child, a boy of three. Mrs. Carter had been a patient at Topeka State for almost three months. She had been admitted on November 29 for evaluation of a progressive disabling disease tentatively diagnosed as amyotrophic lateral sclerosis. She was further disabled by two hip fractures that had failed to mend properly, and by a severe mental depression. The hospital was discharging her that afternoon. There had been no improvement in her physical condition, and a recent psychiatric diagnosis had described her as a hysterical personality with neurotic or psychotic potentialities, but the hospital felt that she would be more comfortable at home with her family. Continued hospitalization seemed useless, and might even be damaging to so young a woman. The only trouble was that the Carters had no

234

regular physician. Might he refer Mrs. Carter and her husband to Dr. Cohen? Dr. Cohen hesitated. It sounded like a discouraging case, but he couldn't very well say no. He told him to go ahead.

"That was Saturday," Dr. Cohen says. "I heard from the Carters on Monday. I called my office from the hospital—Stormont-Vail Hospital—as I always do after my morning rounds, and my nurse gave me the morning calls and messages. One of the calls was from Joseph Carter. His wife wanted to see me—sometime that day, if possible. Well, right then was as good a time as any, so I asked my nurse to call and say I'd be over directly. I got there around ten o'clock. It was a fairly new house on an unpaved road in a kind of development way out on the north side of town. Carter was at work by then, and a neighbor girl opened the door. They had got her in as a combination nurse and babysitter. She took me into the bedroom. Mrs. Carter was lying there flat on her back in a hospital bed. She was a nice-looking woman with pretty black hair, but her face was as white as a sheet, and she was nothing but skin and bones.

"I introduced myself and sat down by the bed, and we talked for a couple of minutes. Mrs. Carter had no particular reason for calling me. I mean, nothing new had happened since Saturday— since she left the hospital. She simply wanted to meet me, and she hoped I could do something to help her. Nobody else had been able to, she said. I said I'd do the best I could. We talked a little more, and then I examined her. It was pathetic. She was really disabled. She was doubly disabled. She was flat on her back because of her fractured hips, but that was only part of it. She was also immobilized by a permanent contraction of the muscles of her legs and abdomen. Her body was pulled as taut as a bowstring. And not only that. Every now and then, she told me, her muscles would suddenly pull even tighter, and she would go into a spasm. I knew what she meant, and I could imagine how it must have felt. It would have been a seizure like the spasms in tetanus or in strychnine poisoning. A powerful convulsion. Those symptoms— the stiffness and the spasms—were manifestations, of course, of the disease that was thought to be amyotrophic lateral sclerosis. Amyotrophic lateral sclerosis is a degenerative disease of the central nervous system. It's somewhat on the order of multiple sclerosis—what they used to call 'Lou Gehrig disease.' Well, I examined her as carefully as I could in the circumstances, and I must say I wasn't particularly impressed by the amyotrophic-lateral-sclerosis hypothesis. One of the usual manifestations of that disease is muscle fasciculations. That's a spontaneous muscular quivering. It's like the deliberate twitch that a horse gives when he wants to shake off a fly. Another, though less frequent, manifestation is a positive Babinski reflex. Babinski's reflex is an upturning of the big toe when the sole of the foot is stroked. A turned-up toe is an indication of damage to the pyramidal tract of the brain and spinal cord. Also, there is usually some spasticity in the lower legs. But Mrs. Carter had a negative, or normal, Babinski, and I found no suggestion of either muscle fasciculations or spasticity.

"So I had my doubts about amyotrophic lateral sclerosis. And yet I couldn't absolutely rule it out. The only certainty was that I needed to know a great deal more about this case than I did. Even the general nature of Mrs. Carter's trouble was not entirely clear. She seemed to be the victim of some central-nervous-system disease, but maybe not. Maybe that was only the way it looked. I remembered that the State Hospital had described her as a hysterical personality. I didn't find her very stable myself. Actually, she was rather hostile. She was more or less hostile all the time I was with her. Still, we talked. We talked about her illness. And the more we talked, the less her hostility bothered me. By the time I left, it hardly bothered me at all. I could understand why she acted that way. I mean, I had an inkling. It wasn't until I dug into her medical history and saw just what she'd been through that I really understood."

Mrs. Carter's trouble began in 1959. One day in early August of that year, she stumbled and fell while getting out of the family car. She wasn't hurt, but the accident unnerved her. It was her conviction that it hadn't been an ordinary accident. There was something wrong with her legs. They had a funny feeling. This impression persisted, and as summer ended and autumn came on she identified the feeling as a stiffness. It was a sudden tightening of the leg muscles, and it seemed to occur at moments of emotional stress. Mrs. Carter had a job at that time as a clerk in a Topeka business office, and she became aware that any little excitement—a teasing remark by one of her fellow-workers—might bring on a stiffening contraction. The spasms lasted for several minutes, and while they lasted her legs were locked at the knee. She could walk only with a painful stiff-legged lurch. Around Thanksgiving, the spasms became more frequent. They also lasted longer, and it seemed to take less and less to bring them on. The telephone, the doorbell, a shout—any unexpected noise would throw her into a spasm, and she found that she was especially susceptible just before a menstrual period. Even a sudden quickening of pace would often excite a seizure. She developed a frantic fear of falling, and refused to ride on escalators or to go through revolving doors. She began to cry at the slightest provocation. Shortly after Christmas—in January of 1960—she called a physician recommended by a friend, and made an appointment for a consultation.

The physician Mrs. Carter consulted was an internist whom I'll call Dr. Warren. He asked her the usual questions and then performed the usual comprehensive examination. The results of the examination were unequivocally normal. There was no evidence of any fundamental physical derangement. It was equally clear, however, that Mrs. Carter was physically disabled. Dr. Warren resolved this perplexity in the standard modern manner. It was his impression, he told Mrs. Carter, that her trouble was functional rather than constitutional in origin. A psychiatric examination was therefore indicated. If Mrs. Carter wished, he would be glad to refer her to a psychiatrist in whom he had every confidence. Mrs. Carter thanked him, took the name of the recommended psychiatrist, and went home.

Mrs. Carter considered calling Dr. Warren's psychiatrist. She discussed the matter with her husband and thought about it for several days. She wanted to call, and yet she didn't. The idea of a psychiatric examination was somehow very disturbing. The days, the weeks, the months went by, and she never made the call. Instead, toward the end of July she telephoned Dr. Warren again and made another appointment. The reason for the consultation was a new set of muscular symptoms. In addition to the spasms that locked her knees, she now had begun to suffer from similar spasms in the muscles of her neck. The muscles there were tender, and they often ached. So did those in her shoulders. Dr. Warren examined her again. The examination confirmed her new complaints. It also further confirmed his impression that her symptoms were psychogenic. He gave her a prescription for phenobarbital to ease her nervousness, and urged her once more to consult his psychiatric colleague. Mrs. Carter said she would.

But she didn't. Nor did she call on Dr. Warren again. With the help of phenobarbital, she continued on her own for three months longer. Then, in November, she consulted another friend and telephoned another physician. I'll call him Dr. Rushing. His impression of Mrs. Carter and of the nature of her illness was much the same as that affirmed and reaffirmed by Dr. Warren. He, too, concluded that what she needed was psychiatric treatment. However, before passing her along to psychiatry, he thought it might be prudent to arrange for a neurological consultation. Mrs. Carter had no objection to that, and a few days later she was admitted for observation to Stormont-Vail Hospital. The observing neurologist returned her to Dr. Rushing with a report that entirely confirmed the latter's understanding of the matter. There was no evidence of any neurological disease—no aberrant reflexes, no abnormal modalities of sensation, no synaptic ambiguities. On the other hand, the neurologist added, there was abundant evidence of "emotional illness . . . lying somewhere in the neurotic range, with components of anxiety, hysteria, and the possibility of a little depression." Psychiatric evaluation was strongly recommended.

Dr. Rushing conferred with Mrs. Carter the following week, and he succeeded where Dr. Warren had failed. Mrs. Carter agreed to let him refer her to the municipal Family Service and Guidance Center of Topeka for psychiatric examination and counseling. Her name was put on the waiting list there, and when the Center called her, early in January of 1961, she responded to the call. The results of the examination were a gratifying justification of the neurologist's apprehension and the suspicions of Dr. Warren and Dr. Rushing. Mrs. Carter was emotionally ill, and the specific character of her illness was diagnosed as a "conversion reaction, or schizophrenic reaction, schizo-affective-type." She was instructed to return to the Center for a psychotherapeutic consultation. She returned for two or three consultations with a designated staff psychiatrist, and then—losing interest or patience or confidence—dropped out of the course. A week or two later, around the middle of March, she called another psychiatrist, a man in private practice, and arranged for an office consultation. Her physical condition by then had conspicuously worsened. The psychiatrist noted that she arrived on the arm of her husband, and was unable to walk across the room without help. He also noted that she "kept her handkerchief over her face at all times" and that her general behavior was "inappropriate." She was, in addition, "quite uncooperative." At the end of the consultation, Mrs. Carter asked for a prescription for phenobarbital. The psychiatrist, detecting in her manner a hint of possible dependence, refused. Instead, he gave her a prescription for mephenesin, a muscle relaxant and a non-addictive drug, and urged her to resume her consultations at the Family Service and Guidance Center. But nothing came of either remedy. Mrs. Carter ignored his advice, and the mephenesin failed to control the crippling muscle spasms. The spasms spread from her legs to her thighs and upward to her abdomen, and the seizures became more violent and more frequent. Early in April, she found it necessary to resign her job. She was practically immobilized by almost daily seizures.

The accident in which Mrs. Carter suffered the first of her two hip fractures occurred on June 21. That morning, as usual, she awakened early, at about six-thirty, and, as usual, asked her husband to help her out of bed. His help had become essential. Her muscles were now so tightly drawn that she couldn't bend at either the waist or the knees. Carter picked her up like a log, swung her gently around, and lowered her feet to the floor. Her heels found a purchase and he raised her stiffly erect. Her body gave a sudden spastic wrench. There was a crack like the sound of a snapping twig, and Mrs. Carter screamed. Carter stood transfixed. Mrs. Carter screamed again, and then began to moan. Carter laid her back on the bed and ran to the telephone and called the Topeka ambulance service. Mrs. Carter was carried into the emergency room of Stormont-Vail Hospital at about seven-thirty. An X-ray examination revealed an intracapsular fracture of the left hip. The bone was set, and fixed in place with a flanged, triangular five-inch length of stainless steel known to surgery as a Smith-Petersen nail.

Mrs. Carter remained in the hospital for almost two weeks. Her hip appeared to be mending normally, and on July 4 she was discharged to convalesce at home.

Mrs. Carter spent the summer on her back in bed. The muscle spasms and the spells of crying continued. Her emotions were stretched as tight as her leg and abdominal muscles, and they were equally sensitive to even the slightest jar. She was still confined to bed when the accident in which she suffered her second hip fracture occurred. That was on October 14, around seven o'clock in the morning. Mrs. Carter had awakened that morning with a soreness at the base of her spine that radiated into her right hip. She asked her husband to massage it. She had experienced this soreness several times before and had found that a gentle massage would relieve it. Mrs. Carter lay on her back, and her husband kneaded her hip and upper thigh. After two or three minutes, she asked him to massage her spine, and moved to turn on her stomach. Her body arched in a spasm—and Carter again heard a crack like the sound of a snapping twig. Mrs. Carter screamed.

An X-ray examination at Stormont-Vail Hospital, to which Mrs. Carter was again conveyed by ambulance, revealed an intracapsular fracture of the right hip. It also revealed that her fractured left hip was unhealed. The Smith-Petersen nail had not been strong enough to withstand the wrench of almost daily muscle spasms, and the bone ends had gradually pulled apart. The attending surgeon had planned to fix the new fracture with another Smith-Petersen nail, but the evidence of the second X-ray immediately changed his mind. He used instead a system of Hague pins. A Hague pin is a stainless-steel bolt with threads at one end to receive a securing nut. The pins chosen by Mrs. Carter's surgeon were about six inches long and just over an eighth of an inch in diameter. He fixed the right hip fracture with three Hague pins, and then removed the loosened nail from the other hip and replaced it with a bone graft and another set of three pins. It was during Mrs. Carter's convalescence from that double operation that a tentative diagnosis of amyotrophic lateral sclerosis was offered as a possible supplement to the continuing psychiatric evaluation. Mrs. Carter remained at Stormont-Vail until November 29. That was when she was admitted to Topeka State Hospital.

A few weeks after her arrival there, she suffered a series of spasms so violent that her fractures were again undone. The spasms were, in fact, so violent that they bent the six Hague pins. The pins still help, but the damage now was irreparable. A normal union of her broken bones could never be achieved as long as her spasms continued, and Mrs. Carter was all but completely helpless.

It took Dr. Cohen several days to root out and review Mrs. Carter's medical history. His findings left him sympathetic but confused. In a memorandum he made at the time, he noted, "Fantastic as it may seem, the possibility must be considered that this patient has fractured both hips during violent muscle spasms of psychic origin. Metabolic bone disease must be considered, and appropriate studies are recommended to rule out this factor. Although the history is against this, a convulsive disorder must be ruled out. Repeat neurological evaluation is thus suggested." Dr. Cohen contemplated this brief patch of diagnostic contradictions, and then, with more hope than expectation, arranged with his colleague at Topeka State Hospital for a thorough reevaluation of the neurological evidence in their file on Mrs. Carter. Meanwhile, he did what he could to make her less uncomfortable. The means he finally settled on was a muscle-relaxant drug known to pharmacology as chlorzoxazone. Its impact, though slight, was perceptible. Chlorzoxazone (in doses of five hundred milligrams three times a day) had no effect on the shackling muscular rigidity, but it somewhat tempered the ferocity of the periodic spasms. That was a small but not insignificant blessing.

A report on the Topeka State review of Mrs. Carter's case reached Dr. Cohen on May 10. It took the form of a letter from his colleague on the hospital staff and (in its essentials) read, "We had an interesting panel discussion. . . . The neurology consultants were unable to make a diagnosis accounting for all the clinical symptoms and signs. There are many features about the patient that did not fit within the frame of the so-called amyotrophic lateral sclerosis group. The patient did not show any atrophy of muscles or muscle fasciculations, and apparently did not suffer from anterior horn [of the spinal cord] degeneration. The hip fractures did not show any degree of healing. The osteoporosis of both hips was still observed. . . . An electromyogram [a recorded depiction of muscular contraction] was normal. Serum sodium, potassium chloride, calcium phosphorous, alkaline phosphatase and acid phosphatase, BUN, Creatinine, uric acid, LDH, LAP, blood sugar, SGOT, SGPT, and CRP were all within limits of normal." Dr. Cohen read the report without elation. Its value was almost entirely negative. Osteoporosis, the one pathological finding, is an abnormal porosity, or rarefaction, of the bones. Bones thus weakened may sometimes fracture spontaneously. There was, however, no reason to believe that osteoporosis was a significant factor in Mrs. Carter's hip fractures. Her fractures were spontaneous fractures, but it was an aberrant force of muscle, rather than a weakness of bone, that brought them about.

Dr. Cohen added the Topeka State report to his file on Mrs. Carter and resumed his diagnostic search. It now took him exclusively to the library. In spite of the lack of neurological evidence, he was increasingly inclined to feel that Mrs. Carter's trouble was basically neurological, and the literature he searched was largely in the field of neuromuscular disorders. His explorations led him through many clinical journals and through the ranks of many clinical investigators, and among those many investigators the name of one turned up so often that it fixed itself in his mind. This was a member of the neurology section of the Mayo Clinic named Donald W. Mulder. There was nothing relevantly revelatory in the writings of Dr. Mulder that came to Dr. Cohen's attention, but they had a decisive impact. He emerged one evening from a Mulder paper with both a sense of resignation and a sudden flash of hope. He faced and accepted the probability that an accurate diagnosis of Mrs. Carter's trouble was beyond him. It might not, however, be beyond the reach of Dr. Mulder.

Mrs. Carter and her husband knew the Mayo Clinic by reputation, and since its reputation is an inspiring one, they responded to Dr. Cohen's proposal with an almost euphoric approval. The only problem was Mrs. Carter's total immobility, but Mr. Carter provided an answer to that. They could make the trip by trailer. Rochester, Minnesota, the seat of the Mayo Clinic, was not much more than five hundred miles from Topeka.

On June 5, Dr. Cohen sat down and wrote an introductory

letter to Dr. Mulder. He had, he said, a "very interesting" patient whom he would like to refer for diagnosis and possible suggestions for treatment. He then related her appalling history—the devastating muscular contractions, the pathological hip fractures, the contradictory diagnosis—and described the treatment she was now receiving. It was his feeling, he went on to say, that she might have an aneurysm pressing on the pyramidal tract of the spinal cord, or a "space-occupying lesion." He ended his letter with a warning that Mrs. Carter "would have to be admitted directly to the hospital" and that she would arrive by trailer.

Dr. Mulder's reply was prompt and eagerly affirmative. It was also brief and to the point. Dr. Mulder was looking forward to seeing "this very interesting patient," and arrangements were being made for her admission to the neurology service at the Methodist-Worrall Hospital, in Rochester, on Monday, June 11. He would keep Dr. Cohen informed of Mrs. Carter's progress.

The Carters reached Rochester on June 10, and Mrs. Carter was admitted to the hospital the following morning. She remained there under observation and examination until July 3. On July 14, Dr. Mulder's progress report came through, and it was indeed a report of progress. It introduced Dr. Cohen to a disease of which he had never heard, and to a drug so new that it was not yet on the market.

Dr. Mulder began with an expression of thanks for the opportunity of seeing Mrs. Carter in neurological consultation. He and his colleagues were very much interested in her problem. It was provocatively reminiscent. Nevertheless, the possibility that she might be suffering from a spinal-cord tumor or spinal-cord lesion "with secondary muscle spasm" was routinely considered. The indicated tests—an X-ray examination of the muscle tissue, an X-ray examination of the spinal cord, and an examination of the spinal fluid—were made. The results, however, were all essentially normal. That returned them to their first impression. It was their conclusion that Mrs. Carter's clinical syndrome might best be classified as being the "stiff-man syndrome." This syndrome had recently been found to respond to a new drug called Valium, and Mrs. Carter had been so treated and with apparent success. He would see that Dr. Cohen received a supply of the drug. He wished

Dr. Cohen and Mrs. Carter well, and hoped to be kept informed of the latter's progress.

Dr. Cohen's decision to solicit help for Mrs. Carter at the Mayo Clinic was more than just a happy one. It was providential as well. The Mayo Clinic was then the only medical center in the world where the stiff-man syndrome could be both readily diagnosed and efficaciously treated. Few physicians even now have ever heard of it. The syndrome is known at the Mayo Clinic because it was there that it was first recognized as an entity. It also was first successfully treated there, and it was named by Mayo investigators.

Its discoverers were two Mayo neurologists—Frederick P. Moersch and Henry W. Woltman. They announced their discovery in a report to the *Proceedings of the Staff Meetings of the Mayo Clinic*, entitled "Progressive Fluctuating Muscular Rigidity and Spasm ('Stiff-Man' Syndrome): Report of a Case and Some Observations in Thirteen Other Cases," in 1956. It was not a hasty announcement. The report began, "In the summer of 1924, an Iowa farmer, aged 49 years, came to the Clinic because of 'muscle stiffness and difficulty in walking.'" It continued:

> His disability . . . had begun insidiously in 1920 with episodes of tightening of the muscles of his neck. Gradually, these attacks had increased in frequency, in severity, and in duration. The tightening had spread to include the muscles of the shoulders and upper portion of the back. In March of 1923, after a fall, which had appeared to have no serious consequences other than to confine the man to bed for a few days, his muscular condition had worsened. His neck muscles had remained rigid most of the time, and his head could be brought forward only with great effort. Also, the abdominal muscles and, to a lesser degree, those of the lower part of the back and those of the thighs had partaken of this same stiffness or tightness. Moreover, the rigidity had been punctuated by intermittent and moderately painful spasms. As might be expected, this behavior of his muscles had interfered with walking. His gait had become slow and awkward and, when spasms had supervened, he might "fall as a wooden man." He had observed that noise, a sudden jar, or voluntary movement often precipitated these spasms. To arise from a seated position he frequently required assistance. . . . Nothing helpful to

diagnosis was learned from routine physical [and] neurologic examination. . . . We could not make a diagnosis, but the unusual condition interested us no end and, to associate it with a memorable and descriptive term that could not be taken by anyone to be final, we nicknamed it the "stiff-man syndrome." In the absence of a diagnosis, and without knowledge of specific treatment, we observed the effects of bromides, of intramuscular administration of magnesium sulfate, and of sedation with barbiturates, but these helped only temporarily. . . . We were not privileged to examine this patient again. . . . He reported last in 1932. . . . He could be on his feet, but he was weak and could take only a few steps unassisted.

This ends our account of that case, but the clinical picture so imprinted itself on our minds that in the course of the following years we recognized the same syndrome in . . . thirteen other cases.

The records of these fourteen cases were similar. There was some variation in rapidity of onset, in degree and extent of muscular rigidity, and in associated spasms. Some patients complained slightly of pain that occurred with the spasms, and in four instances pain was of major importance. A critical review of the records suggested no common cause. . . . Of our fourteen patients, ten were males and four were females. The age of onset of the illness varied from twenty-eight to fifty-four years. . . . It is worth noting that the malady frequently was considered to be functional, especially in its early stages. Of our fourteen patients, four came to us without previous diagnosis. In five cases, a diagnosis of "functional condition" had been made by the referring physicians, and one of these patients had been given several electric-shock treatments to no avail. We, too, considered the possibility of a functional disorder in these five cases, and in several we pursued psychotherapy, including hypnosis in one case, before realizing our error. The previous diagnosis made in the remaining five cases was chronic tetany [a convulsive muscular disorder of metabolic origin] in two, and, respectively, dystonia [a disturbance in muscular tonicity], stroke, and arthritis in three. . . . In six cases the muscles of the trunk were first affected, in four cases the muscles of the neck and shoulders, and in the remaining four, the muscles of the limbs. Of these latter four cases, the legs were first involved in three, and a leg and the ipsilateral arm in the fourth. In all instances, the affliction spread to include other muscles. . . . Routine physical examination of the patients did not help toward diagnosis. Neurologic examination of the patients demonstrated only fluctuating muscular rigidity and spasm. . . .

Thus our story ceases for the present. The threads are there but, in spite of their being woven into a fairly constant pattern, the completed design awaits added study. Whether the rigidity occurred reflexly by way of the spinal cord, or whether it represented involvement of the basal ganglia, we could not decide. . . . Because of the fluctuating intensity of symptoms and because four patients had reducing substances in the urine, a metabolic basis for the malady should be considered.

The completed design of the stiff-man syndrome still awaits added study. It is generally accepted that the disease has its seat in the spinal cord, and that both the creeping rigidity and the volcanic spasms are brought about (like the convulsions in strychnine poisoning and in tetanus) by a disturbance in the polarizing elements called synapses, which separate one cell from another in the neuron chains along which nervous impulses travel. This disturbance, it is thought, manifests itself as a suppression of synaptic inhibition, and a kind of neuromuscular anarchy results. The nature of that fundamental disturbance, however, remains a total mystery. The years since the publication of "Progressive Fluctuating Muscular Rigidity and Spasm" have produced just two real certainties about the stiff-man syndrome. One of these, the discovery of a Mayo Clinic neurologist named Frank M. Howard, is that a drug variously known as diazepam, Valium, and 7-chloro-1, 3-dihydro-1-methyl-5-phenyl-2H-1, 4-benzodiazepin-2-one has the power to throttle its symptoms. The other is that the stiff-man syndrome is not a phenomenon peculiar to the American Middle West. Clinicians have reported cases in other parts of this country and in Britain, Germany, and Spain. In the spring of 1962, when Mrs. Carter made her instructive visit to the Mayo Clinic, the number of cases of stiff-man syndrome on record was twenty-three. She brought the total up to twenty-four.

Dr. Cohen was out of town when Mrs. Carter returned from the Mayo Clinic. He didn't see her until the day he received Dr. Mulder's revelatory letter. Mrs. Carter was another revelation. Her response to diazepam had been complete. The muscle spasms had ceased, and her leg and abdominal muscles were normally relaxed. Moreover, for the first time in almost three years she was able to make herself comfortable.

"Not only physically comfortable," Dr. Cohen says. "She also seemed to be more comfortable in her mind. She was beginning to stop just lying there and waiting for the next spasm to hit. She was beginning to hope. And so was I. With those terrible spasms under real control, her fractures would finally have a chance to mend. She would probably always be a cripple. That was almost certain. But she might someday be able to walk a little. It all depended on diazepam. The only trouble was that diazepam wasn't on the market yet. It didn't become generally available in this part of the country until about 1964. Mrs. Carter had a supply on hand. Dr. Mulder had fixed the dosage at fifteen milligrams four times a day, and he had given her enough tablets to last for three or four weeks. After that, it was up to me. I wrote to the people who made it—the pharmaceutical firm of Hoffmann-La Roche, in Nutley, New Jersey—and they wrote right back. They were very much interested in the case I described, and they would be glad to provide me with a regular supply of Valium—that's their brand name for diazepam—for experimental clinical use.

"Which they did. They worked out the amount I needed, and every month or so they sent me something like five hundred five-milligram tablets, and I rationed them out to Mrs. Carter. I followed the dosage set by Dr. Mulder. It was fairly heavy. Sixty milligrams a day is a lot of diazepam. But it takes that much to do the job in the stiff-man syndrome. And it did a wonderful job. Mrs. Carter continued to respond. Her hips began to knit, and in less than a year she was up and walking with the help of a walker. Her progress was all I had hoped for. There was only one incident —one interruption. That one was plenty, though. I don't know if you've ever seen a Valium label, or one of the ads for Valium. There's a paragraph there headed 'Side Effects.' The last sentence reads, 'Abrupt cessation after prolonged overdosage may produce withdrawal symptoms similar to those seen with barbiturates, meprobamate, and chlordiazepoxide HCl.' The reason for that paragraph is a number of experiences very much like mine. And mine was one of the scares of my life.

"It happened in the second year of treatment, in December

1963. I don't know how it happened—and it doesn't matter. But there was a slipup here or there or somewhere, and we ran out of diazepam. I sent an airmail letter off to Hoffmann-La Roche, but I wasn't particularly worried. I didn't think that a couple of days off diazepam would seriously revive her symptoms. And they didn't. She seemed to be all right—for a day or two. She was much the same as ever. She then began to act a little anxious, and there was some tremor and twitching. I still wasn't really worried—only a bit uneasy. Then, all of a sudden, I got a call from Mr. Carter. His wife was having convulsions. For a moment, I thought he meant a return of the stiff-man spasms. But it wasn't that. I realized a moment later that he was describing a status-epilepticus seizure, and I told him I'd get out there as fast as I could. Status epilepticus is a series of epileptic-like seizures, and it represents a real medical emergency. The seizures often come so fast the patient has no chance to breathe. There are several drugs that are more or less effective in controlling status epilepticus. The drug I used was sodium pentobarbital. It worked well enough. Then I called an ambulance and got her to the hospital. She had no more seizures that day or that night, and the next morning a new supply of diazepam arrived by special-delivery airmail.

"So it turned out to be just an incident. The effect of diazepam is practically immediate. There was no harm done. There was no setback. There were no aftereffects. Mrs. Carter continued to improve. In a few more months, she could walk around the room by holding on to the furniture. Then she was doing the cooking again, and even a little housework. And then she got to the point where she could walk just leaning on her husband's arm. They even go out now and then. The last time I saw her, she was talking about getting a job."

[1968]

CHAPTER 17

The Hiccups

———————————⟨◆⟩———————————

AMONG THE SEVERAL PATIENTS who consulted Dr. Heinz B. Eisenstadt, an internist, at his office in Port Authur, Texas, on the morning of February 13, 1945, was a sixty-year-old oil-refinery worker whom I'll call Eliot Warren. Warren's appointment identified him as a new patient, and, as was usual in such cases, his medical history was recorded by a nurse in a cubicle off the reception room. It showed that he had undergone a hernia operation in 1940, and that he suffered from hives (after eating certain foods), hay fever (in season), asthma, and a frequent need to urinate. This visit, however, had nothing to do with any of those afflictions. His present complaint, he told the nurse, was what he took to be an attack of indigestion. He had been troubled for almost a week with flatulence and heartburn. Dr. Eisenstadt had the nurse's report on his desk when Warren was shown into his office. He could see no cause for serious concern in either Warren's past or present problems, and an immediate freehand examination confirmed that first impression. Warren's allergic susceptibilities were essentially unimportant, his asthmatic symptoms were a manifestation of a mild emphysema, his urinary difficulties were the natural consequence of a moderate (and, in a man of sixty, more or less normal) enlargement of the prostate gland, and his indigestion was probably simple indigestion. Dr. Eisenstadt explained these observations to Warren, and then turned him over to a technician for a definitive appraisal—a chest X-ray, an electrocardiogram, and the standard laboratory tests. Such an appraisal, he said, was merely prudent. He was confident that Warren had nothing to worry about. Meanwhile, he added, he would draw up a prescription to ease his stomach and a diet to keep it easy.

Dr. Eisenstadt didn't expect to see Warren soon again, and he didn't. Warren had not been a memorable patient, and Dr. Eisenstadt almost at once forgot him. Warren remained forgotten for almost exactly four years—until March 1, 1949. On the morning of that day, he reappeared at Dr. Eisenstadt's office with what sounded like the same complaint as before. Also, he had the hiccups. He had been hiccuping off and on for several weeks. Some of the spells had lasted as long as two or three hours, and he was beginning to get worried. He had tried all the home remedies that were known in his home, but none of them had worked. When the hiccups stopped, they simply stopped. Warren added that he had had a similar experience back in 1940. That was the year of his hernia operation, and, as well as he could remember, the hiccups had happened around that time. Dr. Eisenstadt made a perfunctory note. He couldn't see any real connection between that experience of hiccups and this. He could, however, see one between these spells and the chronic indigestion about which Warren had consulted him in 1945. Indigestion—gastric irritation—is the usual cause of hiccups. But his first concern was for Warren's comfort. He wrote out a prescription for what he hoped would be a curative combination of codeine, phenobarbital, and belladonna. He then reviewed Warren's diet. That seemed to confirm the cause of the trouble: Warren had drifted away from most of the 1945 recommendations. Dr. Eisenstadt put him firmly back on a proper bland regimen.

That was a Tuesday. Six days later, on Monday, March 7th, Dr. Eisenstadt received a telephone call from Warren. The reason for the call was only too apparent. Warren had the hiccups. Dr.

Eisenstadt told him to come at once to the office, and he was ready for him when he arrived. He gave him an intravenous injection of a respiratory and central-nervous-system stimulant called nikethamide. Nikethamide is a powerful drug, and it had a powerful effect on Warren. He gave a gasp—an enormous gasp—and his hiccups stopped. The attack had lasted for five or six hours, and the relief he now felt was exquisite. It enabled him to think of other things—other problems. He reported to Dr. Eisenstadt that he still had trouble urinating. In fact, he thought, it was worse than before. Dr. Eisenstadt examined his prostate. Four years had made a difference. It was considerably enlarged. Dr. Eisenstadt gave him a prostatic massage, and that seemed to help. Warren left the office in good spirits.

Two weeks went by. Dr. Eisenstadt heard nothing more from Warren, and he found his silence gratifying. The nikethamide injection had apparently had a lasting impact. But it hadn't. Warren's hiccups returned on the morning of March 24th, and that afternoon he was back in Dr. Eisenstadt's office. Dr. Eisenstadt did as he had done before. He gave Warren an injection of nikethamide, and again the hiccups stopped. But this time they hardly stayed stopped at all. Warren was back again the next afternoon in the clutch of another seizure. Dr. Eisenstadt's confidence in nikethamide was shaken but not yet shattered. He gave Warren another injection, and it worked as it had before—exactly as before. It stopped the hiccups, but only for a matter of hours. They returned the following morning. Nevertheless, Dr. Eisenstadt tried nikethamide once again. He knew it would give Warren at least some relief, and he hoped it would do more than that. If it didn't, he decided, Warren would have to go into the hospital. He would need the kind of treatment that only a hospital can provide. The nikethamide failed to recover its enduring original power, and the hiccups were back the next morning. That was March 27th. Dr. Eisenstadt called St. Mary's Hospital and made the necessary arrangements, and Warren was admitted there that afternoon for observation and treatment of persistent hiccups.

A hiccup (or, as medical pedants sometimes prefer, singultus) is the strangulating result of a spasmodic contraction of the diaphragm. It occurs when the massive intake of air thus involuntarily induced is abruptly checked by a sudden, arbitrary closure of the windpipe. The name of the phenomenon derives from the sound of that explosive interruption. In this onomatopoeic respect, the hiccup resembles the cough, the sneeze, and the belch, and it is also, like those similarly spontaneous spasms, a physiological commonplace. There, however, the similarity ceases. The cough, the sneeze, and the belch are all protective reactions. They are an essential part of the body's defensive apparatus: they clear the throat, they open the nose, they ease the bloated stomach. Hiccups serve no useful purpose. They are purely pathological. At best, they are merely innocuous. At worst, they can be, and often have been, fatal.

The immediate cause of the hiccup spasm is a reflex set in motion by an abnormal stimulation of the conductors that control the diaphragm and the opening (which science calls the glottis) at the mouth of the windpipe. These conductors are the phrenic and the vagus nerves. The stimulation that excites these nerves may be direct or it may have its origin in the central nervous system. Almost any disease, including (particularly in women) psychogenic disorders, thus has the power to precipitate an attack of hiccups, and, for the same reason, hiccups are a not uncommon aftermath of serious surgery. Hiccup spasms, being reflex actions, occur with metronomic regularity, but the tempo may be fast or slow. In dangerous attacks (those that persist for forty-eight hours or more), the beat is always fast. Persistent hiccups usually appear in tandem with some serious disease or condition. The severity of an attack of hiccups is determined by its duration, and it is persistence—hour after hour of jolting, jarring, breath-taking, sleepless spasms—that makes hiccups dangerous.

The treatment of hiccups involves the interruption of the perpetuating reflex. Once its regular rhythm is broken, the spasms generally cease. Simple hiccups—the hiccups that follow the bolted meal or the ultimate drink—respond to simple devices. There are many such devices, and most of them are very old. Some understanding of the cause and cure of simple hiccups is probably as old as the hiccups themselves. Plato, in the fourth century B.C., enlivened the Dialogue that he called the "Symposium" with a sudden attack of the hiccups: "The turn of Aristophanes was next, but either he had eaten too much, or from some other cause [he had been 'drowned in drink' the day before], he had the hiccough." Aristophanes is advised by Eryximachus, "Let me recommend you to hold your breath, and if after you have done so for some time the hiccough is no better, then gargle with a little water; and if it still continues, tickle your nose with something and sneeze; and if you sneeze once or twice, even the most violent hiccough is sure to go." A few minutes later, Aristophanes announces, "The hiccough is gone. . . . I no sooner applied the sneezing than I was cured." Sneezing was the remedy most favored by Hippocrates. He seems, moreover, to have understood why it worked. "If sneezing is produced," he notes in the clinical testament known as "Aphorisms," "the singultus being temporarily suppressed, the singultus will be cured." The first-century Roman encyclopedist Pliny also recommended sneezing. "To sneeze," he notes in his "Natural History," "is a ready way to be rid of the yex or hiccough." Sneezing was one of several similarly effective remedies proposed by the eighteenth-century German physician Valentino Krauetermann. In a book called *Der Thueringische Theophrastus Paracelsus, Wunder- und Kraueterdoctor, oder der curieuse und verneunftige Zauber-Arzt,* he notes, "Some cure [the hiccups] by unexpectedly frightening the patient. Some say to rub the little finger in the ears; some hold the breath or sneeze." Other standard remedies long listed in the folk pharmacopoeia include a cold compress on the back of the neck, a glass or two of cold water drunk slowly, and a sharp pull on the tongue. All of these several remedies are empirical remedies. They were discovered by some happy accident, and they have survived because—though for reasons unknown to the discoverer (the phrenic nerve, for example, runs up the side of the neck)—they more or less consistently work. The most reliable of the empirical hiccup cures is a refinement of Eryximachus's first recommendation. It is also ingeniously simple. The patient, instead of holding his breath, merely breathes for two or three minutes into a paper bag. Breathing and rebreathing the air in the bag increases, first, the amount of carbon dioxide in the bag, then the carbon dioxide in the lungs, and, finally, the cardon dioxide in the blood. This emergency arouses the respiratory centers in the brain to defensive action. They move to eliminate the dangerous concentration of carbon dioxide by quickening and deepening the contractions of the diaphragm, and the hiccup spasms are tripped and broken.

The dyspeptical hiccup remedies have no effect on hiccups of more complicated origin. They are too feeble to interrupt the spasms that spring from powerful provocation. Persistent hiccups give way, if at all, only to overwhelming pressures. The most overwhelming of these maneuvers is surgical—one of the phrenic nerves (usually the left) is exposed and blocked. Another approach is chemical. This includes the administration of such variously potent drugs as anti-spasmodics, muscle relaxants, respiratory stimulants, and central-nervous-system depressants. A third approach is an absolute refinement of the paper-bag technique. The paper bag is here replaced by a machine that produces a mixture of five to ten per cent carbon dioxide in oxygen. The patient, masked and closely attended, breathes that near-toxic air for several minutes (but no more than ten) every hour until his hiccups cease—or until he feels a warning wave of dizziness. It was to receive this often magisterial treatment that Eliot Warren was admitted to St. Mary's Hospital on the afternoon of March 27, 1949.

Warren spent a week at St. Mary's. The carbon-dioxide-inhalation treatment was at first only briefly effective, but then the intervals between attacks began to lengthen. They grew from hours to a day to days. By the seventh hospital day—on Saturday, April 2nd—it was clear that the seizure was over, and Warren was discharged that afternoon. Dr. Eisenstadt saw him out with a comfortable combination of relief and satisfaction. He was relieved that Warren's hiccups had finally relented, and he was satisfied that he knew their probable cause. He didn't think it was indigestion again. These hiccups were too persistent for that. But the hospital had offered a clue. A series of diagnostic tests and examinations showed that Warren's general debilities now included an incipient cerebral arteriosclerosis. His arteries were beginning to harden. It was Dr. Eisenstadt's guess that Warren had recently suffered a little stroke. Little strokes—strokes so slight that they do no perceptible damage—are not uncommon in men past sixty. Warren's arteriosclerotic condition favored such a stroke, and such a stroke could easily have produced the neural excitation necessary to set off a prolonged attack of hiccups. Dr. Eisenstadt closed his record of the episode with that tentative explanation.

Warren faded once again from Dr. Eisenstadt's mind. He was recalled, but only for a moment, in the spring of 1951. Dr. Eisenstadt had been away on a short vacation. When he returned to his office, he found among the reports left by his locum tenens a note on a visit from Warren. Warren's complaint was hiccups—intermittent hiccups for three days' duration. The doctor had prescribed, apparently successfully, a sedative. Two more years went by. Then, on June 22, 1953, Warren turned up again. But it wasn't hiccups this time. The symptoms that promoted his visit were swollen ankles, shortness of breath, and a recent gain in weight. Dr. Eisenstadt's interpretation of these conspicuously dropsical signs was conventional. In view of Warren's arteriosclerotic history, they almost certainly pointed to congestive heart failure. At the moment, he thought, it was not an unduly dangerous condition, but he prescribed the conventional treatment: digitalis, once a day. He then asked Warren about his other, established complaints. Warren thought they were much the same. Two years ago, not long before his last visit, he had suffered a painful attack of prostatitis, and a urologist he consulted had performed an alleviative transurethral resection—but that was all. What about hiccups? Warren shook his head. He hadn't had a real hiccup in months. He thought they were gone for good.

Warren spoke a bit too soon. Three weeks later, on July 12th, Dr. Eisenstadt got a telephone call from Warren's urologist. Warren was back in St. Mary's Hospital. His prostate was again inflamed, and he had been admitted the day before for a cystoscopic (or direct) examination to evaluate the nature of the trouble. The cystoscopy had been reassuring—no sign of any serious disease. But shortly after the operation Warren had begun to hiccup, and he had been hiccuping ever since. Would Dr. Eisenstadt, as Warren's family physician, come over and lend a hand? Dr. Eisenstadt would, and did. He treated Warren first with carbon dioxide, and then, when that failed to firmly subdue the spasms, with a respiratory stimulant called pentylenetetrazol. Pentylenetetrazol, after almost a week, brought the attack to an end. But what had caused this attack? Warren's general condition seemed much as usual. Dr. Eisenstadt was at a loss for several days. He finally decided to attribute the attack to the stress and strain of the cystoscopic examination.

Another interlude occurred. Warren came to Dr. Eisenstadt's attention just four times in the course of the next twelve years. He saw him once in 1955, once in 1958, and twice in 1962. Three were office calls, and one was a hospital visit. The 1955 consultation was for a sudden recurrence of the hiccups. It was not a vigorous attack, and Dr. Eisenstadt treated it successfully with a muscle relaxant called quinidine. The cause of the attack appeared to be a return of Warren's chronically recurrent indigestion. It was an attack of indigestion—including heartburn, nausea, and vomiting —that brought Warren into Dr. Eisenstadt's office in 1958. Dr. Eisenstadt satisfied himself that it was indeed an attack of indigestion, and then treated Warren with a soothing drug and another warning word on diet. He also took advantage of the occasion to give him a comprehensive checkup. This confirmed that Warren's several ailments were still progressing at an unhurried rate commensurate with his age. It also added a new debility to the list. Warren now had a mild and easily controllable diabetes mellitus. The first of the 1962 visits was brought about by another prostate operation—a transurethral re-resection. Dr. Eisenstadt's role was that of a clinical consultant to the urologist. He determined that Warren had the stamina to endure such an operation, and then stood by in case an attack of post-operative hiccups broke out. One did, but he brought it quickly to heel with Dramamine. The other 1962 visit occurred only two weeks later. It was a routine post-operative consultation, and Dr. Eisenstadt's findings were entirely routine.

Warren turned eighty in 1965. He was still active enough for his limited needs and notions, but the burden of ailments that he carried now was considerable. Dr. Eisenstadt examined him in February of that year and found that he was suffering from general arteriosclerosis, congestive heart failure, coronary heart disease, emphysema, chronic indigestion, prostatic hypertrophy, diabetes, hay fever, phlebitis (in the left leg), and gallstones. None, however, was alarmingly advanced, and most of them were held in tolerable check by drugs. The drugs that performed these services were also notably numerous. Dr. Eisenstadt ran down the list. It included digitalis, an aluminum hydroxide stomachic, a diuretic (to control the edema resulting from his congestive heart failure), an antihistamine (to control his hay fever), tolbutamide (to control his diabetes), a choleretic (to control his gallstones), and sulfamethizole. This last was news to Dr. Eisenstadt. He was aware that Warren's urologist had prescribed sulfamethizole at various times in the past. The sulfonamides have always (since their first appearance in the late nineteen-thirties) been the drug of choice in the control of infection in urinary-tract disorders. But now he learned that Warren had not confined his use of sulfamethizole to the periods immediately following his prostatic operations. He took the drug whenever he felt or feared a recurrence of prostatic pain. He sometimes took it every day. Dr. Eisenstadt opened his mouth to remonstrate, and then changed his mind. He didn't approve of this casual consumption of sulfamethizole, but he could see that it probably performed a salubrious psychological service. It was probably almost as necessary to Warren's well-being as any of his other drugs. Dr. Eisenstadt completed the examination in a generally optimistic frame of mind. For a man of Warren's age and afflictions, he was in satisfactory shape. The only problem was his hiccups. Their persistence was inexplicable. He may have been right in attributing Warren's first attack to a burst of indigestion. He may have been right in attributing the second to a little stroke. He may have been right in attributing others to the stresses and strains of surgery. And yet he didn't think so. He couldn't believe that so many different attacks had sprung from so many different sources. He couldn't believe in anything as arbitrary as that. He thought there was probably a single underlying cause. But he couldn't think what it might be.

Warren's hiccups lay unaccountably quiescent for just over a year. Then, in the spring of 1966, they unaccountably returned. The attack began on May 12th. None of the usual home or office remedies had any prolonged effect, and on May 15th Warren was again admitted to St. Mary's Hospital for observation and treatment. The treatment included carbon-dioxide inhalation, intravenous injections of the respiratory stimulant pentylenetetrazol, and, finally, intravenous injections of a tranquilizer called chlorpromazine hydrochloride. The observation took the form of an allergy investigation. Dr. Eisenstadt was still convinced that all of Warren's hiccup attacks were the work of a common cause, and it now occurred to him that the cause might be some food, some drink, or some drug. The investigation followed the standard elimination procedure. Certain frequently allergenic foods—milk, eggs, corn, wheat—were successively eliminated from Warren's diet. Then, after an interval, they were successively and abundantly restored. The results were noted. They were negative. Warren had no allergic reaction to any of the tested foods. Neither deprivation nor plenty had any effect on his hiccups. Dr. Eisenstadt then turned his attention to Warren's diet of drugs. The drugs that he took every day—digitalis, aluminum hydroxide, tolbutamide, antihistamine, the choleretic, and the diuretic—were one by one withdrawn. The results were the same as those of the food-allergy tests. Warren's hiccups continued. They continued through the elimination tests, they continued in spite of repeated carbon-dioxide inhalations, they continued in spite of the pentylenetetrazol injections. They were stopped at last by several commanding injections of chlorpromazine hydrochloride. That was on May 29th, and Warren's endurance was almost at an end. He had endured three weeks of almost continuous hiccups.

The episode had also shaken Dr. Eisenstadt. It left him with an uneasy view of the future. Warren's persistent hiccups were becoming more and more persistent and less and less susceptible to treatment. He dreaded the next attack.

The next attack began on April 6, 1967. Warren was then making his home with a married daughter, and it was she who notified Dr. Eisenstadt. He responded by coming at once to the house. He found Warren exhausted and in bed—the hiccups had kept him awake all night—but otherwise much the same as before. His only notable bedside finding was that Warren was now wearing (on his urologist's prescription) an indwelling catheter to relieve his urinary difficulties. The hiccups were, as always, inexplicable. Dr.

Eisenstadt considered his diminishing armamentarium, and gave Warren an intravenous injection of chlorpromazine hydrochloride. Chlorpromazine was the drug that he had used with success in the last persistent attack. Its effect this time was similarly, but not equally, successful. It lasted only overnight. Warren's hiccups then gradually returned—gradually and, as if some authoritative trace of chlorpromazine still lingered on, in a muted form. The spasms were weak and widely spaced. Dr. Eisenstadt prescribed an oral dose of Dramamine. The muted spasms subsided, but after a couple of restful hours Warren began to hiccup again. However, Dramamine was still effective, and it remained effective against a succession of recurring mild attacks. Then, on April 14th, Warren was shaken by a violent seizure, and it was necessary for Dr. Eisenstadt to administer another chlorpromazine injection. That drug was once again effective, and Warren once again experienced an overnight remission and another week of generally mild and easily subdued atacks. By the end of the week, the Dramamine tablets had begun to lose their suppressive power, and Dr. Eisenstadt revised his prescription to Dramamine suppositories. This more forceful treatment prevailed for another week, and then it, too, began to weaken. On April 29th, the violent hiccups violently reappeared. They yielded again for several hours to intravenous chlorpromazine, but when its hold relaxed they erupted as violently as before. Dramamine suppositories had no effect on this attack. It was brought under control with chlorpromazine in suppository form. But only momentarily. Another, more severe attack occurred on April 30th, and this was followed three days later by another. That attack was intractable, and on Thursday, May 4th, after two days of unbroken hiccups, Warren was admitted once more to St. Mary's Hospital. He reached there more dead than alive. Four weeks of almost continual jerking had exacerbated most of his chronic ailments, and his heart was enlarged and beating hard. He was groggy from lack of sleep, and weak from lack of food. The hiccups that kept him awake had kept him from eating, and he had lost some twenty pounds of weight. He was also in pain. All of his muscles were stretched and sore, and he hurt at every gulping, strangulated breath. His condition at admission was described as critical.

The first hospital attempt to hobble Warren's hiccups involved the once-triumphant carbon-dioxide-inhalation treatment. It gave him only a few short spells of relief. The next treatment was an intravenous injection of nikethamide. His hiccups continued unimpeded. A lumbar puncture was then proposed. A lumbar puncture is usually performed to obtain a quantity of cerebrospinal fluid for diagnostic analysis, but the operation was recommended now for therapeutic purposes as well. It was hoped that an examination of the fluid would suggest the cause of Warren's hiccups, and that the operation itself would excite a remedial reaction in the central nervous system. The lumbar puncture was half successful. It didn't explain the hiccups but it stopped them. The remission lasted twenty-four hours, and then the spasms started up again. Another lumbar puncture was tried, but this time nothing happened. Warren continued to hiccup. The news of his trouble had spread by now throughout the Jefferson County medical community, and on May 10th Dr. Eisenstadt was approached by a colleague who was also a hypnotist. The hypnotist offered Warren his salubrious powers of suggestion. Dr. Eisenstadt considered, and agreed. He didn't think that hypnotism would do much good. He didn't think that Warren's hiccups were psychogenically inspired. Psychogenic hiccups seldom interfere with sleep. But it could hardly do any harm. The hypnotist appeared at Warren's bedside at nine o'clock the following morning, and he stayed there most of the day. He then wrote a short memorandum and left it for Dr. Eisenstadt. It read, "Patient hypnotized and taught how to relax. Second technic: to forget how to hiccup. Third: improve bowel habits. Fourth: improve sleep pattern. The patient was very coöperative, and I feel that he responded well to hypnotherapy. He said he may want me to come back. Thanks for letting me see this fine gentleman." But Warren went on hiccuping. A desperate remedy composed of promethazine hydrochloride (an antihistamine), meperidine hydrochloride (or Demerol, a narcotic analgesic drug with certain antispasmodic powers), and oxygen inhalation produced a restful respite, but— as so often before—it was only temporary. Surgical intervention involving the phrenic nerves was next considered. That, however, wasn't possible here. The action of the diaphragm is directed by two phrenic nerves, and in Warren's unfortunate case both of these nerves were involved in his spasms. To block them both would also block his breathing. Dr. Eisenstadt and his hospital consultants consulted once again. There was almost nothing left to try. And then, while they were consulting, the crisis resolved itself. Warren's hiccups spontaneously stopped. His general condition at once began to improve, and on May 20th, the seventeenth hospital day, he was judged sufficiently recovered to go home.

Warren was at home for just two days. He was discharged from the hospital on a Saturday, and on Monday he was readmitted. His hiccups had intractably returned. All of the standard remedies were tried, but only one was more than momentarily effective. That was oxygen, and even it gave only an hour or two of relief. Dr. Eisenstadt sat down with Warren's chart and re-read its entries. The reading confirmed his belief that there were no more untried drugs to try. Nor were there any new techniques or devices. He reconsidered and once again discarded the possibility that Warren's hiccups might have their seat in one or another of his many chronic diseases. Except when exacerbated by the hiccups, all of Warren's diseases were pretty well under control. He reviewed the series of allergy tests that had been performed in 1966. The results still looked as conclusive as they had a year ago. There was nothing in Warren's diet that could possibly cause his hiccups. The same was true of the drugs he took. Dr. Eisenstadt checked them off—digitalis, aluminum hydroxide, tolbutamide, antihistamine, a diuretic, a choleretic, sulfamethizole. He stopped and looked again at the chart. Sulfamethizole was on the list of Warren's drugs, but it hadn't been included in the allergy tests. There had been no reason to suspect it. Its use was too occasional. It wasn't part of Warren's daily regimen. But now he began to wonder.

Dr. Eisenstadt returned the chart to the record room and went into the ward and had a word with Warren. Warren told him what he wanted to know. He was taking sulfamethizole. He had been taking it for the past two or three days. His prostate had been acting up again. Dr. Eisenstadt went to a telephone and put in a call to Warren's urologist. He explained what he had in mind. It wasn't a hunch. It wasn't even a notion. It was just that sulfamethizole was the only unknown factor, the only uninvestigated drug. The urologist listened, and unenthusiastically agreed to indulge Dr. Eisenstadt in his whim. He would see that Warren was taken off sulfamethizole for a couple of days. There were other, though less satisfactry, drugs that could replace it if the need arose. He would make the necessary arrangements at once. Dr. Eisenstadt thanked him and crossed his fingers and waited. He wasn't kept in suspense for long. Warren was separated from sulfamethizole—from all and any sulfonamide drugs—in the late afternoon. Late the following afternoon, his hiccups began to subside. They continued to slow and slacken, and in the early evening of the second day they finally stopped altogether. The urologist extended the sulfonamide ban, and entered an antibiotic substitute in the order book. Another day went by, and then another. By the end of the week, it was certain. The attack was definitely over, and on Sunday, June 4th, Warren was discharged to convalesce at home.

Warren's recovery left Dr. Eisenstadt in a state of hamstrung exultation. He thought he had found in sulfamethizole the root of Warren's endlessly recurring hiccups. The evidence was everywhere. Warren's last attack had followed a self-prescription of sulfamethizole, and the elimination of sulfamethizole had been followed by a remission. That plainly projected a cause-and-effect relationship between sulfamethizole and the hiccups. Nor was that all. The presence of sulfamethizole—or of some other sulfonamide drug—could at least be assumed in all of Warren's persistent attacks. Hindsight seemed to show that they had coincided with either self-prescription or surgical prescription of that drug. It was even possible to link it with Warren's first attack—the outbreak of hiccups that followed his hernia operation back in 1940. Nineteen-forty was before the development of antibiotics. The only drug then available for use in the routine prevention of postoperative infection was one of the sulfonamides. Reflection also suggested that sulfamethizole had the power as well as the opportunity to precipitate Warren's attacks. It was true that none of the sulfonamides had ever before been implicated in a case of persistent hiccups, but most of them were notorious for their manifold side effects, and these included a malevolent impact on the central nervous system. In a man as variously debilitated as Warren, that impact could easily detonate a violent attack of the hiccups. And yet. None of this was proof. It was merely a structure of supposition. Warren's remission wasn't necessarily attributable to the elimination of sulfamethizole. It could have been simply spontaneous.

Whatever its nature, Warren's remission continued. He looked and felt and was in better health than he had been in for more than a year. His only remaining complaint was his perennially progressive prostatic hypertrophy, and toward the end of July the urologist judged—and Dr. Eisenstadt concurred—that his general condition was robust enough to withstand another transurethral re-resection. Warren re-entered St. Mary's Hospital on July 24th, and the operation was performed the next morning. The following day, Dr. Eisenstadt received a telephone call from the urologist. He was calling to report on Warren. The operation itself had gone very well, but now, he was sorry to say, a complication had developed. Warren had the hiccups again. He had been hiccuping for several hours and responded to none of the conventional remedies. Dr. Eisenstadt's heart sank. He thanked the urologist and said he would see what he could do and started to hang up—and had a sudden thought. The urologist was still on the line. By the way, Dr. Eisenstadt said. He spoke as casually as he could. What drug were they using to control post-operative bladder infection? Drug? the urologist said. They were using sulfamethizole. That was the usual drug in such . . . Memory struck him, and he stopped. He cleared his throat. But if Dr. Eisenstadt preferred, he would change his orders to some non-sulfonamide drug. As he had before. Dr. Eisenstadt said he thought it might be worth trying.

It was. Sulfamethizole was stopped and Warren's hiccups stopped, and he never took any more sulfonamides and he never hiccuped again.

[*1969*]

CHAPTER 18

A Woman with a Headache

—————————◆—————————

A WOMAN I'LL CALL Mildred Anderson—Mrs. Harold Anderson —was admitted to Temple University Hospital, in North Philadelphia, on the afternoon of Friday, January 19, 1968, for observation and treatment of a severe and persistent headache. Mrs. Anderson's admission was arranged by Dr. Albert J. Finestone, an internist and a clinical professor of medicine at Temple University School of Medicine, to whom she had been referred by her family physician, and she was shown to a two-bed room on the fourth floor and made as comfortable as possible. That was around two o'clock. At five, an interne on Dr. Finestone's service named Mary E. Moore dropped in for the opening diagnostic interrogation.

Dr. Moore introduced herself. She sat down and smiled and asked Mrs. Anderson how she felt. Mrs. Anderson said she felt pretty good. She hesitated. As a matter of fact, she felt fine. It was a funny thing, she said. It was almost embarrassing. Her headache was gone. In the two or three hours that she had been in the hospital, it had completely vanished. She didn't understand it at all. It was almost as if the hospital had scared it away. Dr. Moore said nothing. She nodded and made a sympathetic sound. But she thought she understood it well enough. Dr. Moore is not only a doctor of medicine. She is also a doctor of philosophy in experimental psychology, and she knew that it was entirely possible that Mrs. Anderson's headache *had* been scared away. Hospitals often have that effect on functional, or psychogenic, disorders. That didn't mean, however, that Mrs. Anderson's headache *was* functional in origin. It was just a possibility. Hospitals often momentarily exert much the same inhibiting effect on the pain of disorders that are fully and ferociously somatic.

Dr. Moore got out her pen and a ruled personal-history form. Mrs. Anderson was a striking-looking woman. Her hair was white, her complexion was rough and florid, and her eyes were large and expressive. She was small and notably thin. Her age, as given on her chart, was forty-one. The chart also noted that she and her husband, a civil engineer, were childless, and owned their own home. Mrs. Anderson shifted her position in bed—and Dr. Moore was startled to see that her spine was twisted and bent in the humpbacked conformation known as kyphoscoliosis. Startled and interested. That explained Mrs. Anderson's size, and possibly more than that. Dr. Moore began the interview. Mrs. Anderson was quietly and politely responsive. Her chief complaint was, of course, a headache. It had first appeared about three weeks ago. She had suffered off and on for many years from what she believed were migraine headaches, but this was nothing like those. There was no nausea, no vomiting, no sensitivity to light. It was simply an excruciating pain that progressed from the back of her head to the top. The migraine headaches had begun in childhood, and she was the only member of her family to be so afflicted. The only drug she ever took was aspirin—until recently. Three weeks ago, her doctor prescribed a drug called Fiorinal for her headache. Dr. Moore nodded. Fiorinal is a popular, non-narcotic sedative and analgesic. However, Mrs. Anderson said, it hadn't done much good. This was the first real relief she had had in all those weeks. It was also her first experience as a hospital patient. Her back was not the result of either illness or injury: she had been born that way. She had never been seriously ill, and she had no known allergies. She drank occasionally, but she didn't smoke. Her ruddy complexion was normal for her. Her skin was naturally very dry.

It was often blotchy, and it tended to redden whenever she was tense or nervous. She had been like that all her life. Was she nervous now? Well, yes—she supposed she was. After all, she had never been hospitalized before.

That completed the historical phase of the interview. Dr. Moore moved from her chair to the bedside, and began the customary routine physical examination. She identified Mrs. Anderson's chronic dermatitis as ichthyosis congenita. She found Mrs. Anderson's eyes, ears, nose, throat, and neck to be essentially normal. There was no ocular evidence of brain tumor or of any intracranial swelling, and no venous distension, and no thyroid- or lymph-gland enlargement. She confirmed her snap diagnosis of kyphoscoliosis. Mrs. Anderson's breasts were normal. Her heart was normal in size and rhythm, and her lungs were clear to auscultation and percussion. There were no discernible abdominal masses, and her liver and spleen felt normal. Her reflexes were satisfactory, as were the results of a careful neurological examination. Dr. Moore added these reassuring but unilluminating findings to the record. She then turned to the order sheet and noted down the several preliminary tests and studies that she wished to have made. They included blood analyses (hematocrit, hemoglobin, serology, blood sugar, kidney function), urinalysis, chest X-ray, spine X-ray, neck X-ray, skull X-ray, brain scan, electroencephalogram, and electrocardiogram. The results of one or another of these should produce at least a glimmer of diagnostic enlightenment. Dr. Moore also asked that a dermatologist be consulted about the treatment of Mrs. Anderson's ichthyosis. She further noted that Mrs. Anderson was to be given codeine as needed (thirty milligrams every four hours) for the relief of her headache, and Nembutal (one hundred milligrams) for sleep. She closed the preliminary report with a preliminary comment: "Impression: (1) Congenital kyphoscoliosis. (2) Congenital ichthyosis. (3) Headache of unknown etiology—probably cervical spine deformity as cause. To be ruled out: Brain tumor or other intracerebral lesion."

Mrs. Anderson spent a generally comfortable night. She slept with the help of Nembutal, but she had no need for codeine. Her headache was still ambiguously quiescent. She was rested but not yet fully relaxed when Dr. Finestone walked in on his rounds the following morning with his entourage of students and internes. Dr. Finestone was roughly familiar with the nature of her case. He had spoken with Dr. Moore the night before, and he had just now read her notes and comments. Nevertheless, like all scrupulous attending physicians, he sat down and saw for himself. He led Mrs. Anderson briefly back through her relevant history, and then appraised by direct examination what her history suggested were the physical essentials. He was interested and puzzled by the disappearance of her headache. But he could see no cause for any alarm, and he ended the visit with a word of sincere reassurance.

The next day—January 21st—was a Sunday. It passed agreeably for Mrs. Anderson. She had a visit from her husband, and there was still no return of her headache. An interne on weekend duty noted that she seemed less tense and restless than reported the day before. The strangeness of the hospital life appeared to be wearing off. On Monday, the first results of the diagnostic studies were reported. They included the standard laboratory tests, the electrocardiogram, and three of the four requested X-ray examinations—chest, neck, and spine. Dr. Finestone and Dr. Moore went over the findings together. None of the reports contained any diagnostic surprises. Mrs. Anderson's chest, heart, kidneys, and blood were normal. The radiologist's report on the look of her neck and spine read: "A marked degree of scoliosis of the dorsal spine with the convexity to the right is seen. . . . Changes in the thorax secondary to scoliosis are also noted. The cervical and dorsal spine reveal no other significant abnormalities. The intervertebral foramina are patent. No osteolytic or osteoblastic abnormalities are seen." (Osteolysis is a dissolution of bone, and an osteoblast is a cell involved in bone production.) Later that day, the dermatological consultant confirmed that Mrs. Anderson's skin condition was indeed a congenital ichthyosis, and prescribed for its correction a regimen of oil baths and rubs.

Two of the three remaining studies were completed on Wednesday. They were the skull X-ray and the electroencephalogram. Dr. Finestone recorded the results on Mrs. Anderson's chart: "EEG & skull films negative." He then added his comments and conclusions: "Pain gone. Likely diagnosis—cervical spondylosis. Doubt intracranial cause." The results of the brain-scan study were reported the following day. They considerably decreased the possibility of any cerebral involvement: "Following administration of technetium 99m pertechnetate, the brain was examined by the scintillation camera in five views (anterior, posterior, left lateral, right lateral, and vertex) after preparation with potassium perchlorate. No abnormalities are noted in any of these views." That was the last of the diagnostic studies, and it seemed to Dr. Moore almost conclusive. It strengthened her impression that there was nothing very wrong with Mrs. Anderson. Even the woman's headache was gone—spontaneously gone—and had been gone for close to a week. Dr. Moore noted on the chart for Dr. Finestone's approval that Mrs. Anderson was now ready for discharge. Dr. Finestone concurred in this judgment, and Mrs. Anderson was discharged from the hospital early on Thursday afternoon. Her case was closed with a final diagnosis: "Headache secondary to cervical scoliosis and nervous tension."

Dr. Moore was with Mrs. Anderson when her husband arrived to take her home. Mr. Anderson was much like his wife—quiet, pleasant, coöperative. He was also, like his wife, a little confused and worried. They didn't understand that equivocal week in the hospital. Dr. Moore undertook to reassure them. She reminded Mrs. Anderson of the many tests and examinations that she had undergone. They were the reason for her protracted hospital stay. She then explained their uniform results. There was no cause for any concern. Just the reverse. The tests had made it clear that Mrs. Anderson was in enviably excellent health. Dr. Moore tried to speak with conviction, and the Andersons were convinced. They thanked her and shook her hand and left the hospital arm in arm. Dr. Moore went on to her other patients. Some of them might never be discharged, and Mrs. Anderson dropped untroubled from her mind.

Dr. Finestone was the first to have Mrs. Anderson recalled to his attention. She was returned to his mind at one o'clock on Friday afternoon by another telephone call. The call reached him at Temple University Hospital, and the caller was Mr. Anderson. He was apologetically distraught. He was calling about his wife.

When he had brought her home from the hospital on Thursday afternoon she seemed to be in good spirits and she said she was feeling fine. He left her at home and went down to his office to finish up some urgent work. When he got back to the house a couple of hours later, she was prostrate on the sofa with one of her terrible headaches. He telephoned their doctor, and the doctor came to the house and gave her an injection of Demerol. That helped her through the night. But the headache came back this morning, and now—just a few minutes ago—his wife had fainted. He had come home from his office for lunch to see how she was. She told him she was feeling sick and dizzy, and that was when she fainted. She was conscious now, but she looked as if she might pass out again any minute. What should he do? Dr. Finestone asked if he had called the family doctor again. No? Then Mr. Anderson should call him, and right away. He was their regular doctor, he lived in the neighborhood, and he had treated Mrs. Anderson only the night before. However, if Mr. Anderson couldn't reach the doctor, he was to call Dr. Finestone again and bring his wife to the hospital. Mr. Anderson thanked him, and Dr. Finestone hung up and resumed his interrupted rounds. He wondered what could have happened to Mrs. Anderson. He couldn't relate it to anything in her known condition of health. It was very strange. It almost sounded hysterical. But she hadn't impressed him as being that neurotic. He finished his rounds, and Mr. Anderson still hadn't called. It was safe to assume that the matter was now in the hands of the family doctor. He looked around for Dr. Moore. It would be interesting to hear her opinion. But she wasn't on the floor. Dr. Finestone went down and changed out of his long white coat and put on his overcoat and went home. He didn't see Dr. Moore again until Sunday. By then it was all over.

Dr. Moore was assigned to overnight duty on Saturday. She reported to the hospital at noon and spent the afternoon on the floor. There were old patients to see and new patients to meet and study. She had dinner in the hospital cafeteria at five o'clock, and then went back to continue with her patients and see them settled for the night. It was an undemanding evening on her floor, and around midnight she went down to the emergency room and joined a couple of other idling internes and the resident on duty there. She had been sitting in their company about an hour—smoking and talking and drinking coffee—when she heard herself being paged. She walked around the corner to the house telephone. The call was not a summons from her floor. It was an outside call. The caller was a young woman and her voice was shrill and excited.

"Is this Dr. Mary Moore?"

"Yes."

"I'm the niece of Mrs. Anderson. One of her nieces. I think you helped take care of her when she was in the hospital?"

"That's right."

"Well, I'm over here at her house. At the Andersons' house. I came over this evening because my uncle called and asked me to help, and something terrible has happened to her. It's awful. She had this terrible headache yesterday, and she passed out I don't know how many times—and now she's lost the power of the tendons in her legs."

Dr. Moore stood silent with the telephone in her hand. She was stunned. She couldn't believe it. Mrs. Anderson had spent a full week under careful observation in a first-class university teaching hospital, and according to the most sophisticated tests and tabulations she was in essentially the best of health. There had been no sign of any serious ailment. But now—just two days later—she . . .

Dr. Moore took a deep breath. "You mean she's paralyzed?"

"I guess that's what it is," the niece said. "She's lost the power of her tendons."

"I think I'd better speak to Mrs. Anderson. Can you get her to the phone?"

"I'm afraid you can't. I mean, it wouldn't do any good. She isn't making any sense."

"Then let me speak to Mr. Anderson."

"My uncle?" She gave a wild laugh. "He's acting just as crazy as she is."

"Oh," Dr. Moore said. But she also felt a kind of relief. If both of the Andersons were affected, it must be something that had happened after Mrs. Anderson left the hospital. It might be some deranging form of food poisoning. It might be drugs. It might be simple alcohol. She remembered that Mrs. Anderson liked an occasional drink. "Do you think they might be drunk?"

"I don't know," the niece said. "I don't think so. I don't see any glasses or bottle or anything." She gave another wild laugh. "My uncle fainted this afternoon. That was before he called me."

Dr. Moore hesitated. She wondered if the niece had been drinking. "How about you?" she said. "Are you all right?"

"I don't know," the niece said. "I guess so. Sure, I'm O.K."

"I hope so," Dr. Moore said. "I want your aunt and uncle at the hospital as soon as possible. Can you get them here? Do you need any help?"

"I don't need any help. My friends have a car. I've got some friends here with me. I guess I forgot to tell you that. They're an older couple I know."

"All right," Dr. Moore said. "Come to the emergency room. I'll meet you there."

"O.K.," the niece said.

Dr. Moore waited at the emergency-room door. It opened and closed on the regular Saturday-night procession of beatings and knifings and car-wreck lacerations. At a little past two, the car with the niece and her friends and her aunt and uncle pulled into the curb, and Dr. Moore sent an orderly out to meet them with a rolling stretcher. She watched him lifting Mrs. Anderson onto the stretcher and the rest of them milling around and trying to help. Mr. Anderson wore striped pajamas under his overcoat, and he seemed to be yelling. The orderly pushed the stretcher up the walk and into the foyer, and Mrs. Anderson lifted her head. Her face was red and her eyes were bright. She saw Dr. Moore, and let out a cry of delight.

"Hi, there, Dr. Moore," she said. "I never expected to see you again. How you doing?"

"I'm fine," Dr. Moore said. "But what about you? What happened?"

Mrs. Anderson laughed.

Dr. Moore asked the niece and her friends to wait, and nodded to the orderly. She led the stretcher down the hall and into an examination booth. Mr. Anderson came stumbling loudly after them. His face was as flushed as his wife's. He flopped down on a chair and leaned loosely back. Dr. Moore sat down on a stool and looked at them. She felt she didn't know them at all. They didn't act or talk, or even look, like the Andersons she knew. She could only think they were drunk—or drugged. But she couldn't think what drugs they might have got to make them act this way. And they didn't smell of liquor.

"All right," she said. "Now tell me what happened. Have you been drinking?"

"Drinking?" Mrs. Anderson said. "Certainly not."

"We haven't been anything," Mr. Anderson said, and laughed.

"You haven't eaten anything unusual?"

"I haven't eaten hardly anything."

"Or taken any drugs?"

Mrs. Anderson let out a wail.

"Then tell me what happened."

"It was my head," Mrs. Anderson said. "You know about my headaches. Well, I got this terrible—"

"Now, wait a minute," Mr. Anderson said. "Wait just a minute. That isn't quite the way—"

"What isn't the way? I think I know—"

"But you're getting it all wrong. It wasn't—"

"Be quiet."

"Don't you tell me to be—"

"I said be quiet."

"Shut up."

"Stop it," Dr. Moore said. "Both of you. There's no reason to get so excited." She considered. They were obviously in no immediate danger. She decided to let the questioning go for a moment. They might be calmer then. And she wanted a moment to organize her own ideas. She stood up. "I'm going to leave you for a minute. Try to relax. I'll be right back."

Dr. Moore went down the hall to the house officers' corner. The resident was with a patient, but there were still two internes there. She told them about the Andersons.

"I just don't know what's going on," she said. "There's something wrong with these people. They're out of their heads. But I don't know why. The only other thing is her face is awfully red.

Except that her face is always red." She stopped. "You know, I just realized something. Her husband's face is also awfully red. They've both got bright-red faces."

One of the internes cocked his head. "Like cherry red?" he said. "Like carbon-monoxide poisoning?"

"My God," Dr. Moore said. "My God—that's it."

The cause of carbon-monoxide poisoning is the inhalation of carbon-monoxide gas. Carbon-monoxide gas is generated by the incomplete combustion of some carbonaceous (wood, coal, petroleum) material. Complete combustion, however, is not a natural phenomenon. It occurs only under the most fastidiously controlled conditions. Thus, for all practical purposes, carbon monoxide is a regular product of fire. Its nature is as insidious as its generation. The presence of carbon monoxide in a room or a street or an automobile is impossible to detect by any means naturally available to man. Its anonymity is as total as that of air. Carbon monoxide is colorless, odorless, and tasteless. It even has the same specific gravity as air. It neither sinks to the ground nor rises away like smoke but mixes and mingles indistinguishably with the atmosphere.

Carbon monoxide, though always dangerous and often deadly, is a poison only in the language of convenience. It is actually an asphyxiant. It deprives its victims of the oxygen they breathe by displacing oxygen in the carrier hemoglobin of the red blood cells. This suffocating displacement is easily accomplished. Hemoglobin, by some hematological quirk, much prefers carbon monoxide to oxygen. Recent investigators have mathematically rendered its preference into odds of approximately three hundred to one. Their calculations suggest that a given concentration of carbon monoxide in the air can successfully compete for the molecular embrace of hemoglobin with anything up to three hundred times its concentration of oxygen. The result of the eager union of carbon monoxide and hemoglobin is a brilliant-red compound called carboxyhemoglobin. Carboxyhemoglobin is the source of the characteristic cherry-red flush of carbon-monoxide poisoning. It also, however, has more sinister powers. It inhibits the release of whatever oxygen has managed to combine with hemoglobin.

Carboxyhemoglobin is a stable compound, but its bonds are far from unbreakable. They readily loosen under the impact of abundant oxygen, and the hemoglobin so released, unharmed by its impetuous encounter, is free to resume its proper physiological functions. That providential frailty of carboxyhemoglobin simplifies the treatment of carbon-monoxide poisoning. It is often treatment enough to remove the victim from the poison air. A few hours of rest will then restore the normal chemistry of his blood. More seriously stricken victims can usually be rallied by the administration of pure oxygen under pressure. Unless, of course, they are already dead or dying.

It takes very little carbon monoxide to contaminate the air. The virulence of carbon monoxide is very nearly unique. A concentration of only two one-hundredths of one per cent (or two hundred parts of carbon monoxide per million parts of air) can kindle in a couple of hours a dull frontal headache, and an exposure of just five minutes to air containing one per cent of carbon monoxide is almost invariably fatal. Moreover, the action of carbon monoxide is ferociously quickened by such environmental factors as heat and altitude, by the presence of debilitating disease like anemia and asthma, and by physical activity. The blood of a man at labor becomes saturated with carbon monoxide about three times faster than that of a man at rest. Mild but perceptible symptoms of illness ordinarily appear when the carboxyhemoglobin level approaches twenty per cent. More conspicuous symptoms—severe occipital headache, nausea, vomiting, dizziness, muscular incoördination, disorientation—develop as the saturation mounts toward forty per cent. At fifty per cent, unconsciousness usually descends, and a saturation of sixty-six per cent (or the conversion of two-thirds of the body's supply of hemoglobin into carboxyhemoglobin) is classically considered fatal.

The sources of carbon monoxide are abundant in the urban Western world. In the United States, they are almost everywhere. Carbon monoxide is perniciously present in the effluvia of all internal-combustion engines, most industrial plants, and many mines, mills, and workshops. There are also many domestic sources: unvented space heaters, floor furnaces, kerosene stoves, gas ranges, camp stoves, and blocked or faulty flues. Among the more familiar fuels, manufactured gas is potentially doubly dangerous, for it not only produces carbon monoxide (like natural gas and the other carbonaceous materials) but actually contains it. Burning charcoal is especially rich in carbon monoxide—so rich that in France, where charcoal fires are widely used for cooking, carbon-monoxide poisoning is sometimes called *folie des cuisiniers.* Another rich source is burning tobacco. The blood of heavy cigarette smokers (those who smoke two or three packages a day) has been found to contain as much as ten per cent carboxyhemoglobin, or almost enough to cause manifest signs of illness. The most insidious source of carbon monoxide is, of course, the gasoline engine. It is also, with an ever-increasing multitude of ever more powerful automobiles on the streets, an increasingly serious one. Automobile (and motorboat) exhaust fumes contain about seven per cent carbon monoxide, and where traffic is slow and heavy the amount of carbon monoxide pumped into the air can easily approach a toxic level. A field study undertaken by the National Air Pollution Control Administration in 1967 has demonstrated that it often does. The study was conducted in ten cities (Atlanta, Baltimore, Chicago, Cincinnati, Detroit, Louisville, New York, Minneapolis, Denver, and Los Angeles) at the peak of the rush-hour traffic. Bumper-to-bumper speeds produce about three times as much carbon monoxide as a cruising speed of forty-five miles an hour. Instruments mounted in a test car analyzed the air at the level of the driver's head. The findings ranged from a low (in Louisville) of sixty-six parts of carbon monoxide per million parts of air to a high (in Los Angeles) of one hundred and fifty-one parts of carbon monoxide per million parts of air. Concentrations of one hundred or more were recorded in four of the other cities: Cincinnati (100), Detroit (120), Minneapolis (134), and Denver (142). New York and Chicago both showed concentrations of ninety-five. The maximum allowable concentration of carbon monoxide for an exposure of several hours (established by the American Standards Association around 1900) is one hundred parts per million parts of air. Within the past few years, however, many investigators have come to believe—on the basis of certain studies on human volunteers which demonstrate that even minute concentrations of carbon monoxide can subtly dull the crucial sense of time and distance—that a concentration of one hundred is much too high for perfect safety, and they have proposed that the maximum he lowered to fifty. In the Soviet Union, the legal (though not necessarily enforced) maximum is eighteen.

It was once generally held that carbon-monoxide poisoning occurred in both acute and chronic forms. Most investigators now deny the possibility of a chronic form of carbon-monoxide intoxication. They distinguish instead between acute and chronic exposure. "Chronic exposure does not produce chronic poisoning," Dr. David H. Goldstein, professor of environmental medicine at New York University Medical Center, noted in a 1963 medical textbook, "but, rather, repeated episodes of mild acute poisoning. Intermittent day-to-day exposures are not cumulative in effect." The incidence of severe acute carbon-monoxide poisoning has declined in the United States in recent years. This is largely attributable to the wide-spread installation of safety devices (fans, baffles, alarm meters) in industrial plants, and to safer home appliances. In New York City, for example, a total of four hundred and twenty cases of serious carbon-monoxide poisoning (a hundred and thirty-one of them fatal) was reported in 1951. The total for 1967 was seventy-three cases, of which four were fatal. Most of these cases were the consequence of dilapidated equipment, sitting in a closed car with the engine running, or a deliberate, suicidal exposure. Less conspicuously clinical cases, on the other hand, are almost certainly increasing. There are no real records of such cases, because they are seldom recognized and reported, but it is probable that thousands of Americans suffer some degree of carbon-monoxide poisoning—a late-afternoon headache, a little lurch of nausea, a creeping irritability—every day. The victims are unsuspecting people who regularly expose themselves to air that, through ignorance or indifference or inadvertence, is perennially polluted. They include automobile mechanics, parking-garage attendants, traffic policemen, newspaper-kiosk keepers, cabdrivers, urban-bus drivers, janitors, commuting motorists, and every now and then, a housewife like Mildred Anderson.

Dr. Moore couldn't doubt that the Andersons' trouble was carbon-monoxide poisoning. She went back to the examination booth in a euphoria of relief. Carbon monoxide answered every question. It explained Mrs. Anderson's interminable headache, it explained the disappearance of the headache after a few hours in the unpolluted air of the hospital, it explained the return of the headache, and the dizziness, the faintness, the weakness, the bizarre behavior. It had to be carbon monoxide, and the source could only be something in the Anderson house. Something that was regularly but intermittently in use. Something like a kitchen range, a hot-water heater, a furnace. That would also explain why Mr. Anderson had only now become sick. He hadn't been sufficiently exposed; he had only been home at night until this weekend began.

"I couldn't doubt it was carbon monoxide," Dr. Moore says, "but I couldn't, of course, just assume it. I had to be sure. I had to document it. There was a senior medical student I knew hanging around, and I grabbed him and asked him to draw some blood from the Andersons for a carboxyhemoglobin-determination test. Meanwhile, I got them both breathing pure oxygen. Then I thought of the niece. I remembered how funny she had sounded. So I rounded her up and got her on oxygen, too. Then I called the lab. The technician who could do the test I wanted wasn't on duty. I got permission to call him at home, and I called him and he moaned and groaned and carried on, but he finally got dressed and came over. A carboxyhemoglobin-determination test takes about twenty minutes, and in twenty minutes we had the confirmation: Mr. Anderson's carboxyhemoglobin level was thirty-nine percent, and Mrs. Anderson's was thirty-seven.

"By the time we got the lab reports, the Andersons were both pretty well recovered. But I kept them at the hospital. I couldn't send them back to that contaminated house. The niece threw off her little touch of poisoning very fast, and I talked to her and her friends before they left. I arranged for them to take the Andersons in until their house had been inspected. They told me the Andersons used natural gas for heating and cooking, and that the house had seemed awfully hot and a little smelly of what they now decided was gas. They said they would get in touch with the gas company the first thing in the morning. I heard the rest of the story a couple of days later. Mrs. Anderson called me. An inspector from the gas company had come out and made a thorough investigation, and my hunch had been in the right direction. The trouble was the furnace. Or, rather, the furnace flue. The inspector had found it practically blocked with fallen bricks. Mrs. Anderson thought she knew how that had happened. They had had their chimney repaired several months before—sometime back in the summer. It had needed pointing. And apparently the mason who repaired it also managed to drop a few old bricks down the flue."

[*1970*]

CHAPTER 19

A Small,
Apprehensive Child

HER EXPERIENCE WAS so exceptional that I'll give her an unex-
ceptional name. I'll call her Barbara Logan. Barbara was then—
in the late spring and early summer of 1968—six and a half years
old. She lived with her mother, a recent divorcée, in a two-family
house in the City Park section of Denver, and it was there, at
around eight o'clock on the night of June 9th, a Sunday, that her
experience began. It began with fever and a spasm of vomiting.
She vomited off and on all night. She vomited all day Monday. She
vomited all through Monday night. On Tuesday morning, she was
still hot to the touch (Mrs. Logan didn't have a clinical thermometer), and she complained for the first time of pain. Her throat was
sore, she said, and there was a sore place under her left arm. Mrs.
Logan felt and found a lump about the size of a golf ball. It was
hard and painfully tender. That alarmed her. She got Barbara up
and into some clothes and telephoned for a taxicab. Mrs. Logan
had no regular physician. She told the driver to take them to
Children's Hospital. That was the hospital nearest her home.

The driver, after a glance at Barbara, delivered them to the
hospital emergency room. The physician on duty there, a woman,

briefly questioned Mrs. Logan, and then turned her attention to Barbara. Her findings, which she noted on the standard chart, confirmed the cabdriver's snap impression: "Physical examination revealed an acutely ill child. Eyes sunken. Looks very miserable. Surprisingly coöperative. Lips and nailbeds cyanotic. Two-inch roughly round left axillary node, which is very tender. Mild generalized abdominal tenderness. Joints not hot or swollen. Right eardrum red. Throat slightly infected. Chest clear. Slight tachycardia [rapid pulse rate], 120. No [heart] murmur. Neck supple. Appears dehydrated. Temperature, 104.4." This last—almost six degrees of fever in so crowded a clinical context—was decisive. The physician made the necessary arrangements for Barbara's immediate admission. She also arranged for certain indicated laboratory tests (blood analysis, urinalysis, throat culture) and a chest X-ray. She did not attempt a comprehensive diagnosis. She merely noted the several apparent infections: otitis media (inflammation of the middle ear), gastritis, and pharyngitis. And added, "Rule out pneumonia."

Barbara was led up to a ward and put to bed. She was wrapped in a cool sheet to temper her fever and given a mild analgesic for comfort. An antibiotic regimen to curb her apparent infections was begun: two hundred thousand units of penicillin every four hours, and four hundred milligrams of sulfisoxazole every eight hours. Half an hour later, she vomited. Then she seemed to feel better, and presently fell asleep. The following day, her condition was, at best, equivocal. The results of the chest X-ray were within normal limits, and any threat of pneumonia appeared to be remote. Her white-blood-cell count, a standard index of infection, was only slightly elevated (to 8,300 per cubic millimeter), and the differential (or constituent) count was essentially normal. The interne assigned to the case noted on her chart, "Temperature, 100. Hydration improved. Patient extremely fussy. Nodes in axilla have increased 3-fold in nite to 15 × 10 cm. mass, which is exquisitely tender. She has had no more vomiting. Taking oral fluids. Primary culture of urine, blood & throat shows no growth. I am not impressed by her response to antibiotic therapy at this time. Will do second blood culture & watch closely."

A week went by. Barbara's condition remained uncomfortably

equivocal. On Monday, June 17th, the interne noted, "Still very tender in axilla, but swelling is down. First blood culture grew Gram-negative rods at 4 days. Second blood culture negative at 5 days. Still has temperature 100." His second entry was a clouded clarification. A rod is a bacillus of cylindrical (or rod-shaped) conformation, and a Gram-negative rod is one that reacts negatively to a staining test developed by the turn-of-the-century Danish physician Hans Christian Joachim Gram. This reaction is a primary characteristic of numerous bacteria. Some, though only some, of these are pathogenic to man. That group, however, includes the agents of brucellosis, glanders, gonorrhea, influenza, plague, salmonellosis, shigellosis, tularemia, typhoid fever, and whooping cough. Later that day, the interne noted on the record that a sample of the cryptic Gram-negative presence in Barbara's blood had been delivered to the nearby laboratory of the Colorado State Health Department for dispatch to the Laboratory Branch of the Center for Disease Control, at Atlanta, for definitive screening and precise identification. He then returned to the bedside with a sudden discordant note: "Patient spiked temperature to 103.4." Confronted by this inscrutable turn, he reinforced the standing regimen with two new varieties of penicillin—potassium phenoxymethyl and sodium methicillin. The following day, he requested an X-ray examination of the left shoulder "to rule out possibility of osteomyelitis." The thought had apparently struck him that a fitful inflammation of the bone might be responsible for both Barbara's persistent fever and the equally stubborn swelling under her arm. If so, his mind was quickly put at rest. The roentgenologist reported on Wednesday morning that he could find no evidence of any bone involvement. Barbara's condition that morning was also reassuring. "Patient feels better," the interne noted. "Ate good breakfast. Tenderness in L. axilla diminished considerably." The sudden improvement continued, Barbara's fever fell to a scant 100 degrees. She continued to eat with appetite, and the tender swelling under her arm continued to subside. On Friday, for the first time, her temperature dropped to normal. She continued free of fever for the next four days, and on Tuesday morning, June 25th, the interne closed his record of the case. "Temperature still normal," he noted. "CBC [complete blood count] WNL [within normal limits]. Patient to be discharged today." She was discharged that afternoon, with a comprehensive supply of sulfisoxazole and supporting penicillins, to convalesce at home.

Barbara's convalescence was a fleeting one. It barely lasted over Tuesday night. She awoke on Wednesday morning with a familiar pain in her armpit. The swelling there had reappeared, and the area was now so sensitive that it hurt to even close her arm. Mrs. Logan was more confused than alarmed. Barbara, after all, had just been discharged from the hospital as recovered from whatever had ailed her. She felt Barbara's forehead. It was reassuringly cool. And Barbara said she was hungry. That surely meant there was nothing seriously wrong. She decided to wait and see. She waited until Thursday afternoon. Barbara was still cool and still able to eat with appetite, but she was also still in pain. Mrs. Logan called a cab and took her back to the hospital. "Glands in axilla have increased," the emergency-room physician noted. "Now is developing enlarged nodes in left side of neck. Child does not look well. Appetite good & no fever since discharge. To return next Wednesday." Barbara did not, however, return the following Wednesday. Mrs. Logan returned her the following day. The enigmatic swellings had increased again in size and sensitivity. "Looks very poorly," the examining physician noted, and, revising his Thursday opinion, he arranged for her readmission. "Suggest surgical consultation for possible incision & drainage." Her temperature then—at eleven o'clock in the morning—was 101.4.

Barbara was assigned this time to a bed in a ward for infectious diseases. She was visited there around noon by an interne on that service. He found her to be "a small, apprehensive child with a painful, swollen left axilla" and confined his diagnosis to the merely descriptive: "Left axillary lymphadenitis." Her indifferent response to antibiotic therapy impressed him even less than it had the interne earlier in attendance. He expressed his dissatisfaction by cancelling the earlier orders. That was the usual step. The next was to mount a new and more aggressive antibiotic attack. But there he stopped, uncertain. The discarded assault was standard in what appeared to be the circumstances of the case. He reflected, and then (with the approval of the guiding resident) stepped in a different direction. Barbara, until further orders, was to be given no medication at all. The nature of those orders would depend upon the nature of the organism that had been cultured from her blood. He would wait until the report on that came through from Atlanta. It was not an easy decision, and it was not an easy wait. Barbara's condition continued as before. Her temperature returned mysteriously to normal, and the painful swellings persisted. June ended and July began. On July 2nd, the operation proposed by the admitting physician was successfully performed, and it had, as planned, the immediate salubrious effect of reducing the monstrous glands. The following day, at two o'clock in the afternoon, the report at last came through. The interne noted it on the record: "CDC called to report blood culture of 6/11/68 as suspect of *Pasteurella pestis.*" That most emphatically answered his question. He could now proceed to treatment with the confidence of certainty. But it far from closed the case. *Pasteurella pestis* is the causative agent of plague.

Plague, as its prototypical name so starkly proclaims, is the oldest and most dangerous of the great epidemic diseases. The weapon with which the Lord punished the Philistines for their victory over the Israelites (and for their acquisition of the Ark of the Covenant) is generally identified as plague. Most medical historians believe that plague was probably the chief constituent of the ambiguous "Plague of Athens" described by Thucydides in his "History of the Peloponnesian War." It was plague that ravaged the Byzantine Empire in the time of Justinian (around 542 A.D.) and, according to the contemporary historian Procopius, killed half of the population. And it was plague that practically decimated Europe in the Black Death pandemic of 1348. Its appearances since then have been less dramatically lethal, but the disease is still far from conquered. Plague was more or less endemic in Europe from the fourteenth century to the end of the eighteenth century (an epidemic in Prussia in 1709 took well over three hundred thousand lives), and it continues to prevail in its classic epidemic form in much of Asia (including Vietnam) and in parts of Africa and South America. It is one of only four diseases that are still accepted by public-health authorities throughout the world as quarantinable. The other diseases whose presence aboard a ship or a plane is sufficient cause to quarantine the craft are cholera, smallpox, and yellow fever.

No disease has inspired a larger general literature than plague. Its literary fruits alone include the "Decameron" of Boccaccio, Daniel Defoe's "A Journal of the Plague Year," and "The Plague," by Albert Camus. The contagion from which the characters in the "Decameron" have fled to a hilltop palace near Florence is the Black Death, and Boccaccio's generally accurate description of the disease at its most relentless indicates the origin of that lurid medieval name. "In men and women alike," he notes, "there appeared at the beginning of the malady certain swellings, either on the groin or under the armpits, whereof some waxed to the bigness of a common apple, others like unto an egg, some more and some less, and these the vulgar named plague-boils. From these two parts the aforesaid death-bearing plague-boils proceeded, in brief space, to appear and come indifferently in every part of the body; wherefrom, after awhile, the fashion of the contagion began to change into black or blue blotches, which showed themselves in many first on the arms and about the thighs and after spread to every other part of the person, and in some large and sparse and in others small and thick-sown; and like as the plague-boils had been first and yet were a very certain token of coming death, even so were these for everyone to whom they came."

The black or blue blotches of the Black Death are multiple tiny hemorrhages of the skin, and occur in both of the two chief forms of plague. These forms are known as bubonic plague and pneumonic plague. Bubonic plague is the classic, and the commoner, form. It takes its name from the inflammatory swellings (so obvious to Boccaccio and so mysterious to the doctors attending Barbara Logan) of the lymphatic glands in the groin and the armpit. These traditionally definitive swellings are called buboes, from the Greek "boubōn," for "groin." Pneumonic plague, as its name declares, is plague in which the lungs are involved. Essentially, it is a complication of untreated bubonic plague. Until shortly after the Second World War, when an effective antibiotic treatment for plague was found in streptomycin and the tetracyclines, pneumonic plague was a common consequence of bubonic plague.

Untreated bubonic plague is fatal in about fifty per cent of cases. Untreated pneumonic plague is always fatal. When plague is promptly and properly treated, however, prompt recovery is the reliable rule. Bubonic plague, though easily capable of the greatest epidemic spread, often occurs sporadically. Pneumonic plague is wholly an epidemic disease, and its appearance is invariably preceded by an outbreak of bubonic plague.

Few diseases have been more portentously explained than plague. Its cause was once (perhaps originally) believed to be a baleful conjunction of the planets Saturn, Jupiter, and Mars. It was also thought (perhaps alternatively) to be caused by other cosmic events—comets, volcanic eruptions, earthquakes. Another, and less fortuitous, explanation attributed plague to the machinations of Jews. ("It was believed that the Jews had poisoned the wells," Guy de Chauliac, physician to Pope Clement VI, noted in his contemporary account of the pandemic of 1348, "and they killed them.") A more persistent view envisioned plague as one of the sterner manifestations of the Wrath of God. This attractively guilt-ridden concept (which inspired the wild-eyed peregrinations of the Flagellants in the fourteenth century) was widely embraced until almost the modern era. Even physicians accepted it, though usually with reservations. A pious seventeenth-century German physician named Johannes Raicus attempted to clarify the matter with a scholarly tract. There were, he pronounced in 1620 in his "Ex Flagello Dei," two different sources of plague. One was divine in origin and the other was a natural visitation. Divine plague, being a punishment inflicted for cause on a discovered sinner, was not infectious. The other was.

By "infectious," Raicus meant "contagious." The truly infectious, or bacterial, nature of plague was demonstrated independently by two bacteriologists—the Japanese Shibasaburo Kitasato and the Swiss Alexandre Yersin—during an epidemic of the disease in Hong Kong in 1894. A French investigator, Paul-Louis Simond, is celebrated as the discoverer of its contagious, or communicable, nature. Simond suggested, in a report to the *Annales de l'Institut Pasteur* in 1898, that the *Pasteurella pestis* of Kitasato and Yersin is not among man's natural microbial enemies. It was his correct assumption that plague is primarily a disease of rats that is accidently conveyed to man by certain fleas. Moreover, as he proposed and as subsequent investigators were able to establish, these fleas prefer the blood of rats to that of man, and it is probable that they turn to man only when rats are scarce. An outbreak of plague in man tends to follow directly upon a decimating epidemic of plague among rats. (The seventeenth-century French painter Nicolas Poussin precociously included among the panicking crowds in his graphic portrayal of "The Plague of the Philistines" the bodies of several dead rats.) The manner in which the flea transmits *P. pestis* to man is also accidental. A flea that has fed on an infected rat ingests a multiplicity of plague bacilli. These bacilli accumulate and eventually block the forestomach of the flea, and in order to swallow newly gathered blood it is forced to regurgitate. Much of this bacilli-laden vomitus inevitably passes into the bloodstream of the host. Plague produced by the bite of a contaminated flea is bubonic plague. Bubonic plague cannot be transmitted by ordinary contact from one human victim to another. Pneumonic plague can. Its accompanying coughs and sneezes are as irresistibly infectious as those of the common cold.

Simond's report on the role of the rat in human plague, like most such pathfinding studies, was at first dismissed as absurd. It then was acclaimed as definitive. It is now merely recalled as a milestone. For there is more to plague than Simond could suppose in 1898. More recent investigation has shown that plague is not, as he conceived, exclusively a rat-borne disease of seaport cities— the morbid consequence of the arrival in a rat-infested city of a rat-infested ship. That is only its classic approach, and one that an almost universal insistence on ratproof ship construction is rapidly rendering historic. The susceptibility of the domestic rat to plague is now known to be shared by many other wholly undomesticated rodents and rodentlike animals. Some seventy equally prolific and comparably flea-ridden creatures—including mice, rabbits, hares, voles, ground squirrels, prairie dogs, marmots, and chipmunks—are more or less hospitable to *P. pestis.* There are pockets of wild-rodent, or sylvatic, plague in the wilds of China and Southeastern Asia, in Africa, and in North and South America. One of the biggest of these enzootic reservoirs lies in the American West. In fact, it *is* the West. The area in which infected animals (and their attendant fleas) have been found embraces the states of Washington, Oregon, California, Nevada, Utah, Idaho, Montana, North Dakota, Wyoming, Arizona, New Mexico, Colorado, Kansas, Oklahoma, and Texas.

Plague is generally thought to have entered the United States with a pack of ailing rats that climbed ashore from a burning freighter on the San Francisco waterfront. Opponents of this notion suggest that plague was here long before its presence was formally noted. San Francisco, at any rate, was the scene of the first American epidemic. The epidemic began with the discovery of a dead Chinese in the rat-infested basement of the Globe Hotel in Chinatown on March 6, 1900, and it lasted, largely because the local authorities tried to hush the matter up, for almost four years —until February of 1904. It was one of the deadliest epidemics on record. One hundred and twenty-one people were stricken, and all but three of them died—a mortality rate of ninety-seven per cent. A second, and only somewhat less lethal, epidemic occurred in San Francisco in 1907, the year after the earthquake and fire. Three other American cities have experienced serious outbreaks of plague—Seattle, also in 1907; New Orleans in 1914 and again in 1919; and Los Angeles in 1924. The Los Angeles epidemic was the last recorded appearance in this country of classic, urban, rat-borne plague. It was not, however, the last appearance here of plague. Since 1908, when an epizootic in ground squirrels near Oakland, California, abruptly announced its presence, sylvatic plague has seized, along with numberless rodents, a number of human victims. One hundred and forty cases, sixty-eight of them fatal, are known. Thirty-seven (or one-fourth) of these have occurred in the past six years, and two-thirds of those recent victims have been children. Seventeen of them—like Barbara Logan— were less than ten years old.

The telephoned report on the nature of Barbara Logan's illness that Denver Children's Hospital received on the afternoon of July 3, 1968, was one of three identically alerting calls that were made that day by the Laboratory Branch of the Center for Disease Control, in Atlanta. The others went to Dr. Cecil S. Mollohan, chief of the Epidemiology Section of the Colorado State Department of Health, in Denver, and to a station of the Ecological Investigations Program of the United States Public Health Service at Fort Collins, Colorado. This last call was taken by Dr. Jack D. Poland, then acting chief (he is now the head) of the station's Zoonoses Section. A zoonosis is a disease of animals that may be conveyed to man. There are many such diseases, and the Zoonoses Section is professionally familiar with almost all of them, but the zoonosis with which Dr. Poland and his staff are principally concerned is plague. He expressed this concern in a matter of minutes with a telephone call to Denver.

Dr. Poland says, "I called Dr. Mollohan. That isn't the way it's usually done, of course. I should have waited for him to call me. The protocol in public health is that a federal agency comes into a local matter on invitation from the local authority—the city or county or state—in charge of the investigation. But we don't stand much on ceremony with plague. I knew Dr. Mollohan would see it that way, and he did. He needed and wanted our help. I told him I'd get our people on it right away. Fort Collins is sixty miles from Denver, but that's no distance in this part of the world. Then I remembered. I said I'd do better than that. I said it so happened that Harry Hill was in Denver that day on a routine tick-fever job, and I'd round him up and send him right over. Harry Hill was Dr. Hill, a young Epidemic Intelligence Service officer assigned to us from C.D.C. I remember Dr. Mollohan laughed. That would be fine, he said, but I didn't really need to bother. Because it also so happened that Dr. Harry Hill was sitting in his office that very minute. They had been talking about tick fever when Dr. Mollohan got his call from Atlanta. So Harry Hill came to the phone, and we talked for a couple of minutes. There wasn't a whole lot to say. He knew what to do. He was a trained epidemiologist. I simply told him to go ahead and do it."

Dr. Hill says, "It wasn't quite as simple as that. There was another matter of protocol. Before I could see the patient, I had to go around to the Denver Department of Health and Hospitals and get permission. Children's Hospital is a municipal hospital. I picked up my wife—she had come down to Denver that morning with me—and I went through the necessary red tape. Then I was ready to begin. I found the interne assigned to the case, and we sat down together. He was shaken. He had just begun his training, and Barbara Logan was his first patient. There can't be many doctors whose first case turned out to be plague. He showed me her chart and gave me what he had on her personal history. Then I saw Barbara. Her clinical picture was certainly compatible with a diagnosis of plague. Anybody could have made the diagnosis— if the possibility of plague had happened to enter his mind. But it hadn't. It very seldom does. Barbara was the third case of plague in Colorado in less than a year, and both of the others were also originally misdiagnosed. One was mistaken for streptococcal sore throat and the other for tularemia. But Barbara was lucky. Or maybe she was just naturally tough. Anyway, they got her started on the right drugs in time—on streptomycin and tetracycline instead of penicillin—and she survived. She made a full recovery. The others didn't. One of them died, and the other ended up with permanent central-nervous-system damage.

"Barbara was too sick and too young for much of a talk, and I didn't stay with her long. I left the hospital and went out to the car, where my wife was waiting, and we drive back across town to the Logan house. Mrs. Logan was at home, and she was friendly and glad to help. What I hoped to get from her was some clue to the source of Barbara's infection. Sylvatic plague is hardly a common disease, but there have been enough cases over the years to establish a characteristic epidemiological pattern. The source, of course, is a wild rodent, and the setting is also wild. It's out in the wilderness somewhere, a place where wild rodents abound. For example, that fatal Colorado case I mentioned was a boy on a ranch in Elbert County who shot and carried home a prairie dog. The other case was an oil-field worker in the mountains north of Grand Junction. The incubation period in plague is from two to six days. Barbara took sick on June 9th. I naturally expected to hear from Mrs. Logan that there had been some sort of outing in the country soon after the first of June. But no. Barbara had hardly been off the block. She had been to City Park, only a few blocks away, on June 5th, and two or three weeks before that she had spent the day with an aunt on the east side of town, in Aurora,

and that was all. If that was true—and how could I doubt it?—
Barbara had been exposed to plague right here in the city of
Denver.

"Which was crazy. Urban plague means rats. But Denver is
unusual among American cities in that it has practically no rats.
A continuing extermination program has just about wiped them
out. However, I asked Mrs. Logan about rats. She said no. There
weren't any rats, she said. There couldn't be any. An exterminator
came to the house regularly. I sat and thought a minute. There had
to be an animal somewhere in the picture, I said. A sick or dead
or dying animal. Mrs. Logan started to shake her head, and
stopped. Did I say *dead* animals? Well, she didn't know, but she
had heard that some dead squirrels had been found in the neighborhood. People had been finding dead squirrels off and on all
spring. That was interesting. It was even promising. Fleas will
desert a host soon after its death, but plague can be contracted
from infected blood or saliva. I asked if Barbara was the kind of
girl who might handle a dead animal. Indeed she was, Mrs. Logan
said. Very much so. She was a very inquisitive child. That was
interesting, too. About these squirrels, I said—I supposed they
were ground squirrels. What some people call chipmunks. Oh, no,
Mrs. Logan said. They were regular squirrels. They were tree
squirrels—like in the park.

"Well, I thanked Mrs. Logan and left. I didn't doubt there were
tree squirrels around. The older parts of Denver are full of trees,
and the Logan street was lined with big old elms. But I had always
thought of plague as a disease of burrowing rodents. I went down
to the car and started to get in, and saw some kids playing in the
yard across the street. I told my wife I'd be right back. I went over
to the kids and said I was an investigator and that I'd heard there
were some dead squirrels around the neighborhood. Did they
know anything about that? They all said 'Huh?' and 'What?,' and
then one of them said sure—he knew where there was a dead
squirrel. Did I want to see it? I said I certainly did, and he led me
back around the house and out a gate and up an alley and over
a fence and out another yard and across a street and around to
another alley and stopped in front of a hollow tree. I looked in the
hollow. I didn't have to see it—I could smell it. But there was

enough of it left for laboratory examination. I went back to the car and told my wife about it and she looked sick, and we drove back to the hollow tree. There was an old fishing creel in the trunk of the car, and I scraped the remains of the squirrel or whatever it was into the creel and covered it up with an old blanket so it wouldn't smell too much. Then I looked around for a telephone and called Dr. Poland and told him what I'd found. He said O.K., bring it in. He didn't sound too excited. My wife and I had dinner and then drove back to Fort Collins. I stopped at the office and unloaded the squirrel or whatever it was and put it—creel and all —in a refrigerator in the lab, and left a note for Allan Barnes. Dr. Barnes is head of the mammalogy-entomology unit of the Zoonoses Section, and a very big man in plague. He'd take it on from there."

Dr. Barnes says, "It was a squirrel, all right—and a tree squirrel. It was the eastern fox squirrel, *Sciurus niger.* From the state of decomposition and an infestation of blowfly larvae, I judged it had been dead about a week. I handed the carcass over to Bruce Hudson in the laboratory to be tested for evidence of plague by his fluorescent-antibody staining technique. It was Dr. Hudson who adapted the F.A. test to plague. And a very good thing he did, too. The squirrel was far too dead to be tested by the standard bacteriological methods. I don't think I nourished any preconceived ideas. I felt pretty much the way Jack Poland felt. I wasn't too excited. I certainly didn't react the way I would have if Harry Hill had brought in a dead prairie dog. And I wasn't about to chase into Denver and start tearing down the Logan house looking for rats. I knew there were very few rats in Denver. I also knew that an eastern fox squirrel had been found dead of plague on the Stanford University campus back in 1966. It was an isolated case. The other campus squirrels tested out negative. But it was a case, a precedent. So I wasn't absolutely flabbergasted when Bruce Hudson walked in and told me that Harry Hill's specimen was positive for plague. It gave me a funny feeling, though. The Stanford case was a totally isolated case. This was different. We not only had a case of plague in an urban tree squirrel. We also had a case of human plague.

"Meanwhile, of course, I'd been talking with Jack Poland and

Harry Hill, and I had also been on the telephone to Denver. The people I mostly talked to there were Cecil Mollohan and Roy Cleere and Douglas McCluskie. Dr. Cleere is director of the Colorado State Department of Health, and Dr. McCluskie is director of the Division of Environmental Health for the city. The lab report was the push we needed, and we arranged for a meeting at Dr. Cleere's office on the afternoon of July 8th. That was a Monday. I went down to Denver that morning and picked up Dr. McCluskie and we drove over to the Logan house. The Logan neighborhood, I should say. We weren't looking for Mrs. Logan. We were looking for more dead squirrels. There were kids playing on the block and women going marketing and old men just sitting around, and we talked to them all. Everybody seemed to know about the squirrels. One man told us he had found a dead squirrel in his yard as far back as May. He tossed it in his garbage can. And we found three dead squirrels. A man took us to one of them, and the kids showed us the others. They looked just as dead as Harry Hill's squirrel, but they weren't too dead to test.

"That sharpened the point of the meeting with Dr. Cleere and the others. One dead squirrel was simply one dead squirrel. But four dead squirrels was a die-off. And a die-off is always suspicious —whatever the cause of death. The other side of the picture, the human side, was fortunately unchanged. A check around the hospitals and clinics had been made, and there were no further cases of plague, or anything that even faintly looked like plague. There was still just Barbara Logan. Moreover, she would be discharged very shortly. The meeting drew up a report to inform physicians about her case and to alert them to the possibility of other victims. It reminded them of the clinical features of plague and pointed out the proper treatment. A general press release was also prepared. It gave the facts of Barbara's case, with a statement from Dr. Cleere to the effect that the situation was cause for concern but not for alarm, and it included a strong warning to the public against handling rodents, dead or alive. We also asked that any dead rodents be reported to the city health department. That about covers the meeting. Except that I was asked to head the field investigation. Dr. McCluskie and I sat down and made plans for a survey that would define the nature and extent of the infection in the animal population. Denver has a great many tree squirrels. The eastern fox squirrel was introduced in 1908. By homesick Easterners, I suppose. Anyway, it prospered. There have also been immigrants. *S. niger* used to be strictly an eastern squirrel. You never saw it west of the Mississippi. But it's been slowly moving west across the plains—living off the wheat fields and nesting in the cottonwood river bottoms—since the late nineteen-twenties. Finally, a few years ago, it joined up with the others in Denver.

"We went to work the following day. The city had the collection facilities. Dr. McCluskie mobilized his Animal Control Division, and the dogcatchers picked up carcasses wherever we had a report and turned them over to us for delivery to the laboratory for examination. Those dogcatchers really had to work. The dead-rodent reports rolled in—the phones rang all day long. Then the laboratory came through with a report on the carcasses Dr. McCluskie and I had found. They were plague-positive, too. So this wasn't anything like Stanford. This was a plague epizootic. Which brought up the crucial question of control. Control, in plague, means ectoparasite control, the eradication of the vector fleas. That was certainly all we wanted in this case. We didn't want to kill the Denver squirrels. But it was a tough nut to crack. We solved it with a system of baited stations rigged up in such a way that the squirrel got a harmless dusting of insecticide when he came onto the station. That took care of the fleas on his body, and also those back in his nest. We had some trouble with bait. Squirrels love peanut butter. But when we baited a station with peanut butter, the first squirrel to show up just settled down and ate and ate until the peanut butter was gone. We finally hit on pine cones impregnated with peanut butter. They carried those away. At the peak of our operation, we had eight hundred stations going.

"The active phase of the investigation lasted about three weeks. It began on July 9th and ran through the rest of the month. By the beginning of August, the peak of the epizootic had passed. We found our last positive on September 18th. And Barbara Logan was still the only human case. The total tally was eight hundred and twenty-one carcasses collected and examined. Six hundred of them were tree squirrels. The others were other animals. None of those miscellaneous animals were positive for plague. Four hundred and ninety-three of the six hundred tree squirrels were found within the Denver city limits, the others on the outskirts. Only the Denver squirrels were plague-positive. The positive squirrels totalled eighty-one. The curious thing was this. We had a big block map of the city set up in Dr. McCluskie's office and we kept a record with colored pins where every squirrel carcass was found. All but six of the positive squirrels were found in the northeast quadrant of Denver—the City Park area, where Barbara lived. That would seem to be where the epizootic began and where it was somehow contained. There was also something else. The other thing was fleas. We collected a number of fleas. We found a few on newly dead squirrels, and the rest we combed off about thirty live and healthy squirrels that we trapped for that purpose. The flea to which *S. niger* is normally host is *Orchopeas howardi*, and we found the expected number of them. But we also found three other kinds of fleas. We found a species that is normally found on ground squirrels, and we found two species that are normally found on rabbits. Let me say that the only infected fleas we found —the only plague-positive fleas—were a few *Orchopeas howardi*. The wild-rodent fleas were clean. Their mere presence, however, was bad news. I'm only thankful that it happened in a city like Denver—a city with practically no rats. Because a flea transfer like that very strongly suggests a wild-rodent intrusion into the urban environment. How this intrusion may have come about I can't say. I don't know."

Neither does Dr. McCluskie. But he is willing to guess. He says, "I think what happened was this. I think some kid caught a ground squirrel up in the mountains and brought it home, and after a couple of days he got bored with it or his parents said get rid of it, and he let it out in City Park. I think it was just an accident like that. I hope so, anyway."

[1971]

CHAPTER 20

The Santa Claus Culture

THE SECOND MONTHLY MEETING in 1966 of the Massachusetts General Hospital's Committee on Infection Control was held at noon on February 23rd in a private dining room in the George Robert White Building, the administrative center of the hospital complex. It was attended by thirteen members. Among them were physicians representing the several hospital services (medicine, surgery, pediatrics, orthopedics, neurology, urology), the chief bacteriologist, the chief of pharmacy, two executive nurses, and the assistant director of the hospital and secretary of the committee, Joseph W. Degen. The principal item of business was a report from Dr. David J. Lang, assistant pediatrician at the hospital and an instructor in pediatrics at Harvard Medical School. Mr. Degen's account of that portion of the meeting read, "Dr. Lang reported on the incidence of *Salmonella cubana* on the Burnham floors. Five pediatric patients have been affected since October, 1965. The prior incidence of two pediatric patients and five adults over the term from April to October had been thought not connected. However, in the absence of finding any specific source for the Burnham episode, and in the presence of certain possible connections via various paths (food, vitamins, persons) of the latest to the earlier cases, there is some possibility of connection. This particular outbreak in the Burnham units seems now to have stopped. No evidence of personnel-contact faults or of any vast breaks in techniques as causes has been uncovered. There was a resultant advantage in the 'sharpening up' of procedures for proper care."

Salmonella cubana is one of some fifteen hundred species of bacteria that compose the genus *Salmonella.* These microbes (whose name commemorates the nineteenth-century American pathologist Daniel Elmer Salmon) produce an acute gastroenteritis known to clinical medicine as salmonellosis. Salmonellosis is almost as common a form of food poisoning as that caused by the ubiquitous staphylococci, but it generally runs a far less commonplace course. When its victims are very old or very young, or are debilitated by some other disease, it is not infrequently fatal. Practically all animals (including rats, snakes, turtles, and insects) are hospitable to the salmonellae. The usual cause of human salmonellosis is infected (and insufficiently cooked) beef, pork, lamb, duck, turkey, chicken, and, particularly, eggs. Other causes include food or drink contaminated by the excreta of infected animals or by tainted equipment. The different salmonella species are distinguished by a serotyping technique perfected by the Danish bacteriologist Fritz Kauffmann in 1941, and they are identified (with a few exceptions) by geographical names that indicate where they were first isolated. Part of the classification process consists of grouping them according to their cell-wall composition. Most salmonellae found in the United States fall into the groups A through E, but there are some forty groups altogether. All of them are pathogenic (the worst being *S. typhi*, which causes typhoid fever), but some are more widely distributed in nature than others. The most widely distributed in this country is *S. typhimurium*; others that are frequently isolated here and elsewhere include *S. newport, S. montevideo, S. anatum, S. oranienburg, S. panama, S. dublin, S. sandiego, S. bareilly, S. tennessee, S. miami, S. derby,* and *S. heidelberg.* One species that is not a member of that cosmopolitan company is *S. cubana*. It was first encountered in 1946 in Cuba, and its recorded appearances outside that country have been relatively rare. In 1970, there were some twenty-four thousand cases of salmonellosis reported in the United States. Only a hundred and sixty-six of these were attributed to *S. cubana*.

Dr. Lang's report on the *S. cubana* outbreak in the Burnham units was the ambiguous result of almost a month of intensive investigation. He had received the assignment at a special meeting of the Infection Control Committee on January 31st. That meeting had been called to consider an urgent memorandum from the chief bacteriologist, Dr. Lawrence J. Kunz. His memorandum read: "(1) Stool of Gail H. on Burnham Six now has Salmonella-like organism which is not in Salmonella groups A-E: *S. cubana*? (2) Patient P. has organism similar to *S. cubana*. (3) Patient F. has *S. cubana* in stools." The identification of *S. cubana* in the first two patients, Dr. Kunz noted, was tentative but probable. There was no question about the third patient. The presence of *S. cubana* had been demonstrated at the leading laboratory of its kind in the East—the New York Salmonella Center, at Beth Israel Hospital in Manhattan. Discussion of the memorandum brought out that all these patients were infants, and all had been on the Burnham floors—the pediatric section of the hospital—for at least a week before the samples were taken for laboratory analysis. None of them had shown any signs or symptoms of salmonellosis at the time of admission. Two of these children were girls, one seven weeks old and the other eight weeks old, and the third was a two-month-old boy. It was added that the boy was no longer a patient. He had died, after a hospital stay of eight days, on January 28th.

Dr. Lang says: "That was when we recognized the outbreak as an outbreak. Those three children in the Burnham Building brought it into focus. They did for me, all right. The Burnham units are my bailiwick. The seven previous cases had been too sporadic to make any great impression. I went down from the committee meeting and looked up the charts of those earlier patients. They didn't seem to have anything in common but an uncommon variety of salmonellosis. There were five females and two males in the group, and they ranged in age from one to seventy years. They had been admitted to the hospital at various times. One came in in

March, two in May, three in September, and one in October. And
they were scattered all over the hospital. They were in Vincent,
in Burnham, in White, and in Baker Memorial—in four of our six
clinical units. Also, according to the records, four of the seven had
shown symptoms suggestive of salmonellosis at admission. That
wasn't what they were admitted for—they all had different diseases—but the symptoms were there on the charts. And a fifth
patient had given a positive stool sample on the second day of
hospitalization. In other words, according to the evidence, five of
those seven patients had come into the hospital already infected
with *S. cubana*. It was just the reverse with the children. It was
just as obvious that they had acquired their infections *after* their
admission. Which meant that this new outbreak, whatever its
source, had its origin somewhere within the walls of the M.G.H.

"I wasn't too concerned about the seven earlier cases. I was
interested—everything connected with a serotype as uncommon
as *S. cubana* is interesting—but they could wait. The immediate
problem was the outbreak here on the Burnham floors. Three
cases of the same unusual thing at the same time in the same
building suggested the possibility of a common source. It also
suggested the rather alarming possibility of an explosive outbreak.
Another possibility was that there might be other cases here we
didn't know about, and this was the question we had to answer
first. It's always helpful to know the scope of a problem. But not
only that. It was entirely possible that the answer might say something useful about the source of the trouble. There were at the
moment three units—three floors—involved. The girls were on
Burnham Five and Burnham Six, and the little boy had been on
Burnham Four. His floor had a certain significance. One reason
was that he was the newest case. Another was that there had been
two Burnham patients among the earlier cases, and both of them
had been on Burnham Four. I was particularly interested in the
little boy's room. I was thinking along the lines of baby-to-baby
transmission, and his room seemed to be a good place for a comprehensive study. It was a room for six, and it had five children
in it now. I ordered stool cultures of them all. Then, for a larger
picture, I ordered cultures of all the Burnham nurses and all the

Burnham food-handlers. A salmonella culture takes about two days to develop. The growth, if any, can then be identified as salmonella. In some laboratories, including ours, the group to which it belongs can also be determined then. Specific serotyping takes about a week. But we would know in a couple of days if the survey had turned up anything that could be *S. cubana*—anything, that is, in Group G, the *S. cubana* group. This was Monday. We would have at least a clue by Wednesday. Meanwhile, we would do what we could to keep the outbreak under control. I sat down with the chief resident and wrote a notice for posting on all the Burnham floors. Then I had a conference with the Burnham chief of nursing. I gave her my ideas, and she drew up a set of emergency regulations."

The notice read: "Recently there have occurred several cases of diarrhea and infection caused by *Salmonella cubana* on the Children's Service. Although this does not represent a major problem or threat at the moment, we are taking certain public-health steps that will prevent the infection from spreading. We have restricted admissions to emergencies or serious problems until we clarify the extent of the problem. We anticipate that by the end of the week we will have a clearer picture of what needs to be done."

The emergency regulations read:

MEMO
To: All head nurses and supervisors—Burnham Units
From: Miss Grady
The following recommendations (outlined by Dr. Lang) are to be effective throughout the Burnham Units until further notice:
A. Strict isolation technique shall be carried out on all patients having loose stools.
B. Protective precautions are to be carried out for *all* patients.
C. General Controls:
   1. Admissions limited to emergency cases.
   2. Cleaning of entire floor by Building Services.
   3. Stool cultures on all patients before discharge.
   4. All nursing staff having symptoms of diarrhea to be sent off duty until report of stool culture obtained.

5. Two rooms in the X-ray Department have been designated for all children having examination.
6. All children leaving Unit for tests in other departments shall be gowned.
7. Personnel transporting all patients from Unit shall be gowned.
8. The services of the evening volunteers shall be suspended until further notice.

Dr. Lang says: "After that, there was nothing to do about the outbreak but wait for the reports on the stool cultures. I had time to think about those earlier cases again. If five of the seven had been infected outside the hospital, *S. cubana* must have been out and around the town. In that case, what about the other Boston hospitals? It might be interesting to hear what they had to say. I sat down and called them up—Peter Bent Brigham, Boston City, Children's, Beth Israel. I called them all. And they all said no. *S. cubana*? Good heavens, they never saw *cubana*. Nobody did. *Cubana* was a very rare bird. All of which left me a bit confused. It was strange enough that we should have all these cases of *S. cubana*, but it was even stranger that nobody else had any. It made me wonder about those five apparently outside cases. Were they actually outside cases? Or had they somehow become infected in the hospital, too? That was a tempting idea. It would simplify things considerably. And yet, of course, it wasn't acceptable. The evidence was all against it. But how could I explain those infections when there wasn't any *cubana* anywhere else in the city? The answer was that I couldn't, and I decided not to try. I decided that one outbreak was all I could hope to handle.

"The first reports on the stool cultures came along, as expected, on Wednesday. Two of the five children in the dead boy's room were positive for Group-G salmonella. And, as serotyping subsequently showed, their salmonella was *S. cubana*. Everybody else —the other children in the room, the nurses, the orderlies, the kitchen people—was negative. I began to get a little excited. I thought I could see the beginning of a pattern. Two of the earlier cases—both of them definitely hospital-acquired infections—had been Burnham patients. So were the three January cases. And now we had two more. That made seven cases clustered in a single building. It was possible that the cluster was just a freak of coincidence. But there was also another possibility. The cluster could also mean that the source of the trouble was right here on my own service. Only, it didn't. A few days later, on Monday, February 7th, I got a call from Dr. Kunz. His laboratory had uncovered another positive salmonella in the Group-G category. The new infection was unquestionably hospital-acquired, and the patient was an adult. He was a man of seventy-two, and he was in the Bulfinch Building. So that was the end of the promising Burnham pattern. We were right back where we had started. The outbreak was hospital-wide. The new case also put an end to the emergency in the Burnham units. I mean, the emergency regulations now seemed needlessly strict, and Miss Grady, the chief of nursing, and I drew up a modified set."

The new regulations read:

1. The Burnham will reopen for all admissions on February 10, but crowding will be avoided absolutely.
2. The two children with positive Salmonella cultures will be transferred to White 12 with pediatric nurse in situ.
3. Strict isolation technique will be maintained as before on all patients having loose stools.
4. Control of visitors will continue as before, and community recreation activities remain suspended. *All* patients will remain restricted to bed area. Maintain handwashing strictly.
5. Stool cultures on all patients before discharge.
6. Regulations persist with regard to personnel who have gastro-intestinal symptoms.
7. *All* bottles will be prepared by nursing personnel, bottles for older children included. Details of this preparation will be given to head nurses.
8. All other regulations (travel to X-ray, gowns on children without diarrhea, etc.) are no longer in effect.

Dr. Lang says: "A hospital-wide outbreak implies a source of infection common to all the hospital units. There has to be a link between the cases. There are various possibilities, including human carriers, but the usual one, of course, is food—either food already contaminated or food contaminated in the course of preparation. In other words, the kitchen. But that didn't look

very likely here. The source could hardly be some already contaminated food or drink. That would mean an explosion—not just
a handful of cases. And it could hardly be a contaminated kitchen.
Each of the clinical buildings at the M.G.H. has its own kitchen.
Then I learned something that I hadn't known before. It was true
that each of the clinical buildings had its own kitchen, but there
was also a special-diet kitchen here that served *all* the buildings.
You can imagine how I reacted to that. A special-diet kitchen
could be the perfect answer. All serious cases at one time or
another get something in the way of special food, and all our
cubana cases were serious cases. I went along on the diet-kitchen
inspection myself. We arranged for all the people there to be
cultured, and then we went through the kitchen. We couldn't have
been more thorough. We looked at all the food and all the equipment and checked over all the procedures. We found a few minor
breaks in technique, but nothing more. A day or two later, the
culture reports came in—all negative. No sign of any kind of
salmonella anywhere in the diet kitchen. So that was another
disappointment, another dead end. The next lead came from Dr.
Kunz."

Dr. Kunz says: "We were talking about possibilities. Possible
vehicles other than food. Salmonella can be transmitted in some
damned weird ways. I remembered an outbreak back in the fifties
that was traced to baby Easter chicks. And that made me think
of the Santa Claus patient. That's an annual practical joke. To me,
it's an annual nuisance, which is probably why I hadn't thought
to mention it to Dr. Lang before. Anyway, there's a tradition here
at Mass. General that Santa Claus turns up every Christmas as a
patient. He usually turns up on the Surgical Service. The way it
works is this. Some nurses and house officers on the Service find
an empty bed and assign it to Mr. S. Claus and make up a chart
and all the rest. They do a complete job. They concoct some crazy
kind of specimen and send it down in Santa's name for analysis.
Sometimes the lab technician will look at the identification and see
the name S. Claus, and that's the end of the joke. But sometimes
she doesn't notice the name and puts the specimen through the
regular procedure. Then the joke is on her. On all of us here in
the lab. The Christmas of 1965 was a little different. The specimen

purported to be a sample of urine. The technician—a girl named Harriet Provine—saw the name, but she wasn't too busy at the moment and so, just for fun, she went ahead and processed it. That was on Friday, and Christmas was on Saturday. On Monday morning, the head technician checked the holiday-weekend cultures, and when she came to Mr. S. Claus she almost went through the roof. It wasn't just the name. It was the culture itself. The Santa Claus culture had grown an organism—a Group-G salmonella.

"The head technician came in and told me what had happened, and then she and I went over and saw Harriet. The rest of the sample, of course, was gone. Harriet had thrown it away. We don't keep that garbage after it's been planted. However, we did know where it came from. I got on the phone to the joker's floor and talked to a nurse who was in on the joke, and she told me how they had made the specimen. She said it consisted of water, an intravenous multiple-vitamin preparation, a pinch of powdered carmine dye for coloring, and a throat swab from one of the patients on the floor. Carmine is a red non-absorbent dye that is used internally in medicine to time and measure bowel action. Well, the recipe sounded plausible. I asked the nurse to send me down another swab from the patient, and went to work making up another specimen of Santa Claus's urine. I didn't use the throat swab in my reconstruction. I wanted that cultured separately. When I finished my specimen, I took it over to Harriet to culture."

Miss Provine says: "But it wasn't the same thing. I told Dr. Kunz that this wasn't it at all. It was the wrong color. It was red. The Santa Claus specimen was yellow. It really looked like urine."

Dr. Kunz says: "I may have got the proportions wrong. But that wouldn't make any difference. The ingredients were the thing. I told Harriet to go ahead and culture it. She also cultured the throat swab. And they both were negative for any kind of salmonella. I hadn't expected anything from the throat swab. After all, it came from a surgical patient. But the original Santa Claus specimen—I couldn't understand it at all. It didn't make any sense. It was totally inexplicable."

Dr. Lang says: "It was interesting, though. I thought it was well worth looking into further. I went up to the floor and talked to some of the jokers. I didn't learn much of anything—except that apparently Miss Provine had been right about the color of the reconstructed specimen. The nurse that Dr. Kunz talked to must have got two hoax specimens confused. The jokers had also faked a blood sample for the chemical laboratory, and that was where they had used the carmine dye. The urine sample had got its color simply from the vitamin preparation. I checked with the chemical lab, and they remembered the blood sample, but they hadn't bothered to test it. They had recognized the joke and thrown the stuff away. It seemed to me that there were still two possibilities —two possible vehicles for the Santa Claus *cubana*. That's what his salmonella turned out to be. One possibility was the water, and the other was the vitamin preparation. I couldn't help but think of water. It had been less than a year since the big Riverside, California, epidemic. That was an epidemic of *S. typhimurium* that caused around fifteen thousand cases of illness, and it was traced to contaminated water. Contaminated municipal water. I don't mean that I suspected Boston city water. My idea was that the water might have become contaminated at some point leading into the hospital. It wasn't a very serious idea. It was extremely farfetched, and I wasn't in the least surprised when it almost immediately collapsed. As soon as I asked about the hospital's water supply, I found that every building had its own connection with the city main. The vitamin preparation seemed to be a little more promising. I got the idea from a paper by Dr. Kunz. The paper had been published back in 1955, but I remembered it. It described culturing salmonella from yeast. Yeast is an unlikely vehicle for salmonella, but Dr. Kunz had shown that it could be one, and yeast is a source of Vitamin B, and Vitamin B was included in the intravenous multiple-vitamin preparation. The fact that Dr. Kunz's reconstructed specimen had been negative for salmonella wasn't necessarily final. It didn't necessarily mean that the preparation was uncontaminated. It could simply mean that the concentration of salmonella was extremely low, and that there was none or not enough in the sample he took for his culture. I made certain of a high concentration. I put fifty vials of the stuff through a millipore filter and then planted the residue in a culture flask. If there was any salmonella there, that would surely show it up. But there wasn't any there. The yeast was just another blind alley. The culture was negative.

"That was around the middle of February. I had been plugging away for two or three weeks and I'd run down every discernible lead, and the result was absolutely nothing. It began to look pretty hopeless. It began to look insoluble. That wouldn't be unheard of, of course. Not by a long shot. A good many epidemiological problems are never fully solved. The Riverside outbreak I mentioned is one of them. They never found the ultimate source of the trouble. They never determined how *S. typhimurium* got into the water. Hospital outbreaks are particularly tricky. A bug can get into a hospital and practically defy detection. In a big hospital— in a hospital like the M.G.H., where you have over six thousand people employed—the pathways can be extremely complex. Everybody I talked to was very consoling. They said I had an impossible problem. They said that I'd never run down the source, that nobody could run it down. I'd done everything that could be done, they said. That was true enough. At least, what I'd done was epidemiologically sound. The outbreak had been reported early on to the Massachusetts Department of Public Health, and Dr. Rubenstein—A. Daniel Rubenstein, the director of its Bureau of Hospital Facilities—had come over and reviewed our procedure and given it his approval. Another thing that my friends all said was that the outbreak seemed to be cooling off. It has probably burned itself out, they said. It's over. So relax. Forget it. They had a point about its cooling off. There hadn't been a new case since February 7th. The old man in the Bulfinch Building was the last one. I tried to take their advice. I had plenty of other work to do at the hospital and in my laboratory and at Harvard. When the time came for me to make my report to the Infection Control Committee on February 23rd, I was almost convinced that all my friends were right.

"But they weren't. They could hardly have been more mistaken. On March 1st, just six days after the meeting, Dr. Kunz's laboratory turned up another case. And that was merely No. 1 for the month. It was the first of a total of five. The first patient was in the White Building—on White Seven. He was a man of seventy-nine, and he had just entered the hospital back in January with

no presenting symptoms that in any way resembled those of sal-
monellosis. So his was clearly another hospital-acquired infection.
So were those of the second, third, and fifth cases. Case No. 2 was
reported on March 16th. He was a teen-age boy on White Five.
The third came along on the following day—a nurse on Burnham
Four. Then, on March 18th, came No. 4, an infant on Burnham
Five who had been cultured on arrival—in the emergency room.
No. 5 was a teen-age girl on White Eleven. She turned up on
March 19th. Four cases in four days! I felt like throwing up my
hands."

Dr. Kunz says: "And all in different places. It was like having
a sniper up in a tower, taking potshots in every direction."

Dr. Lang says: "But then it really did cool off. March went out
like a lamb. There were no more cases that month, and there were
none in April and none in May. And there were none in the first
half of June. I really thought it was over. A good thing, too. My
wife was bloody sick of hearing about *S. cubana*, and for three
months she got a relief. I didn't talk about it, but I didn't forget
it. I put it out of the forefront of my mind and concentrated on
my virus lab and on making rounds and on teaching, but I was
too involved to give it up. It was my investigation, it was my
responsibility—it was even more than that. It was my fascination.
I never really gave up. I certainly never stopped running down
possible leads. I think I must have known in my heart that this
was just another hiatus.

"One idea I had was that the spread of the infection within the
hospital might be attributable to sporadic carriers. It was obvious
that the nurse on Burnham Four had been infected by one of her
patients, and she could easily have carried the infection on to
somebody else if our routine culturing hadn't picked her up. What
I had in mind was hospital personnel that once in a while moved
out of their regular bailiwick. Every now and then, a nurse will
special on another floor. Or a surgeon will answer a consultation
in another building. And the X-ray people are always going somewhere. I checked up on everybody who had had any contact with
any of the cases. That turned out to be a lot of people, and it took
a lot of time, but it was no good. I drew a blank again. Another
lead had to do with powdered milk. The government's Center for

Disease Control, down in Atlanta, puts out a monthly bulletin called *Salmonella Surveillance*, and the June issue had a report from the Oregon State Department of Health about two cases of *S. cubana* infection in infants that had been traced to contaminated instant nonfat dry milk. It was *S. cubana* that caught my eye, of course. But the vehicle was provocative, too. I began to think that I was finally on to something. Powdered milk or nutritives containing powdered milk are used extensively in hospitals. I went down and got out the charts and orders on our cases —and there it was. Powdered milk or some nutritive additive had been prescribed for practically all of them. I rounded up some samples of the various products and sent them down to Dr. Kunz. Then I got on the telephone to the manufacturer. And that was the end of that. I knew that the manufacturer had a reputation for maintaining a high standard of quality control, but I hadn't known just how careful they were until I talked to the plant. They told me that they cultured all their products before they shipped them out. And Dr. Kunz confirmed what they said. All my samples were negative."

Dr. Kunz says: "We confirmed it, all right. But this thing was beginning to get on my nerves. We kept testing all this garbage that Dr. Lang kept sending down to the lab. We cultured every child who was discharged from Burnham. We cultured around three hundred hospital employees. We cultured God knows how much food and drugs. And the results were always the same. It didn't seem reasonable. *Cubana* ought to be showing up somewhere. I began to wonder if maybe we were doing something wrong."

Dr. Lang says: "It *was* a hiatus. The outbreak opened up again on June 15th. That was a Wednesday. On Wednesday morning, Dr. Kunz called up to report another case, and that afternoon he called me again and reported still another. They brought the grand total up to twenty. One of the new cases was a baby girl on Burnham Six, and the other was a man of thirty-nine on White Seven, and the records showed that both of them could have become infected only in the hospital. I ran around and gathered the same old information once again. I talked to the internes and the nurses and the residents. There was nothing else I could think of to do, and, as always, it came to nothing. There was no link, no connection, no rational explanation. I met with Dr. Rubenstein. He and his department were giving us every kind of coöperation, but they were as stumped as we were. Dr. Kunz and I were beginning to think that what we needed was some help from the Center for Disease Control. Their people have the training and the facilities to really dig into problems like this. But it wasn't up to us to ask them. The invitation would have to come from the State Health Department. And then we had another lull—another hiatus. It lasted exactly six weeks. It ended on July 27th, a Wednesday, at about one-thirty in the afternoon.

"I had just got back from lunch, and I was working in my office. The telephone rang and it was Dr. Kunz. We now had a total of twenty-one cases. His people had grown another culture of Group-G salmonella. The patient was another infant—a four-month-old boy. He had been a patient on Burnham Four since June 26th, and the information was that his infection was hospital-acquired. I hung up and sat back and looked at my notes. I remember thinking that here was an opportunity for a really special study. This little boy was an isolated case—the first new case in weeks. He was a crib child and therefore not very mobile —no wandering around or playing with other kids. And, if only because of his age, his diet would be relatively simple. So I went up on the floor. I started with his chart. It didn't tell me much. He had been admitted to the hospital with a general diagnosis of failure to thrive. Since then he had lost weight, and on July 24th he had developed diarrhea. His condition now was fair. I went over to the floor nurse's desk and got out the order book. An order book is a record of the physician's specific instructions for the care of the patient. It covers medication, diet, tests—everything. I found the boy's page, and read through the entries. There was a request to check on vital signs every four hours, and a diet warning about a possible milk allergy. Diet was limited to strained foods and meats; d-xylose, a non-fermenting sugar used in a test procedure; and a milk substitute called Nutramigen. Two drugs were prescribed—a multiple-vitamin preparation and an oral iron preparation. There was an order for a urinalysis, and for four stool tests. The stool tests were a test for fat and fibres, a test for trypsinenzyme activity, a routine culture for pathogens, and a carmine dye transit-time test. All the tests had been done—the stool-culture request was obviously the source of Dr. Kunz's salmonella report. But what interested me was the use of carmine dye. That lit me up like a light bulb. I don't know why, exactly. It made me think of the Santa Claus specimen, but we had ruled that out of the picture. I think it was just the coincidence. I had hardly even heard of carmine dye until the Santa Claus case, and here it was again. That was enough to arouse my curiosity.

"I got a nurse to open the medication closet, and I took a sample of everything the boy had been given—d-xylose, Nutramigen, vitamins, oral iron, carmine dye. The first information I wanted was what these drugs contained and how they were made. I carried my samples down to the pharmacy in the Burnham basement and showed them to the chief of pharmacy and his assistant. When they came to the carmine dye, they looked at the capsules and said the stuff had been purchased from an aniline-dye company in New Jersey. My heart sank down to my heels. Aniline dyes are synthetic dyes, and synthetics do not usually harbor salmonellae. I asked if carmine was an aniline dye. The chief wasn't sure, but his assistant, who had been around a long time, said he didn't think so. Carmine was made from something called cochineal. The chief got out a copy of the *Merck Index* and looked up carmine dye. The other pharmacist was right. It defined carmine as a pigment made from dried cochineal. But what was cochineal? The chief went back and got a copy of the *Dispensatory of the United States of America*, and we looked it up in that."

The entry reads:

> Cochineal consists of the dried female insects *Coccus cacti* Linné (Fam. *Coccidæ*), enclosing the young larvae. . . . The cochineal insect is indigenous to Mexico, Peru, and Central America, and in general appearance resembles a wood louse. The red dye found in the remains of the female insect has long been esteemed by the old races in these subtropical countries. Indeed, not only did they appreciate its value, but in order to increase the supplies, the cacti with the insects were successfully cultivated many years before even Cortez landed in Mexico in the early part of the sixteenth century. . . . The insect

feeds upon various species of the *Cactaceæ*. . . . It was spread into other parts of South and Central America and has been introduced into the West Indies, East Indies, Canary Islands, Southern Spain, Algeria, and is said to be found in Florida and California. The cultivation of cochineal is rather simple in a tropical climate; all that is necessary is to have the cochineal insects and the proper cacti. . . . The insects are 'sown' on the cacti in the open fields, where fecundation takes place. After this, the females attach themselves to the plant, and when their bodies have become swollen from the development of the enormous number of eggs, they are scraped off and killed either by boiling water or by the fumes of burning sulfur. . . . Powdered cochineal is very dusky to very dark red. It contains fragments of muscle fibers; portions of the chitinous epidermis with wax glands; fragments of larvae with coiled proboscides; occasional claws and segments of the legs; and fragments of antennae. . . . During 1952, a total of 83,713 pounds of cochineal was imported into this country from the Canary Islands, Peru, and Chile. . . . Cochineal was at one time supposed by some to possess anodyne properties, and used in whooping cough and neuralgia. At present, it is employed only as a coloring agent.

Dr. Lang says: "That really lit me up. I knew I had found the explanation. I was sure of it. There were two particular points. One was that carmine dye is ground-up insects. What could be a better vehicle than that? The other was that the insect is indigenous to Central America. I know it's ridiculous, but I saw an association: Central America, Cuba, *cubana*. I thanked the pharmacists and gathered up my samples and carried them over to Dr. Kunz's office."

Dr. Kunz says: "Ground-up insects—it seemed possible. I wasn't really excited. We had been through so many dry runs. I just for the first time wasn't bored to tears. But I turned everything except the carmine over to the girls. I planted the carmine myself. And it was the only sample that grew anything. I planted it on August 1st, and on August 3rd it grew a culture that tested out as Group-G salmonella."

Dr. Lang says: "That was good enough for me. I didn't wait for the New York Salmonella Center to identify the serotype as *S. cubana*. Which it did, of course, toward the end of the following week. We knew that the carmine dye was contaminated. But that didn't solve the problem unless the *cubana* patients and carmine could be linked. There were fourteen hospital-acquired cases in addition to the little boy on Burnham Four. I found that carmine-dye tests had been prescribed for ten of them. The four other hospital cases were no embarrassment. One of the four was the Burnham nurse, and her infection had almost certainly come from one of her patients. As for the others, the fact that carmine wasn't noted in the orders didn't really mean a thing. I was willing to assume that they had been given carmine or were secondary cases. I assumed it from their histories. They all appeared to be suffering from some sort of gastro-intestinal dysfunction, and carmine isn't always entered in the orders. It isn't required to be, because it isn't a medicine or what we call a charge drug—a drug for which the patient is charged.

"It took a little longer to explain the six infections that must have been acquired outside the hospital. One thing that had to be clarified first was the nature of the carmine contamination. Carmine dye is dispensed at the M.G.H. in capsules that are filled here at the hospital. Could the carmine have been contaminated in the course of that operation? Dr. Kunz got the answer to that by culturing carmine from the sealed jars in which it reached the hospital. To be absolutely sure of his results, he made his tests in the sterile room in my virus laboratory, where I do tissue cultures. There was no possibility there of any outside contamination. Well, the carmine from the sealed jars grew *S. cubana*. That naturally raised the question of the other local hospitals. They used carmine, too. Why hadn't they been getting any *cubana* infections? Dr. Rubenstein and his associates at the Massachusetts Department of Public Health were able to suggest an answer to that. They turned the answer up in the course of an intensive investigation they mounted as soon as they got our carmine-dye report. They found the explanation in the hospitals' laboratory procedure. The usual approach to salmonella detection in those laboratories was serologic, but their diagnostic process embraced only Groups A through E. A salmonella in Group G could escape detection. It wouldn't even be recognized as a salmonella. So it was entirely possible that our twenty-one cases of *S. cubana* were not the only cases in town. They were merely the only cases diagnosed as such. But how did our outside cases get their infections? My answer is only a guess—it couldn't be anything else—but I'm inclined to think it's the truth. Our experience set in motion a series of investigations by various state and federal agencies. The Center for Disease Control and the Food and Drug Administration were particularly active. They found carmine dye contaminated with *S. cubana* throughout the country, and several outbreaks identical with ours. At that point, of course, the sale of carmine was halted, and all hospitals and other users were warned about its dangers. The investigators also found that the use of carmine dye was not limited to hospitals—or even to medicine. It was also used as a coloring agent in numerous foods and drugs. The investigation showed that the American manufacturer sold carmine to twenty-eight food companies, ten spice companies, thirty-three pharmaceutical companies, seven cosmetic companies, and fifty-six less specialized companies, and the contaminated products they found included candy, chewing gum, preservatives, seasonings, meat, ice cream, and tomato extracts. Incidentally, the presence of carmine dye in these products was not noted on the label. The labeling law applies only to *artificial* coloring agents. Well, I think that answers the question. Not every person exposed to salmonella gets sick, but those cases of ours were highly susceptible people. I mean, they were already sick."

Dr. Kunz says: "We had an explanation for everything except my Santa Claus specimen. I think I can explain how the original specimen was contaminated. Carmine dye was not one of its ingredients, but it was the main ingredient of the blood sample that the jokers also made. I talked to them again, and it seems probable that a swab that was used to stir the blood specimen was later used to stir the other specimen. So there *was* a certain amount of carmine in the original Santa Claus specimen. But there was much more carmine in my reconstructed specimen, and that culture was negative. I don't know why. Maybe the carmine I used was the last of an earlier, uncontaminated supply. I don't know. I can't explain it. It's inexplicable."

The case was closed at the September meeting of the Committee on Infection Control. The secretary's account of that portion of the meeting read, "A follow-up report on salmonella was presented by Dr. Lang, who reviewed the investigations carried out within the hospital and in conjunction with the F.D.A. and the C.D.C. The source of hospital-acquired *Salmonella cubana* was traced to carmine red, which has been discontinued for clinical use. The chief of pharmacy is to circulate a statement to the staff regarding the discontinuance of carmine red, and he awaits direction from the F.D.A. on how to process the stock on hand. The Committee feels that to sterilize the present stock is perhaps hazardous, and that it should be discarded. At the moment, carbon is being used as a substitute for carmine red."

The conclusion of the investigation at the Massachusetts General Hospital was not quite the end of the matter. There remained the question of how the carmine dye had become contaminated. The natural assumption was that the contamination occurred in the course of processing at the plant of the American manufacturer. An early finding by the government investigators seemed to confirm that supposition. They found that although the manufacture of carmine dye included three processes employing heat (leaching, precipitation, and drying), the heat employed was seldom intense enough to destroy salmonellae. Another finding, however, suggested another explanation. A bacteriological examination revealed that recently imported stocks of dried cochineal at the plant were crawling with *S. cubana*. It thus seemed possible that the insect *Coccus cacti* was itself the source of the contamination, and this baleful possibility was presently supported by word of similar findings at the plants of the leading manufacturers in Britain and in West Germany. It was also determined that all these manufacturers—American, British, and German—were supplied by dealers in both Peru and the Canary Islands.

The entomological implications of these revelations changed the course of the investigation. They moved it from the national to the international scene. In June, 1967, two C.D.C. investigators —Steven A. Schroeder and L. Ariel Thomson—were dispatched to Peru to make a thorough study of the cochineal industry there. Dr. Lang and Dr. Kunz were invited to make a similar study in the Canary Islands. They accepted the assignment, and carried it out in August. The results of the two field studies were summarized by Dr. Schroeder in a subsequent report.

His conclusion read: "In Peru and in some areas of the Canary Islands, the cochineal insect grows wild on cactuses . . . while in parts of the Canary Islands, there are actual plantations where the insects are cultivated. The insects mature during the dry season, and in Peru are harvested by Indians, who then sell the insects to local merchants. The merchants then spread the insects on canvas cloths and allow them to sun dry on the streets or in yards, often adjacent to animal feces and flies. After a week or so of drying, the insects are put into sacks or tin cans and are sold at irregular intervals to brokers for the three or four large Peruvian cochineal exporting firms. . . . Dr. Thomson and I collected numerous samples of insects on cactuses, insects prior to being dried, while drying, and after drying. Of the more than fifty samples analyzed, only two, both of dried insects, were positive for salmonellae. The serotypes identified were *S. newport* and *S. enteritidis*, both of which are quite common throughout the world. Similarly, Drs. Kunz and Lang examined twelve samples from the Canary Islands, all of which were negative for salmonellae. It would appear therefore that salmonellae are not intrinsic to the cochineal insect, but are introduced, possibly through fecal exposure during the drying process. It seems reasonable to speculate that a batch of insects containing *S. cubana* contaminated machinery used in carmine-dye production, resulting in continuing contamination of the dye product with this same serotype. . . . Terminal heat sterilization [in processing] seems to have eliminated the salmonella hazard of carmine dye."

[*1971*]

CHAPTER 21

The Prognosis for
This Patient Is Horrible

AT AROUND TWO O'CLOCK on the afternoon of Tuesday, September 12, 1978, an eleven-month-old boy named Chad Shelton, the only child of Bruce Shelton, a television repairman, and his wife, Sallie Betten Shelton, was admitted to Immanuel Medical Center, in Omaha, Nebraska, for evaluation of persistent vomiting. Chad, his parents told the admitting physician, had been vomiting off and on for two days—since early Sunday evening. They added that they, too, had become sick Sunday evening, with severe abdominal cramps, diarrhea, and vomiting, but had now pretty well recovered.

The determination of the cause of an ailing infant's illness can be a serious diagnostic challenge. The diagnostician, being unable to elicit any account of how the patient feels or where he hurts, can make a judgment only on the observable and measurable signs of abnormality. The admitting physician at Immanuel Medical Center noted and recorded that Chad was "irritable," that his "right tympanic membrane was red," and that his tonsils were red and somewhat swollen. On the basis of these rudimentary findings, together with the information provided by the Sheltons, he recorded three tentative diagnoses: gastroenteritis, otitis media (inflammation of the middle ear), and tonsillitis. He also, as is usual in such ambiguous cases, sought the opinion of a consultant. The consulting physician's observations were entered on Chad Shelton's chart the following day. He observed that the patient was "somnolent through the evening, and this morning was noted to be poorly responsive." He noted what appeared to be multiple "bruises." Preliminary laboratory tests were generally normal, with two striking exceptions. One showed abnormal liver function. The other was the blood-platelet count. Platelets are protoplasms intricately involved in the salvational coagulation of blood that normally follows trauma. A normal platelet count ranges from a hundred and fifty thousand to three hundred thousand and upward. Chad's platelet count was nineteen thousand. That would seem to explain the "bruises." They were hemorrhages. The consultant noted his preliminary impression: "This may be a Reye's syndrome." Reye's syndrome, an entity of recent recognition, is a disease of still uncertain origin that largely afflicts young children and is characterized by vomiting, central-nervous-system damage, and liver damage. The production of platelets is a function of the bone marrow, and a low platelet count may reflect defective production or disordered distribution. The latter can be the result of a rush of platelets to a damaged organ—for example, the liver. The consultant recommended that more definitive tests be made and that the patient be transferred to the intensive-care unit of Children's Memorial Hospital.

Chad was admitted to Children's Hospital late that afternoon. He arrived there in a coma. It was noted on his chart that "within an hour after admission, the child's respiratory status began to deteriorate and it was necessary to place him on a ventilator. . . . A repeat platelet count at 4:30 P.M. revealed a platelet count of 18,000 [and] support was begun with platelets and whole blood. . . . During the evening and early morning hours, bleeding problems became increasingly difficult to control. The child's condition continued to deteriorate, and he was pronounced dead at 4:30 A.M. the morning of September 14th." An autopsy was performed. It revealed an "essentially complete necrosis of the child's hepatic [liver] cells, with very little fatty infiltration." The opinion of the pathologist was that "this pattern is more consistent with a toxic ingestion of an unknown agent rather than Reye's syndrome or other infectious etiologies." The final diagnosis reflected his opinion. It read, "1. Severe acute hepatic necrosis secondary to a toxic ingestion of an unknown agent. 2. Disseminated intravascular coagulation. 3. Cerebral hemorrhage secondary to #2. 4. Cerebral edema secondary to #1 and #2. 5. Terminal renal failure."

That was the beginning, but only the beginning. Shortly before noon that day—Thursday, September 14th, the day of Chad Shelton's death—a man named Duane N. Johnson, aged twenty-four and a trucker by trade, was admitted to Immanuel Medical Center by way of the emergency room. He was brought to the hospital by ambulance from the office of his family physician. He had collapsed in the waiting room there, and when he reached the hospital he was comatose. His wife, Sandra Betten Johnson, accompanied him. She told the admitting physician that her husband had become ill on Sunday evening. He had had an attack of chills, then diarrhea, then vomiting. He vomited several times on Monday and again on Tuesday. Yesterday, Wednesday, he had a severe nosebleed. This morning, he felt even worse—he was still vomiting, his head ached, light hurt his eyes, he was exhausted—and he arranged to see their doctor. Mrs. Johnson was frightened and confused. Her husband had never been sick a day in his life. Now he was lying there unconscious. And not only that. Sherrie, their three-year-old daughter, was also sick. Not as sick as Duane, but she had complained of stomach pains, and she had vomited several times. The last few days had been a nightmare. Mrs. Johnson didn't know what was happening. Her sister Sallie and her husband had also been sick this week—sick to their stomachs, like Sherrie. And only last night—early this morning—Chad, her sister's little baby, had died at Children's Hospital. They said he might have been poisoned. The admitting physician pricked up his ears. Chad? Was her nephew named Shelton? That's right—Chad Shelton. Did the doctor know about him? The doctor said he did. He said it was he who had admitted him to the hospital here on Tuesday. The doctor stopped and reflected. He reminded himself that Chad had suffered multiple hemorrhages. And Johnson had had a nosebleed. He asked himself if there might be some connection here. And Mrs. Johnson had said that their daughter was sick. He asked Mrs. Johnson to bring her daughter around to the hospital. He thought he ought to take a careful look at her.

Johnson remained comatose. The results of the admitting physician's preliminary examination were both unrevealing and alarming. The pupil of Johnson's right eye was "dilated and fixed," he wrote in his report. "Left pupil was pinpoint. Evidence of some conjunctival hemorrhage bilaterally. There was some blood in the pharynx." The physician again felt that a second opinion would be helpful. The consultant's findings, refined by a series of laboratory tests, fully justified the admitting physician's alarm. He noted on Johnson's chart, "There is no motor movement. There is no response to painful stimuli. . . . He is on a respirator. He has had an intracranial hemorrhage. . . . A CAT scan shows an intracerebral hematoma." Johnson's platelet count was a mere six thousand. An S.G.O.T. test was performed. This is a test that determines the concentration in the blood of an enzyme whose excessive presence is indicative of liver damage. A normal S.G.O.T. count is from five to eighteen units. Johnson's count was nine hundred and ten. The consultant concluded his report, "The patient, I think, has essentially gone into . . . a neurological situation from which he cannot be retrieved." Nevertheless, in the hope of retrieval, Johnson was transferred late that day to another hospital, Bishop Clarkson Memorial Hospital, where a technical procedure not available at Immanuel Medical Center could be performed. He was examined at Clarkson by a second consultant. It is usual for a physician confronted by a hopeless or near-hopeless case to note on the patient's chart some easy euphemism like "The prognosis is guarded." Johnson's condition jolted the consultant at Clarkson into the open. He concluded his report, "The prognosis for this patient is horrible."

Meanwhile, as requested by the physician who had admitted her husband that morning, Sandra Johnson returned to Immanuel Medical Center with her daughter, Sherrie. Sherrie was still in pain, still vomiting. She was admitted there at around two o'clock in the afternoon. The preliminary physical examination revealed a scattering of small intradermal hemorrhages on her eyelids and on her lower legs. Her liver was found to be tender and somewhat enlarged. Her platelet count was thirteen thousand. Her S.G.O.T. was seven hundred and two. An exchange blood transfusion was ordered. Following that, in the late afternoon, Sherrie was moved to Children's Hospital and placed in the intensive-care unit there.

Mrs. Johnson saw Sherrie settled at Children's Hospital. There was nothing more that she could do. She then visited her comatose husband at Clarkson Memorial Hospital. There was nothing that she could do there, either. She went home. But at least she did not go home to an empty house. Her second sister, Susan Betten Conley, was then staying with the Johnsons. The two distraught young women talked—about Duane, about Sherrie, about Chad. It was hard for them to believe that this was happening. Nothing in this terrible day seemed quite real. They later drove over to the Sheltons' house. The Sheltons were not as well recovered from their gastrointestinal troubles as they had tried to persuade themselves. Chad's pathetic illness and then his shattering death had distracted them from their own illness. Now they realized that they were far from well. Sallie Shelton, especially, felt poorly. She had abdominal pain, diarrhea, and nausea. Shelton and the three sisters talked. It was suggested that maybe Sallie should be hospitalized. Susan and Sandra left. They felt even more bewildered after talking with their sister and brother-in-law. They couldn't understand why they themselves were not sick—why they alone of the two families, the two households, were well. Sandra drove back to Children's Hospital. Sherrie was asleep, and her condition was described as stable. Sandra drove on to Clarkson Memorial. Her husband was still in a coma. There had been no improvement in his condition. He was almost certainly dying. She settled down to an all-night vigil.

Sallie Shelton spent a restless night. She awoke the next morning—Friday, September 15th—feeling very definitely ill. As she and her husband were dressing, the telephone rang. It was Sandra Johnson. Duane was dead. He had died about an hour ago, without recovering any degree of consciousness. That decided the Sheltons. They drove to Clarkson Memorial Hospital. Mrs. Shelton was examined in the emergency room. Her son's death and its cryptic nature were remembered. She was admitted for observation and testing. Then, as a precaution, it was decided to also admit her husband. The indicated tests revealed that Bruce Shelton's S.G.O.T. was mildly elevated (a hundred and twenty-five units) and his platelet count was a hundred and twenty-three thousand, or a little low. Sallie Shelton's condition was found to be more serious. She was still nauseated, still diarrheic, she had a headache, she was running a fever, and she was noticeably lethargic. Her S.G.O.T. level was eighty-five, and although her initial platelet count was a hundred and sixteen thousand, only a little lower than her husband's, subsequent evaluations showed an ominous downward trend.

Later that day, with Mrs. Johnson's permission, an autopsy was performed on Duane Johnson. The immediate cause of death was found to have been a cerebral hemorrhage. The pathologist's report also noted an almost total lack of platelets, and massive liver damage "of unknown etiology."

A memorandum dated September 18, 1978, from J. Lyle Conrad, director of the Field Services Division, Bureau of Epidemiology, Center for Disease Control, in Atlanta, reads:

> On September 15, 1978, Alan Kendal, Ph.D., Respiratory Virology Branch, Virology Division, Bureau of Laboratories, C.D.C., received a call from Paul A. Stoesz, M.D., State Epidemiologist, Nebraska, concerning two recent deaths in a group of families in Omaha, Nebraska. . . . Dr. Stoesz related that 2 people, an 11-month-old child and a 30-year-old [sic] man, had died within the past 2 days of an illness characterized by vomiting and diarrhea. Clinical information on the child indicated a death from hepatic failure. No information was available on the cause of death in the man, although an autopsy was being performed. . . . Both toxic and infectious etiologies are being considered as possible causes for these deaths.
>
> Dr. Stoesz, on behalf of Henry D. Smith, M.D., Director of Health, Nebraska State Department of Health, and Warren Jacobson, M.D., Director, Douglas County Health Department, invited C.D.C. to assist in an investigation of the situation. . . . After further discussions about potential etiologies for the outbreak, Dr. Conrad then contacted . . . John P. M.

Lofgren, M.D., E.I.S. [Epidemic Intelligence Service] Officer
in Jefferson City, Missouri. . . . Dr. Lofgren departed for
Omaha the evening of September 15.

"Yes," Dr. Lofgren says. "I got Dr. Conrad's call at about three
o'clock in the afternoon. Omaha and Jefferson City are not that
close together, but apparently I was the nearest E.I.S. officer to the
scene. Anyway, I got the call and went home and packed and took
off. I drove the rest of the day and part of the night. I got to Omaha
—to a motel room that the doctors there had reserved for me—
at about 2 A.M. There was a message waiting for me. There was
to be a big meeting the next morning in the conference room at
Clarkson Memorial Hospital, and one of the local doctors would
pick me up. Which he did. At the meeting, there were about thirty
people—the attending physicians, house officers and medical students involved in the case, lab people and pathologists, hospital
social workers, the staff of the county health department, and the
state epidemiologist and his staff. We settled down to work in good
order. We had the two autopsy reports and the charts on the three
surviving patients. It was a strange case, and very wide open. But
there were a few conclusions that we could be comfortable with.
It seemed clear that we were dealing with a disease that was not
epidemic, that was limited to just the Johnson and the Shelton
families. Then we defined the disease. Our case definition required
these symptoms: vomiting, an increased S.G.O.T., and a decrease
in platelets.

"The state and county epidemiologists had made a good beginning. A setting had begun to take shape. The Johnson home
seemed to be the site of the trouble. The outbreak had its origin
there on the afternoon of Sunday, September 10th, sometime between three and four o'clock. The two families had not been
together in about a week until then. But that afternoon the three
Sheltons—Bruce, Sallie, and the baby, Chad—dropped in on the
Johnsons and Susan Conley. They visited about an hour. At about
three-fifteen, Sandra Johnson went to the refrigerator and took out
a white plastic pitcher of lemonade. She added ice and filled some
glasses. Bruce Shelton took a couple of swallows from his glass
and then poured about three-quarters of an inch in a glass for little
Chad, and Sallie Shelton finished off the rest. Sandra didn't like

lemonade, and she drank none. Neither did her sister Susan. Duane Johnson and the little girl, Sherrie, both drank some of the lemonade. It was suggested that Duane might have drunk two glasses. The Sheltons left to make another call and then started home. On the way home, Bruce and Sallie began to feel sick to the stomach. A few minutes after they got home—at about six o'clock —Sallie vomited. That made her feel a little better. Then, at about seven o'clock, Bruce vomited, and then little Chad. Then Sallie vomited again, and she and her husband vomited again and again during the next four hours. But Chad vomited only that once that night. The two Johnsons—Duane and his daughter, Sherrie—had much the same experience. The investigation had shown that Sandra Johnson had made the lemonade. She had made it a day or two before Sunday—maybe as early as the previous Thursday. But she had made it as she always did—a packaged mix with water and sugar. It was uncertain whether all the lemonade was drunk or whether some was left and thrown out. In any event, the pitcher was empty. The fatal lemonade was gone.

"I say 'fatal' because, as unlikely as lemonade sounds as a cause of poisoning, we were satisfied that the outbreak was an outbreak of poisoning, and that the lemonade was the vehicle. There had been some toxic material in it. The onset of illness was compatible with poisoning by some organic poison. The incubation period was all wrong for an infectious disease. Much too short. Later, after the meeting, I went out to the Johnson house and had a look around. It was a lower-middle-class house on low ground and in bad repair. The plumbing was poor. The house had already been carefully searched, and I was provided with samples of everything that could be even remotely connected with the trouble. One of these possibilities was some firecrackers. Firecrackers contain yellow phosphorus, and its taste could have been masked by the lemonade. There was no indication of how the phosphorus might have got into the lemonade. So that's where we stood. We had a clear clinical syndrome and a likely vehicle. But we didn't have any idea of what the toxic agent might have been. The answer, if we were going to get one, would seem to be up to the laboratory people. John Wiley, the Douglas County epidemiologist, was very helpful. We arranged for samples of everything found in the Johnson house that could be analyzed and sent them off to C.D.C. We also sent off blood and urine samples taken from all the patients, and frozen liver, brain, lung, kidney, and spleen specimens from Duane Johnson. That was about the end of my role in the investigation. I went back to Jefferson City and wrote up my report."

The samples gathered for Dr. Lofgren by Mr. Wiley and his staff were received at C.D.C.—at the Toxicology Branch of the Bureau of Laboratories—in three installments, on September 20th, 21st, and 25th. It was a comprehensive and a very considerable collection. It numbered thirty-four items, including a packet of twenty firecrackers. Animal experiments were at once begun. A group of laboratory rats were fed (by gavage) various materials found in the Johnson kitchen—tap water, sugar, lemonade mix. Other rats were injected with material taken from the several patients. The plastic pitcher in which the lemonade had been made was treated with a citric-acid solution in the hope of extracting some minuscule remains of the lemonade, and the solution was fed to another group of rats. The firecrackers were anatomized. They were found to contain only an insignificant quantity of yellow phosphorus. The laboratory animals were sacrificed at intervals during the next week or so, and their kidneys, livers, and other organs and tissues were examined for eloquent pathological changes. None were found. Liver tissue obtained from Johnson at autopsy was further analyzed for the presence of selenium, a substance that in large concentrations has a toxic affinity for the liver, and for arsenic. The results were essentially normal. Urine samples taken from Bruce and Sallie Shelton at the peak of their illness were analyzed for evidence of a dangerous herbicide called paraquat. The results again were negative.

The toxicological examination of the various samples and specimens relating to the Omaha outbreak was monitored and its results were evaluated by a research medical officer in the Toxicology Branch of C.D.C. named Renate D. Kimbrough. Dr. Kimbrough, a native of Germany and a graduate in medicine of the University of Göttingen, is the wife of a research chemist and the mother of three children. She is also a pathologist and a

toxicologist of national distinction. She found the laboratory results, for all their negativity, both useful and interesting.

"One thing was particularly noteworthy," Dr. Kimbrough says.
"The liver was the only affected organ. That eliminated a good
many possible poisons. Most toxic chemicals that cause severe
liver damage also cause damage to other parts of the body. As a
matter of fact, it is unusual to find only liver damage—to find the
liver destroyed and none of the other organs affected. There were
also other limiting factors to consider. One was that the poison
had to be something that was easily soluble in water—in lemonade. Another was that it had to be more or less tasteless and
odorless. There was no indication that the Johnson lemonade had
either a funny taste or a funny smell. Well, those factors eliminated a number of other compounds. In fact, they narrowed the
field to a group of readily modifiable hydrocarbons called alkylating agents. This was not an area in which I felt very much at home,
but I knew someone who did. I knew an expert. I put in a call to
Ronald C. Shank. Dr. Shank is associate professor of toxicology
in the Department of Community and Environmental Medicine at
the University of California at Irvine. I told him my story and
what I needed. Could he give me a list of water-soluble alkylating
agents? No problem. He gave me a list of eight—methyl methane
sulfonate; dimethyl sulfate; dimethylnitrosamine; N-methyl-N'-
nitro-N-nitrosoguanidine; 1, 2 dimethylhydrazine; methyl chloride; methyl bromide; and methyl iodide. Then I went to work. It
was another process of evaluation and elimination. I ruled out
methyl chloride, methyl bromide, and methyl iodide almost at
once. They are all weak alkylating agents, and they are lethal only
in very large amounts—amounts too large to go undetected in a
glass of lemonade. Moreover, the initial impact of those agents is
on the brain, so the initial effect is mental confusion. That had not
been noted in any of the Omaha cases. I could also rule out 1, 2
dimethylhydrazine. It causes severe damage to the red blood cells,
and no such damage was noted in any of the Omaha reports. Then
I eliminated methyl methane sulfonate. The kind of liver damage
it produces is quite different from that observed in Duane Johnson
and Chad Shelton. The same was true of dimethyl sulfate and
N-methyl-N'-nitro-N-nitrosoguanidine. And the latter, again, is

lethal only in very large amounts. That left dimethylnitrosamine.

"I think I knew almost at once that dimethylnitrosamine was the answer. It perfectly met all the required criteria. It is a liquid, and it is well miscible with water. It is largely odorless and tasteless. It is extremely toxic in very small amounts. The lethal dose for a medium-sized adult is less than two grams, and for a small child about one-third of a gram. A third of a gram is about seven drops, or less than half a teaspoonful. And dimethylnitrosamine is peculiarly liver-specific. It attacks the liver and only the liver, and the lesions it causes are quite distinctive. I studied the textbook lesions caused by dimethylnitrosamine. Then I examined under the microscope the liver specimens taken at autopsy from Duane Johnson and Chad Shelton. The Johnson and Shelton lesions were identical with the textbook examples. Now, let me move ahead for a moment. I was satisfied that the poison involved was dimethylnitrosamine, but I wanted to be more than that. I wanted to be absolutely sure. This was not an accidental poisoning. Everyone involved in the matter was certain that the poison had been deliberately added to the lemonade. It was a case of murder. Well, I called Dr. Shank again. Dimethylnitrosamine is very rapidly metabolized and excreted—within a couple of days of ingestion. So there was no possibility of turning up any trace of it in the liver samples. Its presence in the liver, however, causes certain chemical changes that can be measured by a high-pressure liquid-chromatography procedure that was recently developed by Dr. Shank. I asked him if he would perform his test on a group of liver tissues. This was to be, of course, a blind test. I supplied Dr. Shank with eight coded vials of material. They consisted of liver tissue taken from Duane Johnson, kidney tissue taken from him, and six liver and kidney specimens taken from cases in our storage file—three of them from alleged cases of methyl-bromide poisoning and three from cases of Reye's syndrome. Dr. Shank reported that one specimen of the eight was positive for dimethylnitrosamine. That was the coded sample of liver tissue taken from Duane Johnson. And that was definitive.

"But all this, as I say, came later. Much later—in August of 1979. So now let's go back to where we were—to October of 1978. I was reasonably satisfied that dimethylnitrosamine was the poison involved, and I acted on that assumption. The next question was: How did it get in the lemonade? And where did it come from? It certainly didn't come from the corner drugstore. Dimethylnitrosamine is not an everyday compound, and its uses are rather limited. It was originally developed in England, as a solvent for use in the automobile industry, and it may have some other highly specialized industrial uses, but it is also known to be a powerful carcinogen. That quality has given it a certain vogue in cancer research. It is widely used to induce cancer in laboratory animals. I thought about that, and I thought about Omaha. Omaha is not a great industrial center; it is a great insurance center. And it is something of a medical center. It has Creighton University School of Medicine and the University of Nebraska Medical School, and it has the Eppley Institute—the Eppley Institute for cancer research.

"I had talked with John Wiley, the Douglas County epidemiologist, a time or two in the course of the investigation. So now I called him again. I told him what I had in mind. I don't believe I actually singled out dimethylnitrosamine. I think I simply said that I was convinced that the poison involved was an alkylating agent, and that it might very well be one used in cancer research. I suggested that it might be a good idea to check and see if anybody connected with the Johnson or Shelton families had any connection with the Eppley Institute. He said he would. And he did. And there was a connection—a very direct, a very real connection."

The criminal investigation of the deaths of Chad Shelton and Duane Johnson was directed by Samuel W. Cooper, the Deputy Douglas County Attorney, together with Lieutenant Foster Burchard, of the Homicide Division of the Omaha Police Department. Much of the field work, and most of the most productive work, was done by a detective in Lieutenant Burchard's command named Kenneth G. Miller.

"It was a strange case," Cooper says. "Our investigation was the third phase of three quite distinct phases. There was first the medical investigation, then Renate Kimbrough's toxicological investigation, and then our homicide investigation. And even our phase was unusual. It was never, from our point of view, a simple case of whodunit. By the time we came into the picture, it had been established that the murder weapon was a toxic substance. So it was more a case of how-he-dunit. It took us a good long time to build up a provable case, but we had both the who and the how, and even the why, in only a matter of days. That was where Ken Miller came in. Miller had been working closely with John Wiley at the Health Department, and Wiley told him about his conversation with Dr. Kimbrough and her suggestion about a possible link between the families involved and the Eppley Institute. Miller was smart enough to take her suggestion seriously. He went back to his office and ran the Johnsons and the Sheltons through the computer file we have on victims of some sort of criminal act. And almost at once he found a lead. It involved the Johnsons—Duane and Sandra—and Sandra's mother and brother. One night in June of 1975, Duane and Sandra—they weren't the Johnsons yet, they were only going together—and her mother and brother went to the movies. Afterward, they were standing together out in front of the Betten house, talking, when a car drove up and a man jumped out and opened fire with a shotgun. One of the pellets hit Sandra's mother, and Sandra's brother was nicked a couple of times, but neither was really hurt. The man drove off, but there was no big mystery about the attack. The man had been a high-school sweetheart of Sandra's. He was jealous and crazed, furious that she had dropped him for another man, and his intended victim may have been Duane Johnson. His name was Steven Roy Harper, and he was a rather familiar type. Good student, quiet, never drank, smoked, or used drugs. The records showed that Harper was arrested, pleaded no contest to a charge of shooting with intent to kill, and was sentenced to one to five years in prison. That was on December 6, 1976. He was paroled on November 16, 1977. Ken Miller absorbed all that and then moved on to the Eppley Institute. It was almost too much. Harper had worked at the Eppley Institute. He had found a job there a few months after his release, and his job was one that put him in the vicinity of various chemical compounds, including alkylating agents, including dimethylnitrosamine. He had held the job for about five months, until August 18, 1978, when he resigned to take a better-paying job as a construction worker. That was the bare bones of our investigation. There was, of course, a great deal more—a lot of legwork, a lot of interviewing of Sandra Johnson and others, a lot of detail. Harper had been in Omaha at the time of the lemonade party, but now he was on a construction job in Beaumont, Texas. Miller and a couple of other detectives and I flew down to Beaumont with a warrant. We arranged for the F.B.I. to pick Harper up, and we took him into custody."

That was on Friday, October 13th, less than a month after the deaths of Chad Shelton and Duane Johnson. After his arrest, Harper made an informal declaration to a homicide detective in Cooper's entourage named Greg Thompson. Thompson's transcript of it reads, in its essentials:

> Harper states that he is still in love with Sandra Johnson, that his life has been miserable for the past four years, and everything built up in him until it came to this point. While working in the Gene Eppley Cancer Care Center [sic], he took a chemical which he called DMNA [dimethylnitrosamine], a carcinogen. . . .
>
> Harper stated that he remembers driving up by the Johnson house, looking and seeing that no one was there, drove past it and parked down the street, around the corner. Harper then got out and walked back up the street, around the corner to the Johnson house, walked all the way around the Johnson house, looking for a way to get in. Harper states that he thought he went in the side door, but he may have went in the window, he can't really remember. Or maybe he just left by the side door. He remembers going into the house, opening up the refrigerator, taking the small vial, which he described to be between two (2) and three (3) inches long and maybe a half-inch (½) diameter, pouring it into the lemonade in the refrigerator. . . . Harper then left the residence.

Harper denied in his statement to Thompson that he had poisoned the lemonade with murderous intent. He told Thompson that "he didn't believe that it [the dimethylnitrosamine] was toxic, that it would only cause cancer." If such was his intention, he may have been not entirely unsuccessful. Of the three surviving victims of his poisoned lemonade, Bruce and Sallie Shelton were discharged from the hospital as fully recovered—he after four days of treatment, she after a stay of sixteen days. Sandra Johnson's daughter, Sherrie, was less fortunate. She was hospitalized for three weeks and then was followed for several months as an outpatient. The most recent record of her condition noted "continuous hepatosplenomegaly [enlargement of the liver and spleen] and elevated liver enzymes, and a liver biopsy obtained three months after exposure showed chronic active hepatitis." A liver so damaged is often eventually hospitable to the development of cancer.

Harper was returned to Omaha. His case was presented at a preliminary judicial hearing, after which the presiding judge charged him with two counts of murder in the first degree and three counts of poisoning. On October 5, 1979, after a three-week trial in which Cooper served as prosecuting attorney and Dr. Kimbrough appeared as a key witness for the state, Harper was found guilty on all five counts and sentenced to die in the electric chair.

[*1982*]

CHAPTER 22

A Contemporary Touch

DR. TAYLOR—David N. Taylor, an Epidemic Intelligence Service officer attached to the Enteric Diseases Branch, Bacterial Diseases Division, of the national Centers for Disease Control, in Atlanta —pushed the telephone away and sat for a moment glancing over his notes. Then he gathered them up and walked down the long hall, the fifth-floor hall, to the office of his superior, Dr. Roger A. Feldman, director of the Bacterial Diseases Division. That was around three o'clock in the afternoon of Wednesday, January 28, 1981. Dr. Feldman, a tall man with a pepper-and-salt beard, a wide smile, and a riveting eye, was at his desk, and he smiled Dr. Taylor into a chair. Dr. Taylor—slim, straight, neatly parted sandy hair, small sandy mustache, steel-rimmed glasses—is thirty-three years old and a product of Kenyon College, Harvard Medical School, and the London School of Hygiene and Tropical Medicine. He took out his notes and made his report. He had, he said, just received a call from an epidemiologist named Frank Holtzhauer at the Ohio State Department of Health, in Columbus. Holtzhauer was calling for Dr. Thomas Halpin, the State Epidemiologist, and his call was a call for federal help in investigating a perplexing outbreak of gastroenteritis in the town of Steubenville. The outbreak had begun on December 10th with the illness and subsequent hospitalization of a five-month-old girl. Since then, in the course of the past six weeks, twelve more cases, both adults and children, had been reported to the local authorities, and it was expected that there were more to come. The nature of the outbreak had been established. The enteritis was bacterial in origin. Laboratory analysis of stool samples of the victims had shown the microörganism involved to be a member of the genus *Salmonella,* and of the species known as *S. muenchen.* But that was all. There was no other apparent link between the several victims.

"Roger listened and smiled and nodded," Dr. Taylor says. "He asked a couple of questions. I knew he would be calling Dr. Halpin for a formal confirmation and for a formal invitation to intervene. But the handwriting was already on the wall. I was going to Steubenville."

Salmonellosis, as the disease caused by the Salmonella organism is properly called, is the commonest single cause of what is commonly called food poisoning. It accounts for at least twenty-five per cent of the numberless outbreaks of mingled nausea and vomiting, abdominal cramps, diarrhea, and fever that occur in this and every other country every year. Its name commemorates the nineteenth-century American pathologist Daniel Elmer Salmon, who first identified the genus, and it is a commemoration of international reach. "Bacteria of the genus *Salmonella,* " Robert H. Rubin and Louis Weinstein, both of the Harvard Medical School, noted in a 1977 monograph, "are perhaps the most ubiquitous pathogens in nature, isolated from, in worldwide distribution, not only man and his domestic animals but also reptiles, wild mammals, birds, and even insects." The usual cause of human salmonellosis is contaminated (and insufficiently cooked) beef, lamb, pork, duck, turkey, chicken, and, particularly, eggs. Other causes include food or drink contaminated by the excreta of infected animals and by tainted equipment. An outbreak in Boston's Massachusetts General Hospital in 1966 was traced to contaminated carmine dye, a diagnostic staining material. The salmonellae are almost as various as they are abundant. Since 1941, when the Danish bacteriologist F. Kauffmann perfected a serotyping technique by which the different salmonellae could be specifically identified, the number of species that comprise the genus grew from a handful to the hundreds. Some fifteen hundred distinct species are now known. The names of these (with two or three exceptions) indicate where they were first isolated—*S. moscow,* for example; *S. panama, S. miami, S. senegal.* Some of these are still found only in their place of discovery, but most have long since achieved a cosmopolitan prevalence. The ten most frequently reported serotypes in the United States (as of 1979) are: *S. typhimurium/copenhagen, S. enteritidis, S. heidelberg, S. newport, S. infantis, S. agona, S. saintpaul, S. typhi, S. montevideo,* and *S. oranienburg. S. javiana* is No. 11. No. 12 is *S. muenchen.*

"*S. muenchen* wasn't much of a clue," Dr. Taylor says. "A really uncommon—a relatively localized—serotype can make things somewhat easier. At least conceivably, it can tell you where to look, and even what to look for as the source of contamination. But *S. muenchen* turns up everywhere—all over the country, all over the world. Around four hundred cases are reported to the C.D.C. every year. So I was prepared for some hard work, for plenty of old-fashioned shoe-leather epidemiology. I should say *we* were prepared. I had an assistant—a fourth-year medical student at Duke who was assigned to the C.D.C. for a term as a sort of interne. A very bright guy named Emmett Schmidt. Emmett and I left the next morning—Tuesday morning—by plane for Pittsburgh. We rented a car there and drove on down to Steubenville. Steubenville is in the eastern part of the state, aross the Ohio River from West Virginia. I come from Ohio. I was raised in Columbus. But Steubenville was an Ohio I had never seen before. It's a mill town—a steel town, down in a deep valley, very old and very run-down. I don't know—maybe it was the time of year, the dead of winter, or because most of the mills were shut down and everybody was out of work—but I've never seen a more depressing place. It took the heart out of me.

"There was a Holiday Inn. We registered there and then drove around to the city health department and met some of the people we would be working with. We met Maurice Pizzoferrato, the Steubenville Commissioner of Health, and two state epidemiologists—Charlene Steris and Robert Campbell—and Janice Schrader, a microbiologist. It was Janice who had identified the serotype as *S. muenchen*. The first thing we learned was that the outbreak was still going on. I've forgotten just how many new cases there were—I didn't keep a daily report card. But I can tell you the total. By the time the outbreak had finally run its course, we had thirty-six confirmed cases. Janice Schrader was a remarkable person. She was doing *all* the laboratory work for the whole area, and she was still able to find time to help us every way she could. She was also a big help in working out our game plan and getting it into action. She seemed to know just about everybody in town. She was involved, she cared about what had happened. Charlene briefed us on the cases—age, sex, date of onset. The incubation period for salmonellosis is about three days. The date of the appearance of symptoms indicates the approximate time of exposure and can often indicate its place and nature. We learned that the outbreak was on the whole pretty severe. There is no treatment for salmonellosis. Antibiotics tend to do more harm than good. But eighty per cent of the children here were sick enough to be hospitalized, and about sixty-five per cent of the adult cases. The age range was enormous. It stretched from a one-month-old boy to a woman of seventy-three. It was hard to know what that signified. The cases were scattered all over town, and only a few of them even knew each other. In such outbreaks, there is always a common denominator—an eating place, a wedding reception, a picnic, a dinner party, a church social. Something in which everybody was involved. This one was a total mystery.

"We formed two teams. I joined up with Charlene, and Emmett worked with Bob Campbell. There was nothing to do but start almost from scratch—to start visiting the households of the patients. I was especially intrigued by the two cases first reported—the five-month-old girl and a twenty-five-year-old man. Because the baby's father—a man I'll call Frank Lowell—was bosom buddies with the second case, whom I'll call Gene Russell. And then there was Case No. 3, a close friend of both Lowell and Russell.

He was a twenty-seven-year-old man I'll call Paul James. Russell was out of work, but Lowell and James both had jobs on a municipal garbage truck. The three of them had been friends since high school. My thinking was this: Young guys, young couples, do things together, so let's see what the Lowells, the Russells, and the Jameses do for recreation. They all lived in the same neighborhood, down by the river. We decided to start with Mrs. Lowell. It's easier to talk to the mother of a sick infant than to a sick adult. The mother cares, the adult tends to shrug it off. Mrs. Lowell was sort of typical—twenty-seven years old, pretty face, overweight. And very nervous. Her house was old and run-down, but it was scrubbed clean. Not a speck of dust. The baby's illness seemed to embarrass her, as though it reflected on her as a mother and housekeeper. She didn't see how a thing like food poisoning could have happened in *her* house. I asked about formulas, about Christmas or holiday foods. There was a famous outbreak of *S. eastbourne* that involved contaminated chocolate Christmas candy. I asked about deli meats—a notorious vehicle. About restaurant meals. All dead ends. The Lowells couldn't afford to eat in restaurants or patronize delis. During the holidays, they had eaten turkey, ham, and some venison. Gene Russell had shot a deer, and dressed it himself at home. They rarely went out. They sometimes played cards with the Jameses and the Russells, or just hung out together.

"So Charlene and I moved on down the street to the Russells," Dr. Taylor went on. "Same kind of household—father, mother, two-month-old boy. Russell was out of work and at home. But this wasn't like the Lowell house. These people were relaxed. Mrs. Russell said that she hadn't been sick, and neither had the baby, even though later tests showed that both had been infected. And Russell himself was the picture of unconcern: 'Gee, Doc, I don't know what happened. I got sick, but I feel O.K. now. What do you think it was, Doc? Could it have been that deer? I shot it out near an old abandoned dump. But, what the hell, it's all over now.' Another dead end. It was the same with the Jameses, around the corner. James was at work and his wife was at home with two children—a boy of five and a daughter of six. James and the boy had been sick, and were treated at the Ohio Valley Hospital. They hung out with the Lowells and the Russells, played cards, drank a little beer. Had a ham for Christmas. That was interesting. I had never thought of ham as a holiday food, but everybody around here seemed to eat it at Christmastime. I filed the thought away. And on we went, from house to house, still fishing, still getting nowhere. But two things did take shape—three, including those Christmas-ham dinners. The first thing was that the cases seemed to fall into three groups. There were the blue-collar cases down in the valley. There were a couple of cases up on the hill, in a middle-class neighborhood. And there were some cases in a different middle-class neighborhood, in a suburb called Mingo Junction. Which, of course, was the reverse of helpful. It simply made things more mysterious.

"The other finding was a little more positive. It was only a statistic, but it had the feel of something solid. This was the age breakdown. The largest single age group in the outbreak was that of twenty to twenty-nine. That group accounted for twenty-eight per cent of the cases. But the national average of salmonella outbreaks in that group is just twelve per cent. That suggested that something a little different was happening here. Why this prevalence of young adults? Was there a preponderance of families of young adults in Steubenville? We decided to find out. So we picked out a set of controls. We selected at random thirty-two households in the neighborhoods of our established cases, and called them up. What was the makeup of the household? And—aha! It was *not* unusual in Steubenville to find a young adult in every family. All our case households included persons aged fifteen to thirty-five, but only forty-one per cent of the randomly selected households included persons in that age range. Well, now we had a common demoninator. Maybe not *the* common denominator, but *a* common denominator. The next question was: What do young adults do? Where do they go? Bars. Fast-food places. We went back to shoe leather, walking the streets. Nothing came of it. These people still didn't have any haunts in common.

"There were two cases in a middle-class neighborhood up on the hill, in a section called Winterville. Both were students—a seventeen-year-old boy and an eighteen-year-old girl—at the local Catholic high school. The boy was in the hospital. The girl had been treated in the emergency room and sent home. We talked to the boy, and he gave us the story of his life. Video games. Pizza parlors. A few private parties. We talked to the girl's parents. The mother had a theory: her daughter had been poisoned by frozen king crab. I thought of the Lowells and the Russells and the Jameses. They had probably never even heard of king crab. And then the girl's mother seemed to finish things off. She said that her daughter and the boy in the hospital moved in entirely different circles and hardly knew each other.

"I'm going to go back a few days now," Dr. Taylor continued. "The morning that Emmett and I left Atlanta, I had had a few words with Roger Feldman, and he showed me a yellow office-memo slip. It said, 'S. muenchen, Michigan.' It was dated about a week earlier. Roger told me what it meant: Michigan had reported an outbreak of S. muenchen and wanted to know if the C.D.C. had had any similar reports. Roger said he had told them about Steubenville. He would pass my reports along to them. O.K. So on the way back down the hill to the Holiday Inn after that wasted day in Winterville, I got to thinking about that Michigan outbreak. S. muenchen is common enough, but still . . . Back at the motel, I called a man I knew in the Michigan State Department of Health named Harry McGee. Harry told me they had twenty-odd cases, all with onset dates much like ours here, and all were in Lansing. Not in East Lansing, the university town, but in Lansing, the blue-collar auto town. They hadn't a clue to the source. Eight of the cases were young adults, and ten were babies —infants—which meant that they were probably in households that included young adults. I began to get a little excited. I thanked Harry and called Roger Feldman. I told him the situation here, that we were getting nowhere. The people were getting tired of us. The health commissioner wanted the case solved and cleared up and ended—he had all the eating places in town on his back. I suggested that a trip to Lansing and a look at those very similar cases might give us a new perspective. Or something. Roger said no. He said to stay where we were. He said the answer was there and that we'd find it. And to let him know when we did. That was on Thursday, February 5th. It was snowing. The charm of motel life fades very quickly. Emmett and I were homesick for our wives, who kept asking when we were ever coming home. We went out in the snow and found a new place to eat and had another awful dinner. Then we went back to the motel. We stared at our data, turning it this way and that, until about 2 A.M. And the only item that meant a thing was all those young adults.

"We started out the next morning on a new tack. I still had ham on my mind—those holiday ham dinners. So we decided to settle the question one way or another. Commissioner Pizzaferrato lent us one of his department's sanitarians, and with him as our guide we undertook a tour of the city's meat markets. We picked up samples of different kinds of ham at each place and Janice Schrader would culture them for possible salmonellae. Most of the markets were ethnic—Polish, Italian, Greek. Steubenville is that kind of town. The proprietors were a little suspicious. They didn't want to get involved in food poisoning. But we got what we wanted. And, all in all, it was a pretty dull tour. There was one incident. It was at the third place we visited. As we were leaving, a young woman came in. Pretty but bedraggled. She was crying, her eye makeup was smeared, and she was acting strange. Stoned. Spaced out. Something. The proprietor went over to her and soothed her, and she left. It was sort of sad, and we talked about it on the way to the next market. Was she drunk? Or was she on drugs? The sanitarian said something about a relationship between unemployment and drugs and alcohol. Looking around Steubenville—those closed mills, all that depression—I could believe him. Anyway, we finished up and took our samples around to Janice. And that, as it turned out, was the end of the ham idea. The cultures all were negative.

"Emmett and I had dinner that night with Janice. We ate at an Italian place she knew about, and for once it wasn't bad, and we sat there after eating, drinking coffee and shooting the breeze about what the heck was going on. We got to talking about those first three families—the Lowells and the Russells and the Jameses. In case you've forgotten, the outbreak was still not over. We were still getting new cases, and all the cases, new and old, were being monitored once a week. Their stool samples came to Janice, and she cultured them. Well, Janice said we might be interested to know that one of the cases had just been cleared. That was Mrs. Russell. For the first time, her weekly sample was negative. The rest of her family was still positive, and so were the Jameses and the Lowells. It *was* interesting. We wondered why her. Janice said that Mrs. Russell was also pregnant. Maybe that had something to do with it. Then we broke up and Emmett and I went back to the motel. I remember that Emmett called his wife and they talked and talked, and he mentioned the woman in the meat market and they talked about drugs. When he hung up, we started talking about drugs. I was thinking of tranquilizers and quaaludes and things like that—drugs in capsules that could get contaminated in processing or packaging or otherwise. It was a thought.

"It still seemed like a good idea in the morning. Janice had mentioned Mrs. Russell, and she seemed as good a place as any to start. We went around to the Russell place right after breakfast, at about nine o'clock. Mrs. Russell received us. Russell was still in bed—and why not? He was out of work and it was a dismal morning. We asked Mrs. Russell once again about food, about mixes, about condiments. We did a thorough kitchen inventory, and it was the kind of kitchen you wouldn't be surprised to find any kind of contamination in. These were real easygoing people —not like Mrs. Lowell. But that was all just thrashing around. Finally, I got down to business and asked her if she or anybody in the family was taking any kind of drugs. She said, you mean like medicine? Oh, no. What about the other kind—illicit drugs? Like, say, quaads? Oh, *no*—certainly not. Then there was a funny kind of silence. Then she said, 'Well, Gene and I and most of our friends, we do smoke a little pot when we're hanging out together. But I stopped last week. I mean, I'm pregnant, so I thought I'd better.' Pot? Marijuana? I was thinking capsules—swallowing something contaminated. Pot was smoking. I didn't know what to think. And then Russell came strolling into the living room. I guess he'd woken up and heard us talking. He was very cool, very relaxed. He said, 'Sure, we smoke a little pot. What else is there to do in this town?' I was still trying to think, to adjust. I asked him very carefully if he happened to have any marijuana on hand —if I could have a sample for laboratory analysis. He looked at me for a moment. Then he said sure. He said, 'Man, I'll roll you a joint.' I told him just a sample for the lab would do. But I was aware of what he was doing. To him and his wife, Emmett and I were some kind of Feds. He wanted to get me involved. He wanted to get me neutralized. Anyway, he just shrugged and laughed, and went off somewhere and came back with a couple of grams in an envelope—about enough for one joint. Emmett and I exchanged a look. We finally, at last, had something concrete. It was a weird idea. I had never heard of marijuana as a vehicle for salmonella. Nobody had. But it was an idea. It was concrete, and I had it in my hand.

"Our next move was going to be a little more difficult. Russell had nothing much to lose—he was unemployed, and who cared if he smoked a little pot—but that wasn't true of most of the other cases. The Lowells and the Jameses were city employees. It was going to be hard to get anything out of them. I decided our best move was through Russell. I explained to him that our interest in marijuana had nothing to do with the law. Emmett and I weren't any kind of police. We had no intention of getting him or anybody else in trouble. We were only trying to get at the source of the outbreak. We rapped like that for a little while, and then I said that we would need to talk to the other cases, including his friends the Lowells and the Jameses. I wondered if he would try to sort of pave the way for us. Would he mind calling Mrs. Lowell? Be glad to. He went to the phone and called her. He was very good, very persuasive. You remember that she was a very nervous, worrying kind of woman. But she agreed to see us. We went right over. She was very stiff and strained. I guess this was as close as she had ever come to a drug bust. But she was making an effort to be calm and sophisticated. She said, well, yes, they did smoke pot. She said, well, yes, they did have some in the house. She went off and came back with about two grams in a plastic bag. She said it came from the same guy that the Jameses and the Russells bought their pot from. She asked me if I really thought that the outbreak was caused by pot. I said it seemed to be a possibility. 'Well,' she said, 'I'm not really surprised. I thought this batch had a kind of funny smell.' That made me smile. But I really wanted to shout. A possibility, of course, was all it was. But it was a possibility that seemed to fit in very nicely with that preponderance of young adults. We were cooking. We were really cooking.

"But down here in this blue-collar valley, down here by the river —this was only one neighborhood, only one part of the outbreak. There was Mingo Junction, and there was the Winterville section, up on the hill. When we had made our first round of house calls, we talked to a young woman at Mingo Junction—Debbie Something-or-other. She was the one confirmed case there, but her brother and her boyfriend were both subclinical cases—positive but asymptomatic. Debbie was twenty-one, a salesgirl in a nut shop by day and a dancing teacher evenings. She never had any reason to go down to the valley. She took sick on December 28th. She lived at home but very seldom ate there. She told us she lived on tacos, submarine sandwiches, and such. When we finished up with Mrs. Lowell, we went out to Mingo, and ran Debbie down again and had a talk. Pot? She said she never used it. Her brother did, though, and so did her friend. She thought she could get us a sample from her friend. We arranged to meet that evening. Then we went on to Winterville. We got nowhere with the two high-school kids. We had to be careful, and they weren't telling: getting caught using pot meant expulsion from school. But I talked with a counsellor at the school, and he told me that while our two kids moved in different circles, the circles they moved in were very far from the best. We met Debbie and her friend that evening, and they had a nice sample for us. I don't know how Emmett and I got through Saturday night. We were really keyed up. I called Janice on Sunday morning and told her what we had, and she agreed to meet us at her lab. Very quietly. This was ticklish business at this point—we didn't know how the Health Department would react. On Monday afternoon, Janice told us that preliminary results showed evidence of contaminated pot—all three samples. By Tuesday, it was definite. She had cultured salmonellae from the samples, and they were salmonellae of a group of twenty-odd serotypes called C/2. C/2 includes *S. muenchen*. On Wednesday, Janice went on to make it certain: our marijuana samples were definitely contaminated with *S. muenchen*. But on Tuesday morning, the C/2 finding was enough. I called Roger Feldman, and he said, 'Well—well, I'll be damned.' "

"Maurice Pizzoferrato had very much the same reaction. Only more so. Roger was naturally pleased that we had solved the problem, and as a professional he was very much interested that we had found a new vehicle for salmonellae. But Maurice! Maurice was euphoric. He had been getting very edgy, very impatient. His lab was tied up, his people were on call to us, and all the eating places in town were on his phone every day and afraid of hearing the worst. And, of course, the press was pressing. Marijuana was an absolutely perfect answer. It took him entirely off the hook. Illicit drugs were no responsibility of his. He wanted the world to know what we had found. He wanted me to call an immediate press conference. And Roger, when I asked him for instructions, agreed. Emmett and I worked up a statement, and the conference was set for ten o'clock on Wednesday morning, February 11th, in Maurice's office at the Health Department. They even had me sitting in Maurice's own big chair at his own big desk.

"It was my début in this sort of thing. All the media were there —the local newspaper, the local radio, the local television, and the stringers for the wire services. I read our statement. I told them that the source of the outbreak wasn't water, it wasn't any eating place, it wasn't any food. I told them—and this is from our prepared statement—that 'our most important lead suggests that a non-commercial product with an unknown distribution is the source of this salmonella. We have tested samples of marijuana associated with three different cases and we have found the identical salmonella which has been isolated from the ill persons. This finding suggests that the marijuana currently in use in Jefferson County has become contaminated with salmonella and represents the primary vehicles of transmission for the illness.' I told them that having diarrhea caused by salmonella didn't necessarily mean that the person was a *user* of marijuana. Many of our cases, I said, were infected indirectly from a person who was a silent carrier, or from environmental sources. The salmonella was in the marijuana. When a marijuana smoker rolled a cigarette his hands became contaminated, and when he put the cigarette in his mouth his lips became contaminated. Then a touch or a kiss or any sort of contact could spread the infection. I said we didn't know yet just how heavily contaminated the marijuana was—actually, it turned out to be *very* heavily contaminated—but even a light contamination would be enough to make a susceptible person sick. And not only that. Pot decreases the gastric acid, and gastric acid is an important defense against infections of all kinds. Regular pot smokers are especially susceptible to infection. Then came the tricky part. Here's what I said in our statement: 'To substantiate our theory that marijuana is the culprit, it is most important that we continue to test marijuana samples from the area. If it were a commercial product, we could just pull it off the shelves and test it—but that is not possible with marijuana. We therefore need the community to help us test additional marijuana samples. People may drop off their samples at the Jefferson County Center for Alcoholism and Drug Abuse . . . or samples may be brought directly to the Health Department. Because we think this is a major health risk, we are testing marijuana free and anonymously. Your sample will be given a number. . . .' And so on. The police had agreed to look the other way for a day or two. Then came the questions. I did the best I could. It was really very exciting. A big story. And not only locally. Both the wire services carried it. It wasn't so much that we had solved the mystery. It was the marijuana. That gave it a contemporary touch.

"That was our last day in Steubenville. There was no reason for Emmett and me to stay on for the windup of the investigation. We flew back to Atlanta that afternoon. I had a day at home—Thursday, February 12th—and then on Friday Roger sent me off to Michigan. I wasn't exactly eager to leave, and yet, of course, I wanted to go. I felt that Steubenville was only one side of the coin. I didn't feel that we had absolutely proven our case. What I wanted, as I had wanted before, was to do a good case-control study. Our studies in Steubenville weren't really precise. The Supreme Court for an epidemiological problem is a case-control study, and I wanted that supreme-court verdict. As I said, my contact in Michigan was Harry McGee, of the Michigan State Department of Health. Nothing had really changed in Lansing since Harry and I had last talked. There was a total of seventeen confirmed cases. The source of the outbreak was still unknown. But now, after Steubenville, we had a lead to work with. The study went like this: We selected thirty-four households to serve as controls. These households matched the case households in neighborhood and in general social and economic status, and they had much the same prevalence of young children and young adults. The one crucial difference was that the controls were households in which there had been no diarrhea illness for at least two months. We did our interviews in person. People respond to a personal visit with trust. We asked a comprehensive set of questions. We asked about restaurant meals. About deli foods. About alcohol. And then about marijuana. The results were very satisfactory. The case households used marijuana over three times more frequently than the control households which was significantly different. We also collected eight samples of marijuana from six households. Only one of them was positive for salmonella, for *S. muenchen.* But that was enough.

"I went back to Atlanta feeling very pleased. The news there made me feel even better. The final reports from Steubenville were in. The public appeal had brought in forty-seven new samples of marijuana, and eight of them were positive for *S. muenchen.* Then came some totally unexpected news: There had been two outbreaks of *S. muenchen* gastroenteritis that were more or less coincident with Steubenville and Lansing—one in Alabama, involving two cases, and another in Georgia, in and around Atlanta, involving twenty-one cases. When the health people there saw our first Steubenville report, they sat up in a hurry. They went back to their cases and interviewed them all over again and collected some samples of marijuana and analyzed them, and the results were positive for *S. muenchen* contamination. The contamination in every instance was very considerable. It was almost incredible —four million organisms to a gram of marijuana. That was so high that it enabled us to make a very reasonable assumption. This was that the contamination could not have occurred by accident, by contamination on the hands of the processors. It must have occurred either in the field, from untreated animal manure used as fertilizer, or by inadvertent contamination during drying or storage, or by direct adulteration of the marijuana with dried manure, to increase the weight and therefore increase the profits. We generally favor the last hypothesis. A good reason for that theory was that *S. muenchen* was not the only contaminating pathogen found in the marijuana. All the samples also showed the presence of such organisms as *Staphylococcus, E. coli, K. pneumoniae,* and *D. Streptococci.* Our only disappointment was that we were never able to determine where the stuff came from. The Drug Enforcement Agency estimates that about seventy-five per cent of the marijuana consumed in the U.S. comes from Colombia, about eleven per cent from Mexico, about seven per cent from Jamaica, and the rest is grown locally. Locally-grown marijuana is consumed locally, and Mexican marijuana is largely consumed in the Southwest. So we can assume our marijuana came from either Colombia or Jamaica.

"There was one last piece of news. Samples of the marijuana collected in Ohio, in Michigan, in Alabama, and in Georgia were passed along to the C.D.C. They were then turned over to a research microbiologist in the microbiology laboratory in the Enterobacteriology Branch. She was Dr. Kaye Wachsmuth. She examined the samples by a very delicate technique developed in 1975 as a research tool by Stanley Falkow and his associates at the University of Washington, in Seattle. What Kaye did was to apply this technique for the first time to an epidemic situation. Put very simply, the cultured *S. muenchen* is broken down and its DNA is extracted and the molecular weight of its parts are measured. These weights are distinguished by a pattern of plasmid banding. Different strains of *S. muenchen*—and every other serotype— have different banding patterns: different, as we say, plasmid fingerprints. Kaye examined all our samples and compared the results with the fingerprints of other—non-marijuana—*S. muenchen* strains. All of the marijuana *S. muenchen* were identical, and distinctly different from the non-marijuana strains. That was the ultimate confirmation. That was the final touch. That put the icing on the cake."

[*1982*]

CHAPTER 23

The Hoofbeats of a Zebra

A LITTLE PAST five o'clock on the afternoon of October 11, 1978, a young black woman shuffled on the arm of a friend into the emergency room of Alvarado Community Hospital, in San Diego, California, and asked to be admitted for psychiatric help. Her name, she said, was Sheila Allen, her age was twenty-four, and her complaint (as later interpreted and standardized and noted on her chart) was "bizarre behavior, with looseness of thought associations and severe depression associated with suicidal thoughts." She was admitted after a brief examination to the psychiatric wing, and made comfortable there in a double room. The following day, and for several days thereafter, she was examined, tested, and variously observed. The results of these evaluations were inconclusive, and on October 16th a member of the psychiatric staff named Robert Brewer was appointed attending physician.

"I went in to see her after rounds the next morning," Dr. Brewer says. "She was sitting on the edge of the bed—sitting there with the help of a nurse. She was tall, with a beautiful figure, a beautiful face, and beautiful, wide-apart eyes. She was also pathetic. She didn't seem to have any strength at all. She couldn't walk. She could hardly sit up. She could hardly lift her arms. I introduced myself and made some getting-acquainted talk. I took her history and did a routine physical and checked her mental status. She was just as weak as she looked. She was well oriented and alert. There was some evidence of conversion hysteria. I finished up with a lot of history and a lot of problems, but no strong impressions in any direction. I was inclined to go functional, but not entirely. I did a residency in neurology, and I always try to keep the organic possibility in mind. I started thinking 'multiple sclerosis.' Her age, for one thing, was right. Multiple sclerosis is a young-person's disease. But I'm a listener. I think that if you listen long enough your patient will usually tell you what the trouble is. So I asked her what *she* thought was her trouble. She said, 'I'm a kook.' I said maybe so, but before we go that road—I'd like you to see a neurologist I know. She almost blew up. I think she might have hit me if she'd had the strength. She said, 'I don't want to see a neurologist. I've seen a dozen neurologists. I'm a kook. I'm in the kook hospital. I want you to fix up my kookiness.' But I wasn't convinced. And that afternoon, I called Fred Baughman, the neurologist I had in mind."

I met Sheila Allen in the spring of 1983, some five years after that pitiful outburst. We met, by prearrangement, in San Diego, in the office of Dr. Brewer's neurological colleague Dr. Fred A. Baughman. She looked good—the picture of health, and beautiful, and entirely free (if she had ever been otherwise) of kookiness.

"Oh, I was," she told me. "I *was* a kook. I had to be, after what I'd been through. If a person can be driven crazy, that was me. But, of course, I wasn't really crazy. I was simply in despair. I had been sick for so long—for almost four years. I was getting sicker and sicker. I was almost helpless. I went to Alvarado Hospital because I couldn't think of anything else to do. I had finally given up.

"I don't know when my trouble actually started. I mean, it came on so innocently. I guess it began in Dallas some time in 1974. No, I'm not from Dallas. I was born in the Chicago area—in Maywood, Illinois. But when I was fourteen, my parents moved to Los Angeles, and I went to high school there. I ran track, and

I was a cheerleader. I've always liked sports. I've always loved to run and dance and bike and everything like that. I went to Cal State, at Northridge, for a year, and I studied physical education. I went to Dallas because I wanted a change. There were no problems at home or anything like that. I just wanted a change. I got a job at a Sears store, demonstrating cosmetics. Then a friend told me that Braniff was hiring flight attendants. I had an interview, and they hired me and sent me to their school—six weeks of emergency procedures, first aid, posture, grammar, how to prepare the meals. I was based in Dallas, and I flew every stop to Chicago and sometimes to New York—all over. I think March of 1974 was when the trouble first began. I was out dancing one night, and my legs gave out on me. I mean, I fell down. But I was able to get right up, and I said it was my high heels. That's what I thought. So I went to lower heels, and then one night it happened again. It was just like the first time. I was able to get right up and go on. Nobody seemed to think anything of it. So I wasn't really worried. But when I had my regular Braniff physical in August, I mentioned it to the doctor. He gave me an extra careful checkup, and passed me. He said I was in great shape. He said I was probably just tired—too much standing. Well, flying is all standing. You hardly ever sit down on a flight. So that made sense. But then my legs began to hurt. I wasn't just tired, I also *hurt*—at the end of a flight, or walking through the airports. Like O'Hare. Or, especially, Dallas. You know how big it is. We were always having to walk from Gate 1 to Gate 22. My legs would cramp. It was a real tight pain. I would have to sit down and rest for a couple of minutes. Then I'd be all right. But all of the girls were always complaining about being tired, so I still didn't think too much about it. Until it began to affect my arms. Just lifting two trays, and my arms would begin to tremble. It seemed like they didn't want to hold. Even a coffee pot was almost too much for my strength. I tried to get more sleep. But I just got tireder and tireder. And I began to almost miss flights because I had to sit down so often along the concourses and rest. So what I did was just get up earlier. If there's one thing I've got, it's will power. I drove myself as hard as I could. But I was getting worried now —real worried. I went to a doctor one of my friends knew. He said take it easy. Stop driving myself so hard. He gave me a prescription for Valium.

"That would have been around the end of 1974. I thought maybe I wasn't eating right. It's hard to eat right when you're flying. All too often after we have served the passengers their lunches or dinners there wouldn't be any food left. Most of the girls carried candy bars for those emergencies. I carried what I called my survival package—tuna fish and peanut butter and crackers and raw carrots and lots of vitamins. A lot of the girls recommended a shot of bourbon at bedtime. I tried that, and it was all right, but I couldn't see that it helped me any. I had to realize that my tiredness was different from the other girls'. So finally—I think it was in October, or maybe November, of 1975 —I tried again. I went to an orthopedic specialist. I told him about my legs, how weak they were—and my arms. He looked me over; he was very thorough. But he couldn't find anything wrong. He said it was probably my job—the standing and the stress and all that. His advice was to quit, to take a leave or something. But I *loved* flying. I loved my job. And I loved the money. I had a little Opel GT sports car. I had a nice apartment. I had a wonderful life. So I kept on working—getting to the airport early enough so I could make it to the gate, and getting back home late—and resting every chance I got. I stopped talking about my problems to the other girls. I didn't want them to say anything. I wanted to keep my job. But I was only fooling myself. It was just too much for me. In February of 1976, I asked for a vacation, and they gave me three weeks' leave. I went to my favorite place—to Hawaii. I relaxed and rested and tried to enjoy myself. The three weeks went by, and I was the same as always. I just didn't have any strength. I went back to Dallas and gave my two weeks' notice. I said I had personal problems. Which was true enough. My sister Enid flew in from L.A., and drove me home in my little Opel—back home to my parents.

"It's hard to explain just how I felt. I was worried about feeling so tired and weak. But I still really thought it would go away. I still really thought I'd get better. Anyway, I couldn't just sit around the house. That isn't my way. I went out and got a job— two jobs, as a matter of fact. I got a daytime job demonstrating cosmetics again. I worked in various stores doing makeup. And at night I worked as a cocktail waitress in a club. I suppose that was kind of foolish. Because I had the same old trouble—the same problem with trays, the same problem with all the standing and walking. I had to wear heels at the cocktail job, and, of course, that made things that much worse. Every now and then I dropped a tray. I could tell when it was coming on—I'd think, There goes the tray. The other waitresses dropped things, too. But they only dropped a glass or something. I dropped the whole tray. But the boss was crazy about me. That made everything O.K. This was in the summer of 1976. But finally the boss got to be too much for me. I had to quit. I had already quit the cosmetics job. Two jobs were too big a load for me, and the cocktail job paid better. When I quit that, I got a daytime job as a hostess in a restaurant at the beach. I guess I knew by then that there was something really wrong, but I wanted to work. I missed the airline income. It's hard to change when you get used to a certain level of living.

"When I first came home to L.A., I had gone to the family doctor. He couldn't find anything wrong with me. Then I met a chiropractor at a party and told him my problem. He checked me out, and couldn't find anything wrong, either. He referred me to a woman psychologist. She gave me an I.Q. test. That only told her that I was bright. So she gave me another test. And then another. She never seemed to try to think anything out—she just kept giving me tests. I decided she was a waste of time and quit. I also quit my hostess job. I had to—I was getting weaker every day. Everything I did hurt. It hurt to comb my hair. My arms were so heavy and weak. It was hard for me to drive my car. Once or twice it was really frightening. I'd try to brake or something, and my foot wouldn't move. One Sunday afternoon I took my little three-year-old niece to the park. When we were driving home, a traffic light up ahead turned red and I started to brake and I couldn't lift my foot. Oh, my God! I thought. I'm going to kill us both. I told my niece to get down on the floor. I hung onto the wheel and we sailed across the intersection. Thank God, there was nobody coming. I don't know how I ever made it home. That was the last time I drove. I was at home now all the time. But I had problems even there. I don't know how many times my legs gave out and I fell down the stairs. They were carpeted, thank God. So I wasn't hurt much. That was going down. Climbing the stairs, I practically had to crawl. My mom was a problem, too. She kept saying I was just trying to upset her. She didn't really mean that. The real reason was that she couldn't bear to think there was something wrong with me. And my sisters. We would be getting ready to go out somewhere, and it took me so long to get ready they'd go off without me. I got so I was crying a lot. I'd try to pick up a glass, and my arm would go limp. And I'd say, 'Oh, no!'—and fall into a chair and just cry.

"But I still hadn't given up. When I quit going to that woman psychologist, my chiropractor friend suggested I see a psychiatrist. I was going out with him some, and he was really trying to help. He was convinced that my trouble was psychosomatic. I didn't know what to think. Some days I was better, and some days I was worse. Some days I could get dressed and go out and everything was almost like normal. Then the next morning I couldn't even fix breakfast. I had a drawer full of prescriptions—Valium, Elavil, Equanil, all those drugs. Every doctor I went to see prescribed something. I tried them all, and I couldn't see any difference. I couldn't see that any of them helped. So I went to a psychiatrist. He was a white guy. Some of the doctors I'd seen were white. Some were black. Anyway, I went to this psychiatrist once a week. We talked. We went over everything I'd been told by all the others. He said I must face it. I had a psychosomatic problem. I liked him; he was a nice man. He made me feel better about myself, which helped. But I didn't really believe what he said. Then I had my family—my mother and my brother and my three sisters—on me. They made it perfectly plain. They said I was crazy. I said to myself that *they* were crazy.

"About that time, in December of 1976, I met a nice guy from San Diego. He was a big guy—six foot six and two hundred and seventy pounds. His name was Ira Watley, and he had been playing offensive tackle for Miami. He'd just got cut. He was going back home to San Diego, and he suggested I come with him—get away from my family. He knew they were driving me nuts. I thought about it. Then one morning I woke up and I almost couldn't get out of bed. But I made it and started down to breakfast, and fell. I fell all the way down the stairs. I didn't know whether I was hurt or not. I hurt all over anyway. I must have looked awful, because my mother helped me up and took me to the emergency room of a hospital a few blocks away. There was a young doctor on duty. He examined me and everything—my arms and legs and all. He said to wait, and went away. He came back with a textbook and he stood there studying it. Then he said, 'I would think you might have myasthenia gravis, but the symptoms aren't right. Myasthenia gravis starts with the eyes and face, with drooping eyelids, and trouble swallowing. You don't have that.' He said he thought I ought to see a psychiatrist. He gave me a prescription for Elavil.

"That made up my mind. I went to San Diego with Ira. He was working, so he could take care of me. He was really understanding. He wanted to get married. I didn't think so, not right then. But I was feeling a little better and getting a little restless. I wanted to do something. Ira suggested I go to school—to a business college he knew about. So I enrolled. That was in February, 1977. But it was the same old story. I wasn't really any better. The school was on the second floor—a walkup—and those stairs were too much. I would go late so people wouldn't see me struggling. It was one step and rest, another step and rest. Some days I could go three steps without resting. I was taking typing. And finally I couldn't do it. I couldn't hold out my arms. It was a three-month course, but I never finished it. After that, I just stayed home. Except to go to the doctor. I had already seen a couple of doctors in San Diego. One was a regular internist. The other was a neurologist. They were like all the rest, psychosomatic, Valium. But Ira kept pushing me to keep trying to get some help. I even went to a doctor in La Jolla who tried to hypnotize me. I wouldn't hypnotize, and that frustrated him. He told me I didn't want to get well. Then I tried an orthopedic surgeon. He asked me to lift my arms. I couldn't do it. He stomped out of the room. He said he couldn't help me because I wouldn't coöperate. Then I tried another psychiatrist. I had four or five visits. The psychiatrists and the psychologists were all alike. What did your last doctor say? I see. Well, I agree. Psychosomatic. I'm going to give you a prescription for an antidepressant. Some of them started with my childhood. Some started now and worked back. I told them I had a normal childhood—a normal middle-class childhood. I told them I didn't hate my parents, and they didn't hate me. They were loving parents. The psychiatrist I went to four or five times, he saw Ira when Ira brought me to his office. I told you Ira is a very big man. So this doctor had a new idea. He asked me if Ira beat me.

"I started getting completely worse in June—June of 1978. Ira was away. The Winnipeg Blue Bombers had signed him on, and he was training up there in Canada. He had arranged everything before he left. He had his father come over and look after me. He sent me his check every week, and one of his friends—Frank or Drake—would take me to the bank and to the supermarket or wherever. Frank was very sympathetic. He had been in Vietnam and had had a hard time there, and he'd had some therapy. He persuaded me to try the state mental-health center. I joined their group-therapy class. I went for a while. But the classes were kindergarten stuff, and I wouldn't take the drugs they offered. Elavil was one of them, and it actually seemed to trigger more weakness. It seemed to actually loosen my muscles. I had some bad experiences even without drugs. I'd sit down in a chair, and when I wanted to get up I couldn't. I'd have to wait for Ira's dad or somebody to help me. It got so I was afraid to cook. I remember one afternoon I had some vegetables on the stove. I left the kitchen and fell, and I couldn't get up. I just lay there smelling them burn. The house was full of smoke when Ira's dad came in and turned off the stove. It was an awful feeling. I wasn't good for anything. I used to sit and meditate and pray. I'd fix my mind on, say, fishing or shopping, and try not to think of anything else. I did a lot of praying. I'd say the Lord's Prayer over and over and over. It helped me, I think. I prayed in bed in the morning, too. I kept a Bible by the bed. In the morning, when I woke up, I'd read or pray, and finally I'd have the strength to get up. One morning, I couldn't comb my hair. I didn't have the strength. I finally had to lay my head on the sink, and that way I could use my arms a little. There was another time. Drake and his brother Lee took me fishing with them out on the park dock. After a while I went to the bathroom. I sat down on the toilet, and I couldn't get back up.

Nobody came in. I yelled and yelled, and finally Lee came in and got me out.

"I think that was about the last time I went out anywhere. I knew I was reaching the end of the line. My muscles were getting weaker and weaker. I had to rest more and more. I knew that pretty soon I'd be helpless. I had to do something before it was too late. I decided my only hope was to get hospitalized. And I knew the best way I could get hospitalized was to talk depression and suicide. That was one thing I'd learn from all those psychologists and psychiatrists. The hospital I picked was Alvarado Community Hospital. It was the nearest one to Ira's apartment. I got Frank to drive me there, and he had to practically carry me into the emergency room. I told my story, and they took me in. I remember the date. I remember it very well. It was Wednesday, October 11, 1978, late in the afternoon. But the date I really remember is the following Wednesday, October 18th, around noon. That was the day I met Dr. Baughman. He came into my room and looked me over and told me what my trouble was. I had myasthenia gravis."

"Well, yes," Dr. Baughman told me. "It *was* almost as quick and easy as that. I was pretty sure the minute I saw her that her trouble was myasthenia gravis. The only other possibility was amyotrophic lateral sclerosis, and she was much too young for that." Dr. Baughman is a slight, wiry man of fifty, with a bang of sandy gray hair and a wide, warm, country-boy smile. He was smiling now. "But it wasn't magic. Myasthenia gravis is a special interest of mine. I trained at Mt. Sinai, in New York, and Mt. Sinai has a rather famous myasthenia-gravis research laboratory. Some important work has been done there. So I learned about myasthenia gravis early, and it is always on my mind. There is a saying about diagnosis—about why doctors often fail to recognize one of the less-common diseases. It goes: When you hear hoofbeats, you don't necessarily think of a zebra. I recognized the hoofbeats of a zebra. That was my only magic. I won't say myasthenia gravis is a common disease. But it isn't a rarity, either. The national occurrence rate is one in twenty thousand. I see my share—

because I'm a neurologist and because I'm aware. I average three to five *new* cases a year. Women seem to be more susceptible than men—particularly young women. Myasthenia gravis is a good descriptive name. The 'my' refers to muscle, and 'asthenia' comes from the Greek for weakness. It isn't as gravis—as serious—a disease as it once was. It was first described in the seventeenth century, and it was named around the end of the nineteenth century, and in those days and up until the middle nineteen-fifties it was very often fatal. There is a treatment now. But, of course, it can't be treated if it isn't diagnosed. That's the problem. In that respect, Sheila was a classic case.

"I remember my first look at Sheila. Bob Brewer had called me and said he had some doubts about a psychiatric patient at Alvarado and would I take a look. So the next day I went up to Four South when I finished my regular rounds. The first order of business is the visual impression. And oh, Lord! She was pathetic—truly pathetic. She was lying in bed and not exactly crying—sort of whimpering. There was a feeling of just hopelessness. Her beauty made it all the worse. I knew the moment I saw her that there was a profound generalized muscle weakness. I called a nurse, and we got her sitting up. She tried to help, but it was a genuine, real weakness. Nothing functional about it. Her face was normal, and so was her speech. There was a slight nasal character, but not much. I had the nurse get her to her feet and walk. It was a definitely abnormal gait; it was a waddle. That indicated a hip-girdle weakness. We have a scale of evaluation. It begins at zero, then trace, then poor, then fair, then good. Sheila's hip and shoulder girdles were poor to fair. Her body and feet were in the good range. The weakness was symmetrical, and there was just no question about it. I knew her history, and I didn't believe a word of all those psychiatric evaluations. This was a serious muscle disease.

"It's sad to think how close she came to an early diagnosis. I'm thinking of that young doctor up in Los Angeles. He suspected myasthenia gravis, but he made the common mistake of going entirely by the book. The books all emphasize that the presenting symptoms are drooping eyelids, facial weakness, and palatal weakness—difficulty in speaking. The classic teaching requires the presence of one or more of those symptoms for a diagnosis of myasthenia. I had one patient who was referred to me by an ophthalmologist. A man had come to him complaining that he was losing his eyesight. The ophthalmologist recognized that the cause of his failing sight was the drooping eyelids of myasthenia gravis. I wish the textbooks were a little less rigid. But the fact is that a mere suspicion of myasthenia is enough, because there's a quick and easy diagnostic test that is almost entirely reliable.

"Myasthenia gravis is a fundamentally mysterious disease. I mean the basic cause is unknown. It is generally thought to be one of the several autoimmune diseases—the consequence of some disturbance in the body's immune system. Antibodies appear in the blood that interfere with the supply of a substance called acetylcholine, which mediates neuromuscular function. I'm putting a highly complicated process in very simple terms. The result of this inhibition is a weakness much like the weakness induced by the poison curare, and the treatment of myasthenia gravis has derived from an understanding of curare intoxication. The site of the physiological defect in both curare poisoning and myasthenia gravis is the neuromuscular junction. In the absence of acetylcholine, the muscular response very rapidly decreases. A period of rest will, at least for a time, restore sufficient acetylcholine to allow for normal function, but only for a limited time. Then the weakness returns. Drugs have been developed that are antagonistic, in varying degrees, to the substance that inhibits acetylcholine. One of these anti-cholinesterase agents is involved in the diagnostic test for myasthenia gravis. Tensilon—or, generically, edrophonium chloride—has the power to restore almost normal muscular function almost instantly, in a matter of moments. Its effect lasts only moments, but a positive response to Tensilon is diagnostic of myasthenia gravis.

"Tensilon was developed at Mt. Sinai in 1952, and I've used it many times. The effect is always startling. I gave Sheila the usual dose—ten milligrams, injected intravenously. I waited a moment, and then checked her arm strength. There was resistance to pressure—maybe eighty to eighty-five per cent of normal. So I asked her to get up and walk. She said, 'You know I can't walk.' I told her to try. She gave me a doubtful look—and sat up. Then she stood up. Then she walked across the room. It was a miracle. It's always a miracle, but this was one of the most miraculous. I'll never forget the look on her face. She was dazed. She was stunned. The tears were running down her cheeks. I felt the way I always do when I see that miracle happen. I felt—I don't know—almost godlike. Then she began to give out. I helped her back to bed. She collapsed. It was all over."

Sheila Allen was discharged from Alvarado Community Hospital on the morning of Thursday, October 26, 1978. That was fifteen days after the day of her admittance and eight days after her dramatic noonday meeting with Dr. Baughman. In the course of those eight days, she was introduced to another, and more durable, anti-cholinesterase agent called Mestinon, and an effective dosage (one sixty-milligram tablet every four hours) was determined. Tensilon is of only diagnostic value. The discharge summary noted: "Discharged to out-patient treatment, to be followed by Dr. Patricia Marrow for supportive psychotherapy (in adjusting to the presence of a chronic debilitating illness) and by Dr. Fred Baughman for control of myasthenia gravis." Her condition, the summary added, was "markedly improved." It was, indeed. The friend who had helped her into the hospital was there to meet her on her departure. She was pleased by his thoughtfulness, she was glad to have his company, but she didn't need his help. She walked out of the hospital with the easy gait of any normal twenty-four-year-old woman. She was, for all practical purposes, a normal young woman, and two weeks later, in early November, she was leading a normal life. She had a job demonstrating cosmetics at a San Diego department store, and she was attending evening classes at a school for real-estate brokers.

Dr. Baughman saw Miss Allen at his office soon after her hospital discharge, and once a month thereafter. At their December meeting, on December 5th, he noted that her response to Mestinon was entirely satisfactory. It was better than that of many other patients in his experience, and inferior to none. Nevertheless, he watched her closely and questioned her closely at their monthly meetings. There is always a chance that Mestinon, or any other anti-cholinesterase agent, may in time weaken in its mastery. There is a surgical procedure that can provide a vigorous supplement to Mestinon therapy. This involves the removal of the thymus gland. The thymus is situated between the chest wall and the windpipe, just below the thyroid gland. Its function has to do with the development and maintenance of the immunological system. The thymus develops rapidly in infancy, grows more slowly until around puberty, and then, in most people, begins to wither away. It has been established that in victims of myasthenia gravis the thymus is abnormally intact, and its functions seem to have been perverted into the phenomenon of autoimmunity. Dr. Baughman decided in the course of the summer of 1979 that Miss Allen would benefit from the removal of her thymus, and he arranged with a thoracic surgeon named David M. Long to perform the operation. Miss Allen was admitted to El Cajon Valley Hospital on September 25th, and underwent a transcervical thymectomy the following morning. The operation was a complete success, and its good results were immediately apparent. Dr. Baughman noted that within less than two hours Miss Allen's muscular powers were stronger than at any time since he had diagnosed her illness. She was discharged, stronger than at any time in recent years, on September 29th.

"Oh, sure," Miss Allen told me toward the end of our talk in Dr. Baughman's office. "I knew that a thymectomy was a serious operation. Dr. Baughman told me all about it. But, of course, I agreed. Whatever he suggested was Gospel to me. He was the Messiah. He *is* the Messiah. I moved back to Los Angeles in January of 1980, but we keep in touch—I'm still on Mestinon; I always will be—and I see him here once a year. It seems to me that I feel better every day. When I moved back to L.A. I had finished my real-estate course, and I went in with my mother and father in their real-estate business. I also did volunteer work for a while in a hospital in the neighborhood. I did physical counselling. Then in 1982 I heard about a new airline opening up with flights between L.A. and Hawaii, and I applied, and they took me on. I'm a senior flight attendant, and I do seven turnabout flights a month. Between trips, I still work in real estate. The only trouble I have now is trying to hold myself back. I don't want to walk— I want to run. I'm *so* full of strength and energy. I guess I'm making up for lost time. I told my new boyfriend about my myasthenia. He said, 'So what?' We dance all night."

[*1984*]

Index